Illustrated Textbook
of
Cardiovascular Pathology

Illustrated Textbook of Cardiovascular Pathology

P Chopra MD FRCPath FAMS

Professor
Department of Pathology
All India Institute of Medical Sciences
Ansari Nagar
New Delhi

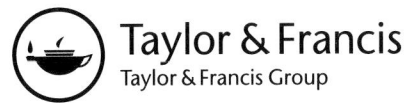

Taylor & Francis Group

LONDON AND NEW YORK

A MARTIN DUNITZ BOOK

© 2003 P Chopra

First published in India in 2003 by
Jaypee Brothers Medical Publishers (P) Ltd, New Delhi, India.
EMCA House, 23/23B Ansari Road, Daryaganj, New Delhi 110 002, India
Phones: 23272143, 23272703, 23282021, 23245672 m\, Fax: +91-011-23276490
e-mail: jpmedpub@del2.vsnl.net.in, Visit our website: www.jaypeebrothers.com

First published in the United Kingdom by Taylor & Francis, a member of the Taylor & Francis Group in 2004. Exclusively distributed worldwide (excluding the Indian Subcontinent) by Martin Dunitz, a member of the Taylor & Francis Group.

Tel.: +44 (0) 20 7583 9855
Fax.: +44 (0) 20 7842 2298
E-mail: info@dunitz.co.uk
Website: http://www.dunitz.co.uk

All rights reserved. No part of this publication may be reproduced, stored in a retrieval system, or transmitted, in any form or by any means, electronic, mechanical, photocopying, recording, or otherwise, without the prior permission of the publisher or in accordance with the provisions of the Copyright, Designs and Patents Act 1988 or under the terms of any licence permitting limited copying issued by the Copyright Licensing Agency, 90 Tottenham Court Road, London W1P 0LP.

Although every effort has been made to ensure that all owners of copyright material have been acknowledged in this publication, we would be glad to acknowledge in subsequent reprints or editions any omissions brought to our attention.

Although every effort has been made to ensure that drug doses and other information are presented accurately in this publication, the ultimate responsibility rests with the prescribing physician. Neither the publishers nor the authors can be held responsible for errors or for any consequences arising from the use of information contained herein. For detailed prescribing information or instructions on the use of any product or procedure discussed herein, please consult the prescribing information or instructional material issued by the manufacturer.

A CIP record for this book is available from the British Library.

ISBN 1 84184 451 9

Distributed in North and South America by

Taylor & Francis
2000 NW Corporate Blvd
Boca Raton, FL 33431, USA

Within Continental USA
Tel.: 800 272 7737; Fax.: 800 374 3401
Outside Continental USA
Tel.: 561 994 0555; Fax.: 561 361 6018
E-mail: orders@crcpress.com

Distributed in the rest of the world (excluding the Indian Subcontinent) by
Thomson Publishing Services
Cheriton House
North Way
Andover, Hampshire SP10 5BE, UK
Tel.: +44 (0)1264 332424
E-mail: salesorder.tandf@thomsonpublishingservices.co.uk

Printed at Gopsons Papers Ltd., A-14- Sec 60, Noida

Author and Contributors

Author

P Chopra
MD FRCPath FAMS
Professor
Department of Pathology
All India Institute of Medical Sciences
Ansari Nagar
New Delhi

Contributors

R Ray
MD Dip RCPath
Associate Professor
Department of Pathology
All India Institute of Medical Sciences
Ansari Nagar
New Delhi

A Saxena
MD DM
Professor
Department of Cardiology
All India Institute of Medical Sciences
Ansari Nagar
New Delhi

Foreword

With significant reductions in morbidity and mortality from infectious and nutritional diseases in developing countries, disorders of the heart and blood vessels have acquired a prime position among human health problems worldwide. Changes in ecology, socioeconomic status and lifestyles have been largely responsible for the increasing incidence of cardiovascular diseases even among large population groups in Asia and Africa. Years back understanding about the pathology of these diseases was limited to study of the involved organs and tissues at autopsy with end-stage changes and secondary complications. Advances in catheterisation and dye injection procedures, fibreoptic visualisations, newer imaging techniques and obtaining small endomyocardial biopsies in patients however, have greatly augmented our knowledge on early pathological changes in cardiovascular diseases and their evolution and natural history. The knowledge on pathology of these diseases has expanded considerably and this information greatly helps the therapeutic and preventive management in individual cases. Information on newer developments in the pathology of cardiovascular diseases would therefore, help not only the students of medicine and cardiology to acquire professional competence but also the pathologists to assess the pathological changes in a patient accurately.

This treatise by Dr P Chopra provides these informations admirably. All forms of cardiovascular diseases are adequately covered with the extensive personal experience and the rich material of the author. The illustrations are excellent supplement to the descriptive aspects of the text. It is noteworthy that rheumatic heart disease gets priority consideration that it deserves in developing countries like ours where it poses a serious community health problem. Heart transplantation and endomyocardial biopsy have received separate identities as due, for the benefit praticularly of the parcticing pathologists. It is also proper that the Chapter on Congenital Heart Disease has been prepared on a clinicopathological basis so that an understanding of the functional anomalies is clear from the pathological alterations due primarily to developmental defects. There is no doubt that this text painstakingly prepared by the author will be of immense value to the education of many in various branches of medical sciences.

NC Nayak
MD, FRCPath, FNA, FNSc, FAMS
Emeritus Professor
Department of Pathology
All India Institute of Medical Sciences
New Delhi
Senior Consultant and Head
Department of Histopathology
Sir Ganga Ram Hospital
New Delhi

Preface

Cardiovascular diseases have emerged as a major problem in India and other developing countries. As yet, only a few centres in India have gathered sufficient experience in these diseases. As a discipline, "Cardiovascular Pathology" seems to have lagged behind as compared to other subspecialties. With the advent of sophisticated techniques for obtaining tissue for diagnosis the pathologist is confronted with an ever widening spectrum of cardiovascular diseases in the laboratory. The pathologist not only must be familiar with the gross and microscopic appearances of commonly encountered cardiovascular diseases and thereby provide appropriate diagnostic support for better management but also be aware of the recent developments for the understanding of these diseases.

The Cardiothoracic centre at the All India Institute of Medical Sciences, New Delhi (India) gets a large number of cases referred from outside. Due to the close collaboration between the pathologist, cardiologist and the cardiothoracic surgeon the Department of Pathology over the years has acquired one of the largest repositories of gross and microscopic material on cardiovascular diseases. With the availability of this precious material it was considered worthwhile to use this rich material and experience in the form of an atlas that will have several illustrations of gross and microscopy pathology. This atlas has been compiled for use by residents and consultants in pathology, cardiology, cardiothoracic surgery, and internal medicine. The atlas would also serve as a guide for undergraduate students in medicine. Therefore, during preparation care has been taken to see that this atlas provides a simple and systematic approach, easy reading and understanding of the disease process.

The unique feature of this book is emphasis on cardiovascular diseases in the developing and tropical countries. An overview of the normal heart provides a basis for understanding the disease process. A simple approach to congenital heart disease evaluation through line diagrams is presented for easy understanding and comprehension. Rheumatic heart disease has been dealt with in detail since morbidity and mortality from this condition continues to be high in India and other developing countries. Chapters on Endomyocardial Biopsy and Cardiac Transplantation illustrate cases all of which have been biopsied at this centre. Chapter on Vascular Diseases lays emphasis on diseases prevalent in this country. Thus almost all the material presented in the atlas is based on our own experience. For completion sake a few inputs have been taken from some colleagues. It is hoped that this compilation will offer a proper insight into important cardiovascular diseases.

P Chopra

Acknowledgement

I am grateful to all staff and residents of Department of Pathology, All India Institute of Medical Sciences, who over the years have in several ways contributed to compilation of the material in this book. I am also thankful to the staff and residents of Departments of Cardiology and Cardiothoracic Surgery, Cardiothoracic Centre, All India Institute of Medical Sciences, who with their persuasive efforts sought permission for autopsies which have importantly contributed to this book. I am grateful to Prof. Veena Malhotra, Head, Department of Pathology, GB Pant Hospital, New Delhi; Prof. Ashok Mukherji; Prof. Sandhya Mani; Prof. Sanjeev Sharma, Department of Cardiac Radiology, Cardiothoracic Centre, All India Institute of Medical Sciences; Dr Manpreet Gulati, Department of Radiodiagnosis, All India Institute of Medical Sciences and to the Department of Pathology, Faculty of Medicine Kuwait University, where I was invited as a Visiting Professor, for generously agreeing to provide some of the illustrations. I thank Dr J Maheshwari who constantly encouraged me to initiate this project.

Contents

1. **The Normal Heart** *1*
   R Ray, P Chopra
2. **Congenital Heart Disease: A Clinician's Perspective** *11*
   A Saxena, P Chopra
3. **Rheumatic Heart Disease** *28*
4. **Valvular Heart Disease** *43*
5. **Infective Endocarditis** *57*
6. **Ischemic Heart Disease** *73*
7. **Endomyocardial Biopsy** *91*
8. **Myocarditis** *108*
9. **Cardiomyopathy** *119*
10. **Cardiac Transplantation** *140*
11. **The Pericardium** *156*
12. **Tumors of Heart** *175*
13. **Diseases of Blood Vessels** *200*

    Index *245*

The Normal Heart

A thorough knowledge of the anatomy of normal heart is an essential pre-requisite before examination of the cardiac system. During postmortem examination, the heart is taken out by midline thoraco-abdominal incision which extends from the neck to the symphysis pubis. The heart is usually removed along with the lungs en bloc which is then separated out from the rest for systematic analysis. Before severing all the connections it is essential to examine and follow the systemic venous drainage and pulmonary veins by blunt dissection. The relationship of the great vessels should be noted carefully. Normally the pulmonary artery lies anterior and to the right of the aorta near the cardiac roof. With the heart *in situ* one should also note the position of atrial appendages. Following this a small nick should be made into the anterior surface of the pulmonary trunk to look for the presence of pulmonary embolus. After excluding any obvious external abnormality one can now safely remove the heart for further detailed examination.

The heart can be opened in one of the following two methods:

Sequential segmental analysis In this method the heart is opened following the flow of blood sequentially exposing the right atrium, right ventricle, pulmonary artery and then the left atrium, left ventricle and aorta by inflow-outflow transvalvular incisions. This dissection is an excellent approach for the demonstration of normal cardiac anatomy, valvular heart diseases and congenital heart diseases. The following sequential incisions should be made to expose the various chambers:

1. An apical incision should be made -2 cm from the apex, parallel to the posterior atrioventricular groove. The size and shape of the ventricular cavities and relative thickness of both the ventricular walls are assessed.
2. Opening of the right atrium is done by joining the superior and inferior vena caval orifices by scissors. This incision exposes the right atrial cavity. An alternative method of exposure includes an incision made 0.5 cm above the inferior vena cava upto the tip of the right atrial cavity.
3. Using a knife, the right ventricle is cut posteriorly through the tricuspid valve 1-1.5 cm away and parallel to interventricular septum, until the first transverse cut through the ventricles is met.
4. The anterior papillary muscle of the right ventricle is identified and the anterior ventricular wall is cut to the right of this structure through the right ventricular outflow tract, pulmonary valve and pulmonary trunk. This cut along with the previous incision exposes the entire right ventricular cavity.
5. The left atrium is then opened by an incision through the left atrial appendage near its base in the midway between the right and left pulmonary veins. The cut is then extended downwards upto the atrioventricular junction.
6. An incision is made by a knife through the atrioventricular valve over the posterior left ventricular wall 1-1.5 cm away and parallel to the interventricular groove. This should be done cautiously so that the chordae tendinea are not damaged.
7. If the anterior mitral valve cusp is normal then a probe should be passed behind this leaflet through the left ventricular outflow tract into the aortic valve orifice. The anterior left ventricular musculature then should be incised carefully

along the probe keeping the anterior mitral leaflet intact. The incision can be extended upwards into the ascending aorta. Prior to this incision, a blunt dissection between the pulmonary trunk and ascending aorta is needed for a neat exposure of the structures.

Alternatively, the heart can be cut by the **"breadloaf technique"** where it is sliced by making several incisions parallel to the posterior atrioventricular groove. This technique is an excellent approach to know the extent of myocardial infarction. However, it is not recommended in cases of valvular heart disease.

The right atrium (Fig. 1.1) On opening, the right atrium is seen to have a smooth posterior part and a rough anterior trabeculated appendage, the junction between which is marked by a well-formed muscle bundle, the **crista terminalis** from which the pectinate muscles arise. Externally there is a groove corresponding to the crista terminalis. This is known as **sulcus terminalis** which is an important landmark to identify the **sinoatrial node**. In complex cardiac anomalies, it is the atrial appendageal structures which remain reasonably constant for identification of right and left atrial chambers. The **right atrial appendage** is triangular, blunt and joins the atrial cavity with a broad base while the **left atrial appendage** is tubular, crenalated and has a narrow base connecting with the cavity. The right atrial septal surface is characterized by **fossa ovalis** which is a depression at the site of foramen ovale – the interatrial communication in the fetal life. This hole shunts oxygenated blood from the right to the left atrium in fetal life and has a prominent rim **or limbus**. The floor of the fossa ovalis is a flap valve of thin partition which is sufficiently large to close the fossa ovalis. However, in approximately 25% of normal hearts, it may not be adherent at its superior margin and a probe can be passed through the right to left atrium producing a condition termed as **probe patency of foramen ovale**. The inferior vena cava opens into the junction of the posterior wall and the floor which is often guarded by a rudimentary valve (**Eustachian valve**). The size of the opening of the **coronary sinus** is variable and it may have a valve (**Thebesian valve**). In about 2% of adult individuals, lace like fibrous tags extend from the margin of the valves guarding the inferior vena cava and coronary sinus. This is known as **Chiari's network** which represents incomplete resorption of the right sinus venosus valve during development. Similar remnants may be seen across the fossa ovalis which represent remnants of the left sinus venosus valve.

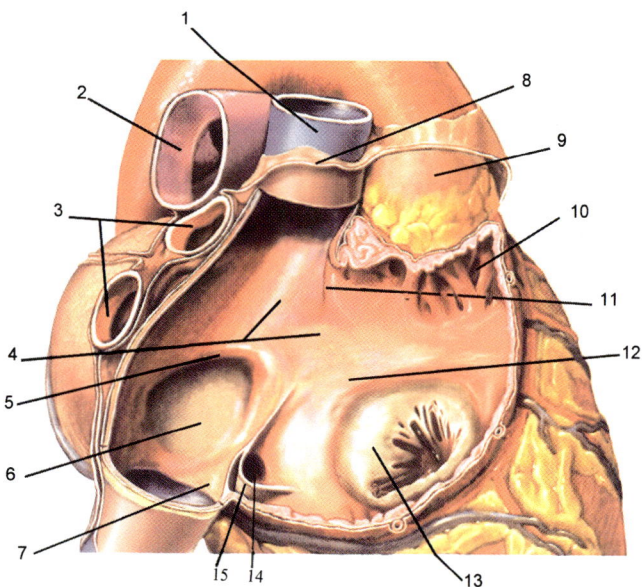

Fig. 1.1: Important landmarks: opened up right atrium

1. Superior vena cava
2. Right pulmonary artery
3. Right superior and inferior pulmonary veins
4. Interatrial septum
5. Limbus fossa ovalis
6. Fossa ovalis
7. Valve of inferior vena cava
8. Pericardial reflection
9. Ascending aorta
10. Pectinate muscles of the right atrial appendage
11. Crista terminalis
12. Membranous septum
13. Septal leaflet of tricuspid valve
14. Opening of coronary sinus
15. Valve of coronary sinus

The Normal Heart

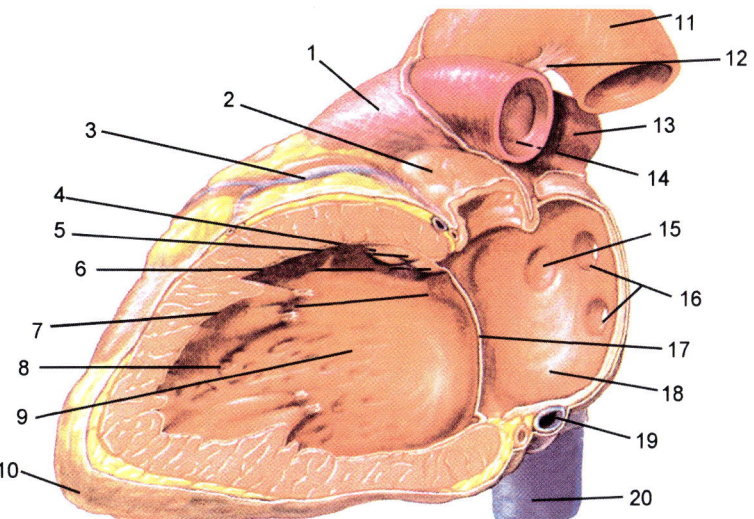

The left atrium (Fig. 1.2) This is the posterior most structure of the heart. The left atrium is entirely smooth walled and receives the four pulmonary veins, two on each side. It is the left atrial appendage which is used for identification of morphological left atrium in complex congenital heart diseases. The left atrial appendage is much smaller than that of the right atrium and is not marked by any specific crista internally or sulcus externally. The trabeculae of the left atrial appendage are less pronounced. The pectinate muscles in the left atrium are confined predominantly within the appendage. The septal surface consists of the left atrial surface of the **fossa ovalis** also known as **fossa lunata**. There is no rim or limbus to the fossa on the left atrial side. However, anteriorly the fibromuscular flap valve is usually plastered with the anterior left atrial wall and the junction is marked by several rough ridges.

Fig. 1.2: Opened up left atrium and left ventricle with mitral valve removed: left lateral view

1. Pulmonary trunk
2. Left atrial appendage
3. Great cardiac vein
4 to 6. Semilunar cusps of aortic valve
7. Interventricular septum—membranous part
8. Trabeculae carnea
9. Interventricular septum—muscular part
10. Apex of heart
11. Aorta
12. Ligamentum arteriosum
13. Right pulmonary artery
14. Left pulmonary artery
15. Valve of foramen ovale
16. Right pulmonary veins
17. Mitral valve (cut edge)
18. Left atrium
19. Coronary sinus
20. Inferior vena cava

1. Left common carotid artery
2. Left subclavian artery
3. Left brachiocephalic vein
4. Arch of aorta
5. Ligamentum arteriosum
6. Left pulmonary artery
7. Transverse pericardial sinus
8. Pulmonary trunk
9. Anterior semilunar cusp ⎫
10. Right semilunar cusp ⎬ Pulmonary valve
11. Left semilunar cusp ⎭
12. Conus arteriosus
13. Septal band
14. Septal (medial) papillary muscle
15. Posterior papillary muscle
16. Chordae tendinea
17. Moderator (septomarginal) band
18. Anterior papillary muscle
19. Inferior vena cava
20. Anterior leaflet ⎫
21. Posterior leaflet ⎬ Tricuspid valve
22. Septal (medial) leaflet ⎭
23. Right atrium
24. Supraventricular crest
25. Right coronary artery
26. Right atrial appendage
27. Branches of right pulmonary artery
28. Transverse pericardial sinus
29. Superior vena cava
30. Right brachiocephalic vein
31. Brachiocephalic trunk

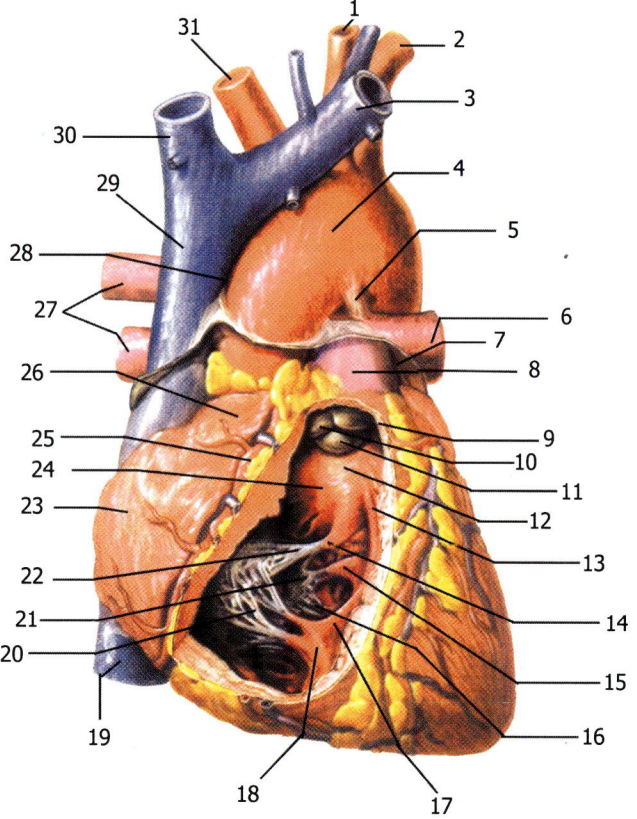

Fig. 1.3: Opened up right ventricle: right lateral view

The right ventricle (Fig. 1.3) The right and left ventricles have discrete morphological features. In the normal heart, the right ventricle lies anterior and to the right of the left ventricle. However, in congenital cardiac malformation, the position of the ventricles may be altered. For these reasons, the ventricles are better distinguished in terms of their morphology rather than their position as the morphologically right and morphologically left ventricles.

The morphologically right ventricle has three portions **(1) the inlet component; (2) the apical trabecular component, and (3) the outlet component.** The limit of the inlet zone is the distal attachment of the chordae tendinea of the tricuspid valve. The apical trabecular part extends inferiorly beyond the attachments of the papillary muscles towards the ventricular apex. The trabeculations are coarser in the right ventricle and on its septal surface there is a prominent muscular band known as **septomarginal trabeculation**. The apical trabecular part is the most constant and characteristic component of the morphologically right ventricle. The right ventricle also has several **septoparietal trabeculations** which extend from the septomarginal trabeculation to the right ventricular parietal wall. Another muscular sling, known as the **moderator band** is prominent and crosses from the septomarginal trabeculation to the anterior papillary muscle and then to the parietal wall. The outlet component of the right ventricle or infundibulum is a muscular tube which supports the pulmonary valve. The inlet and outlet components are separated by a prominent muscular bar known as **crista supraventricularis.**

The Normal Heart

The tricuspid valve The normal tricuspid valve has septal, antero-superior and inferior leaflets. The valve usually lacks a distinct fibrous annulus as seen in the mitral ring. Instead, the valve fibrosa blends with the adipose tissue of the atrioventricular sulcus. Each commissure is tethered by a fan-shaped chordae arising from the apex of the papillary muscles. The commissures are not always supported by the corresponding papillary muscles. The major anterior papillary muscle is the largest and usually springs directly from the body of the septomarginal trabeculation. At the point of insertions of the papillary muscles and chordae, the right ventricular inlet blends with the coarsely trabeculated component of the right ventricle. The most important distinguishing feature of the tricuspid valve is the direct attachment of chordae from the septal leaflet into the septum. In the morphologically left ventricle, chordal attachments to the interventricular septum are never seen.

Pulmonary valve The pulmonary valve has three cusps of approximately equal size which are semilunar in shape. Two of the cusps face the aortic coronary cusps and are known as right-facing and left-facing pulmonary cusps. The third cusp is called the non-facing cusp. The free edge of each cusp is thickened at its center to form nodule Arantii. Sometimes the valve cusps can have small fenestrations which are of no pathological significance.

The left ventricle (Figs 1.2 and 1.4) The left ventricle also has an **inlet, apical trabecular** and **outlet** components. Unlike the right ventricle, the inlet and outlet portions are not demarcated by the muscular cuff of the crista supraventricularis. The inlet extends from the atrioventricular junction to the a tachment of the papillary muscles. The most characteristic feature to decide the morphological leftness is the fine trabecular nature of the apical component. The septal surface of the left ventricle is smooth as it does not have a septomarginal trabeculation or a moderator band. Another characteristic feature of the left ventricle is that the mitral va ve never possesses chordal attachments to the septum. The **membranous** part of the **interventricular septum** is best identified from this chamber, which lies between the right coronary and non-coronary cusps. The outlet component of the left ventricle is

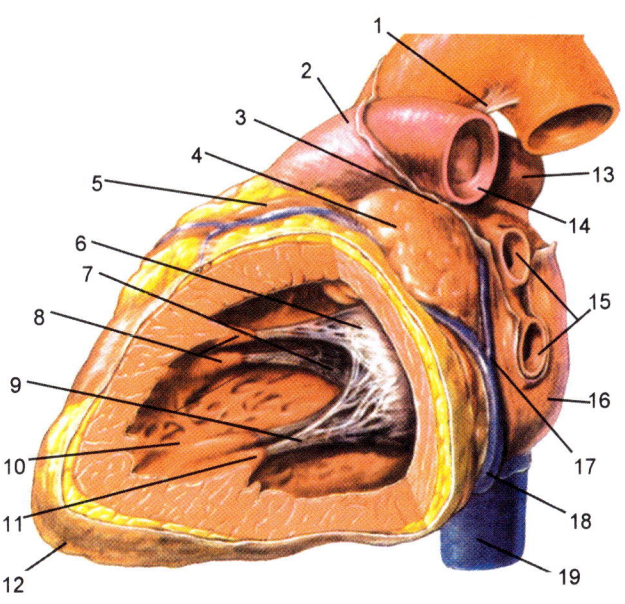

Fig. 1.4: Opened up left ventricle: left lateral view

1. Ligamentum arteriosum
2. Pulmonary trunk
3. Transverse pericardial sinus
4. Left atrial appendage
5. Left anterior descending artery
6. Posterior (mural) leaflet of mitral valve
7. Anterior (aortic) leaflet of mitral valve
8. Anterior papillary muscle
9. Chordae tendinea
10. Apical trabeculations of left ventricle
11. Posterior papillary muscle
12. Apex of heart
13. Right pulmonary artery
14. Left pulmonary artery
15. Left pulmonary veins
16. Left atrium
17. Oblique vein of left atrium
18. Coronary sinus
19. Inferior vena cava

(Figs 1.1 to 1.4 Courtsey: ADAM Student Atlas of Anatomy, Williams & Wilkins, 1996, Editor Todd R Olson pp. 82-84, 88-90)

deficient posteriorly so that the aortic and mitral valves are in fibrous continuity.

The **interventricular septum** is predominantly muscular with a small component of apical membranous septum. The membranous septum is part of the fibrous skeleton of the heart which supports the atrioventricular musculature. Because of the more apical placement of the tricuspid valve in comparison to that of the mitral valve, the septal leaflet of tricuspid valve divides the membranous septum into atrioventricular and interventricular components. The muscular septum has inlet, trabecular and outlet portions. Again, on account of more apical attachment of tricuspid valve than that of the mitral valve, this septum is divided into atrioventricular and interventricular components. This atrioventricular muscular septum should not be confused with the atrioventricular membranous septum as discussed earlier. Attachment of the septal leaflet of the tricuspid valve separates the inlet of the right ventricle from the outlet of the left ventricle. The trabecular part of the interventricular septum has coarser trabeculations on the right ventricular aspect. The outlet component of the interventricular septum is considerably small. It should be mentioned here that the posterior wall of infundibulum beneath the pulmonary valve is not a part of the septum. It separates the infundibulum from the outside of the heart. The outlet septum separating the ventricular outlets lies below the distal part of the infundibulum. With increasing age, the septum becomes sigmoid and the interventricular component of the membranous septum increases.

The mitral valve The mitral valve has two leaflets, the anterior or aortic and posterior or mural leaflet which are separated by the posteromedial and anterolateral commissures. The anterior leaflet is triangular which has fibrous continuity with the aortic valve leaflets. The posterior leaflet is quadrangular, has three scallops and takes up two-thirds of the annular circumference. The posterior leaflet throughout its length is attached to the mitral annulus while the anterior leaflet is in fibrous continuity with the aortic valve, the two valves sharing a common annulus. The anterior leaflet has a rough and clear zone and the posterior leaflet, similar to the tricuspid valve has a basal zone. The leaflets are supported by two groups of papillary muscles situated in the posteromedial and anterolateral positions.

Aortic valve The aortic valve is a semilunar valve which has three cusps two of which are named according to the origin of the two coronary arteries as right coronary and left coronary cusps. The remaining one is known as non-coronary cusp. The coronary arteries arise from the sinuses located behind the semilunar cusps. The free edge of each cusp is thickened at its center to form a nodule. The aortic root is the area occupied by the semilunar cusps. The anterior mitral leaflet is in fibrous continuity with the adjacent aortic cusps where the aortic and mitral valve rings are fused together. The cusps may be unequal in size. Sometimes the aortic valve may be bicuspid which may lead to calcific aortic stenosis. The two coronary arteries usually arise from the center of the sinus and are of approximately equal size. Occasionally the right coronary artery may have two ostia one of which is for the first conal artery.

The conduction system (Fig. 1.5) It includes the **sinoatrial (SA) node**, the **atrioventricular (AV) node**, the **bundle of His** and the **bundle branches** with the terminal ramifications. SA node is a cigar-shaped structure lying immediately subpericardially within the terminal groove on the lateral aspect of the junction of the superior vena cava and the right atrium. As the SA node is grossly invisible, the entire block of tissue from the suspected area should be taken and serially sectioned either parallel or perpendicular to the long axis of the vessel. The node usually has a single large nodal artery which serves as an important landmark on histological sections.

The AV node is arranged as a continuous axis which extends from the atrioventricular septum, penetrates the atrioventricular membranous septum and divides on the crest of the muscular interventricular septum. The atrial component of the AV node is contained exclusively within the Koch's triangle. This triangle is demarcated by the septal leaflet of the tricuspid valve, eustachian valve, and the tendon of Todaro. The apex of the triangle denotes the point at which the common bundle of His penetrates the membranous septum to reach the left ventricle. It then emerges in the subaortic outflow tract beneath the commissure between the non-coronary and right coronary leaflets of aortic valve. The axis branches on the crest of the muscular septum. The left bundle branch then fans out in a continuous cascade splitting into anterior, septal and posterior divisions towards the ventricular apex. The right bundle branch turns back through the interventricular septum as a cord like structure before crossing in the moderator band and ramifying into the right ventricular myocardium. Thus the tissue excised for the study of the conduction system must include the atrioventricular septum, the membranous septum and the rest of the interventricular septum.

Coronary artery circulation In the normal heart, only two of the three aortic sinuses give rise to coronary arteries. The two aortic sinuses that usually support the coronary arteries are always adjacent to the subpulmonary infundibulum. The third sinus is the **nonadjacent/nonfacing** sinus. The right

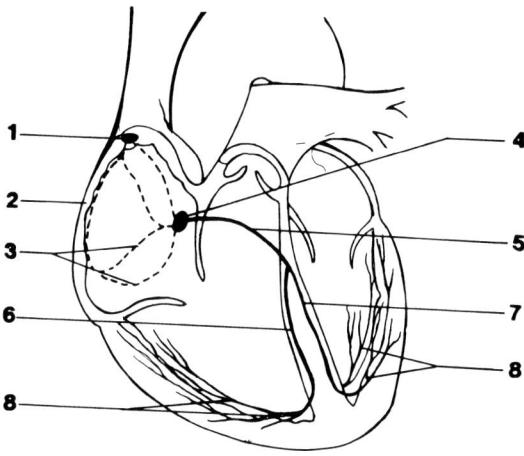

Fig. 1.5: The conduction system

1. Sinoatrial node
2. Right atrium
3. Internodal pathways
4. Atrioventricular node
5. Atrioventricular (AV) bundle
6. Right branch of AV bundle
7. Left branch of AV bundle
8. Purkinje fibers

coronary artery (RCA) emerges from the right sinus. The proximal course of the RCA is almost at right angle to the aortic sinus from which it emerges. The artery gives rise to infundibular and a series of anterior, middle and posterior atrial arteries that run upward to supply the atrial musculature. One of these branches usually the anterior one is prominent and forms the artery to the sinus node in 60% of cases. Other branches variable in number, run downward from the right coronary artery to supply the right anterior wall of the ventricle. These are generally called the right anterior ventricular branches. Of these the infundibular and acute marginal arteries have specific names. As the right coronary artery passes along the diaphragmatic surface of the heart, it reaches the crux in 90% of individuals where it gives off the artery to the AV node and the posterior descending artery. The **dominance** is determined by the artery that gives rise to the posterior descending and AV nodal artery.

The main stem of the left coronary artery (LCA) after its origin from the left hand facing aortic sinus runs a very short course behind the pulmonary trunk. Within 2.5 cm or so, the main stem branches into left anterior descending (LAD) and left circumflex (LCF) arteries. In one-third of individuals, the stem of the left main coronary artery trifurcates. The branch between the anterior descending and circumflex branches is called the intermediate branch. The first septal perforating artery is a relatively large branch which takes origin from the anterior descending branch close to the origin of the first diagonal branch. This branch can greatly enlarge in coronary atherosclerosis. LAD runs directly into the interventricular groove giving oblique branches and diagonal branches to the ventricle. The first diagonal branch is usually a small branch to the right ventricular infundibulum. In cases of occlusion of the LAD, this branch may link with the counter part of the right side to form the ring of Vieussens. The other branches are the septal perforating arteries which run perpendicularly into the substance of the muscular septum. Beyond the first diagonal artery the LAD runs intramyocardially for some distance. The usual course of LAD is then across the apex of the heart, where it turns toward the cardiac base of the posterior interventricular groove. The circumflex artery after its origin passes beneath the left atrial appendage to enter the left atrioventricular groove. In 10% of cases the circumflex artery is much larger giving the posterior descending artery and the artery to the AV node. In this pattern, known as the **left dominance**, the circumflex artery gives rise to the posterior descending artery and the artery at the crux to the AV node. It then continues into the right AV groove to supply the diaphragmatic wall of the RV. It is one of the superior atrial branches of the circumflex artery which in 40% of the population provides the artery to the SA node.

The posterior interventricular artery (90% from RCA and 10% from LCF) runs in the posterior interventricular groove and gives rise to a series of perforating arteries that run forward to the muscular septum often connecting with the branches of the anterior interventricular artery. The posterior descending artery then terminates at the apex connecting with the terminal branches of LAD. In a small percentage of cases, the terminal branches of the circumflex and right coronary arteries descend parallel to either side of the posterior interventricular groove which is known as the **"balanced pattern"**.

Histology of the heart The normal cardiac myocyte has a diameter of 10 to 15 μm. It has a single central nucleus. The cytoplasm, in addition to the organelles contain lipofuscin pigment, the amount of which increases with age. The myocardium has syncytial like arrangement of cardiac myocytes which take origin from the fibrous skeleton of the heart. The Purkinje fibers, present in the subendocardial location of all heart chambers are more prominent in the sections from the ventricles. They are larger than the normal cardiac myocytes and have a vacuolated cytoplasm and central nucleus.

The atrioventricular valve leaflets have a fibrous core (**lamina fibrosa**) which is continuous with the valve ring on one side and chordae tendinea on the other side. Over this layer, lies a loose connective tissue zone known as **lamina spongiosa**. A thin fibroelastic layer covering the spongiosa is continuous with the atrial and ventricular subendocardial layers and are known as **"atrialis"** and **"ventricularis"** respectively. The former contains more elastic tissue. The valve leaflets are avascular and a thin layer of endothelium covers the fibroelastic structure of the leaflets.

The semilunar valves also have a dense **lamina fibrosa** and a loose **spongiosa**. They have a thin fibroelastic layer beneath the endothelial lining. The elastic tissue strands are more prominent over the ventricular aspect of the valve than on the arterial side of the cusp. The normal semilunar valve cusps are avascular.

Electron microscopy of cardiac myocytes The myocytes have a syncytial arrangement and they are separated from each other by intercalated discs. At subcellular level the myofilaments are arranged in bundles as myofibrils with intervening mitochondria and sarcoplasmic reticulum. The sarcomere, the functional unit of cardiac contractile mechanism is formed by the organization of the myofibril. The sarcomere is delimited on each side by a Z line with thick and thin filaments in between arranged perpendicularly to the Z line. The thick filaments contain myosin which form the A band. The actin filaments or the thin filaments with the regulatory proteins troponin and tropomyosin extend from the Z line up to the A band through the I band. The force of contraction is generated from the interaction of these myofilaments. The extent of overlap between the adjoining thick and thin filaments decides the amount of force that can be generated for myocardial contraction.

SUGGESTED READING

1. Anderson RH, Becker AE: *Cardiac Anatomy: An Integrated Text and Colour Atlas*. Churchill Livingstone, Edinburgh, 1980.
2. Anderson RH, Becker AE: Normal cardiac anatomy. In Robertson WB (Ed): *The Cardiovascular System Part A* (3rd edn) Churchill Livingstone. **10**: 3-26, 1993.

APPENDIX

Various weight and measurements of adult heart.

Weight

    250-300 g   (0.45% of body weight in males)
    200-250 g   (0.4% of body weight in female)

Wall thickness

    Atria – 1-2 mm
    Right ventricle – 3-5 mm
    Left ventricle – 10-15 mm

The wall thickness of right ventricle is measured 2 cm below to the pulmonary valve and that of left ventricle is measured 2 cm below the mitral valve. The measurement should exclude the trabeculated subendocardial muscles.

Valve circumference

    Aortic valve – 7.5 cm (6-7.5 cm)
    Pulmonary valve – 8.5 cm (7-9 cm)
    Mitral valve – 10 cm (8-10.5 cm)
    Tricuspid valve – 12 cm (10-12.5 cm)

2 Congenital Heart Disease: A Clinician's Perspective

INTRODUCTION

Significant changes have occurred in the diagnosis and treatment of various congenital heart diseases (CHD) over the last 20 to 30 years. The recognition of different types of CHD especially the complex ones has markedly improved, largely due to the technology of echocardiography and Doppler. There is also a shift from palliative to definitive surgical procedures and these operations are now being performed in infants and neonates with the hope that long-term results would be better.

According to worldwide figures, about 0.8% of children born every year have some form of congenital heart disease. This incidence is not likely to be much different in India. Going by the current birth rate of about 29/1000/ year in this country, the total number of children born with CHD will approximate 1.8 lakhs every year. Left to right shunts like ventricular septal defect, atrial septal defect and patent ductus arteriosus constitute about 35-40% of all cases with CHD. The incidence and the profile of CHD have not changed over the last several decades.

ETIOLOGY

Development of heart is an interaction of genes, environment and chance, resulting in a complex series of biochemical events. It has been observed that embryos with severe cardiac defects are generally aborted in the first trimester and those with relatively less severe malformations survive to live birth.

The etiology of congenital heart disease remains unknown in large majority of cases. In approximately 10% of cases, an etiologic basis attributable to genetic factors is identifiable. In the rest of 90% of cases, the etiology is best explained by a genetic-environmental interaction (multifactorial inheritance) in which the contribution of genetic and environmental factors are of variable importance.

Chromosomal abnormalities Chromosomal anomalies are found in about 5-8% of children with congenital heart disease. It is likely that with the availability of newer, more sophisticated methods of chromosomal analysis, one will be able to identify minor aberrations in chromosomes more often in congenital heart disease patients. The common chromosomal syndromes associated with congenital heart disease are trisomy 21 (Down's syndrome: atrioventricular septal defect), trisomy 18 (Edwards' syndrome: ventricular septal defect, patent ductus arteriosus), trisomy 13 (Patau's syndrome: ventricular septal defect), XO (Turner syndrome: coarctation of aorta), etc.

Single mutant gene abnormalities Like chromosomal abnormalities, this also results in a clinical syndrome involving many systems. The examples include association of atrial septal defects and common atrium with Ellis-van Creveld syndrome, pulmonary stenosis in Noonan's syndrome, cardiomyopathy in Friedreich's ataxia, aortic valve disease in mucopolysaccharidosis, etc. Most of these lesions have a multifactorial inheritance.

Genetic-environmental interaction The etiology of majority of congenital heart diseases has been postulated to genetic-environmental interaction or as having multifactorial inheritance. An environmental trigger in the form of an **infection** or **drug** at a vulnerable period of cardiac development in fetus results in congenital heart defect in a hereditary predisposed individual.

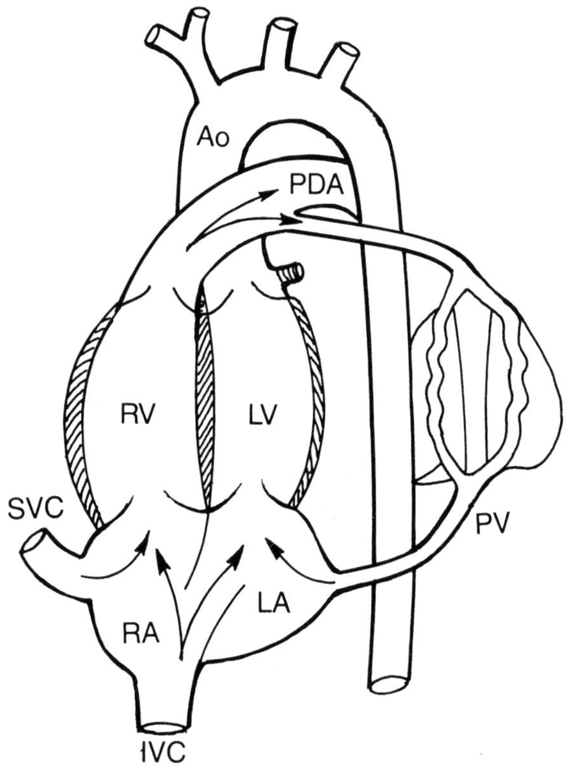

The potential **cardiovascular teratogens** include drugs like alcohol, hydantoin, trimethadione, lithium, retinoic acid and thalidomide. Some maternal conditions like infections (Rubella), diabetes, lupus erythematosus also act as teratogens resulting in congenital cardiac malformations.

In summary, our understanding of etiology of cardiac malformation remain primitive, although rapid progress is being made in this field. There is lack of information on the complete process of transformation from abnormal genome to phenotypic expression. Further information on etiology would aid in counseling, prenatal diagnosis and hence ultimately in prevention of birth of children with congenital heart disease.

FETAL CIRCULATION AND CHANGES AT BIRTH

In order to understand the influence of various congenital heart diseases on a newborn, knowledge of fetal circulation is essential (Fig. 2.1). The basis of this understanding mostly comes from animal studies.

Umbilical vessels act as connecting links between the fetus and placenta. Umbilical arteries carry blood from the fetus to the placenta and umbilical vein which has a higher PO_2 in turn takes blood from placenta to the fetus. The umbilical venous blood reaches the inferior vena cava partly through the hepatic circulation and partly through ductus venosus bypassing the liver. Therefore, inferior vena cava has a highly oxygenated blood. About one-third of this blood is directed into left atrium through patent foramen ovale due to the particular relationship of inferior vena cava opening to the foramen ovale. The rest of caval blood mixes with the inflow from superior vena cava and enters the right ventricle and then the pulmonary artery. The oxygenated blood which reaches left atrium from inferior vena cava is further passed into left ventricle and then pumped into ascending aorta, thereby, giving supply to the heart and brain. On the other hand, 90% of the mixed blood from pulmonary artery is shunted through patent ductus arteriosus (PDA) into the descending aorta. The blood going to the descending aorta supplies the rest of the fetus and umbilical arteries. Very small amount of blood

Fig. 2.1: Diagrammatic representation of fetal circulation. Ao—Aorta, IVC—Inferior vena cava, LA—Left atrium, LV—Left ventricle, PDA—Patent ductus arteriosus, PV—Pulmonary vein, RA—Right atrium, RV—Right ventricle, SVC—Superior vena cava

passes through the isthmus (i.e. part of aorta where arch and descending thoracic aorta join).

Hence, fetal circulation is adjusted in such a manner that highly oxygenated blood reaches the heart and brain, and this is facilitated by three communications namely ductus venosus, patent foramen ovale and patent ductus arteriosus (Fig. 2.1).

Changes in Fetal Circulation at Birth

Some immediate changes occur in circulation within a few minutes after birth. The gas exchange function is transferred from placenta to the lungs which expand immediately at birth. Clamping of umbilical cord removes the low resistant circuit of the placenta, thereby increasing the systemic vascular resistance and decreasing the inferior vena caval return to the heart. On the other hand, with onset of respiration, there is abrupt decrease in the pulmonary vascular resistance and increase in the pulmonary blood flow. These changes result in eventful closure of the three communicating channels, i.e. ductus venosus, patent foramen ovale and patent ductus arteriosus.

Due to the nature of fetal circulation, some of the complex congenital heart defects may not cause any disturbance during fetal life leading to normal fetal growth and development, e.g. transposition of great arteries, coarctation of aorta, ventricular septal defect, atrial septal defect, etc. In these types of defects, changes in fetal circulation after birth may make the newborn symptomatic, e.g. sudden deterioration in a baby with transposition of great arteries or severe coarctation of aorta with closure of ductus arteriosus. On the other hand, some other cardiac defects affect the heart growth during fetal life, e.g. in a case of mitral atresia, very little blood flows to left ventricle and aorta, therefore, the left ventricle is hypoplastic and isthmic hypoplasia of aorta or coarctation of aorta may also be associated. In conditions like tricuspid and pulmonary atresia, the right ventricle is small, aorta is large and therefore association with coarctation of aorta is very rare.

Congenital Heart Diseases

Congenital heart diseases (CHDs) can be classified in many ways, the simplest being to use clinical classification. According to this classification the various CHDs are divided into two major groups:

Acyanotic CHD This includes (a) Left to right shunts like atrial septal defect, ventricular septal defect, patent ductus arteriosus, etc. and (b) Obstructive lesions such as pulmonic stenosis, aortic stenosis, coarctation of aorta, etc.

Cyanotic CHD This is also further divided into several subgroups as is discussed later.

LEFT TO RIGHT SHUNTS

This group includes:
1. Atrial septal defect
2. Ventricular septal defect
3. Atrioventricular septal defect or endocardial cushion defect
4. Patent ductus arteriosus
5. Others like aortopulmonary window, coronary arteriovenous fistula.

Atrial septal defect

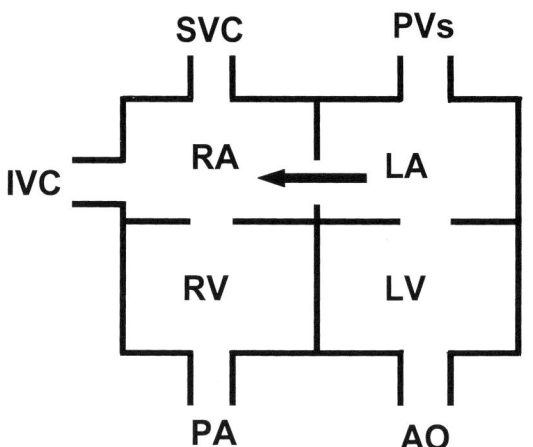

Fig. 2.2: Line diagram showing atrial septal defect: Ao—Aorta, PA—Pulmonary artery, IVC—Inferior vena cava, LA—Left atrium, LV—Left ventricle, PVs—Pulmonary veins, RA—Right atrium, RV—Right ventricle, SVC—Superior vena cava

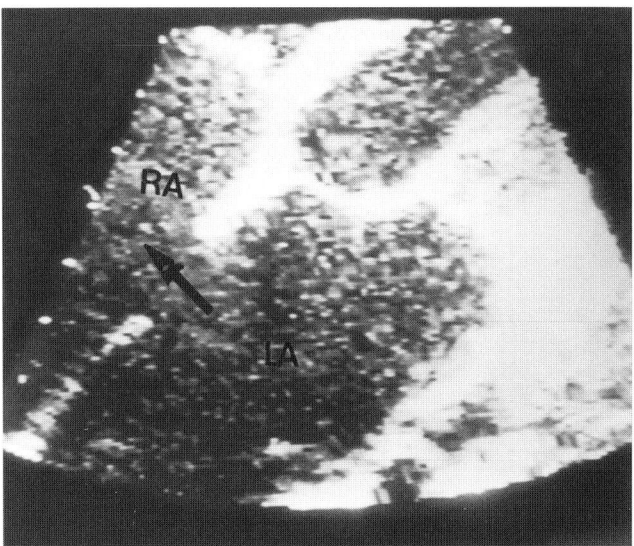

Fig. 2.3: Echocardiogram showing a defect in the atrial septum in region in fossa ovalis (arrow). LA—Left atrium, RA—Right atrium

ATRIAL SEPTAL DEFECT

Atrial septal defect (ASD) constitutes about 6-7% of CHD and is seen twice more often in females. The defect usually occurs in isolation (Fig. 2.2). It is a relatively benign lesion and does not increase the morbidity or mortality associated with congenital extracardiac anomalies. Patients are often asymptomatic or mildly symptomatic. Rarely, an infant with isolated ASD may be symptomatic with growth failure, recurrent chest infections, congestive heart failure and pulmonary hypertension. Such babies must be extensively evaluated to look for any associated conditions like left ventricular inflow obstructions.

Examination reveals hyperactive impulse, mild left parasternal lift and a wide and fixed second heart sound. There is an ejection systolic murmur at the base due to large flow across the pulmonary valve. A mid-diastolic murmur at lower left sternal border is due to increased flow across the tricuspid valve.

ECG shows right axis deviation and incomplete right bundle branch block due to right ventricular volume overload. In cases with primum ASD, the QRS axis is to the left.

X-ray chest reveals cardiomegaly, right atrial enlargement, dilated pulmonary segment and evidence of increased pulmonary blood flow. Echocardiography demonstrates a dilated right atrium and right ventricle, the actual septal defect is also seen and its site and size can be determined (Fig. 2.3).

Management

Usually the lesion is well-tolerated in infants and the surgery can be deferred till 3-4 years of age. It is perhaps best to close it before the child starts going to school. The surgical mortality is close to zero in most of the centers. Recently there are reports of transcatheter closure of ASD using occlusive devices.

VENTRICULAR SEPTAL DEFECT

Ventricular septal defect (VSD) is the most common CHD, seen as an isolated defect in 20% of cases with congenital heart disease (Fig. 2.4). The prevalence may go down in adults due to the phenomenon of spontaneous closure in some of these.

The defect may be single or multiple. The site of VSD is used to classify these defects into perimembranous (which is the most common location seen in nearly 80% of cases), infundibular or supracristal (beneath the pulmonary valve), inlet and muscular (seen in 5-20% of cases, could be multiple). The primary variable that determines the physiologic state of the patient is the defect size which varies from very small which are of no consequence to large nonrestrictive defects resulting in elevation of pulmonary artery pressure. The magnitude of the left to right shunt across the VSD can be assessed reasonably well by clinical examination including an X-ray chest and ECG.

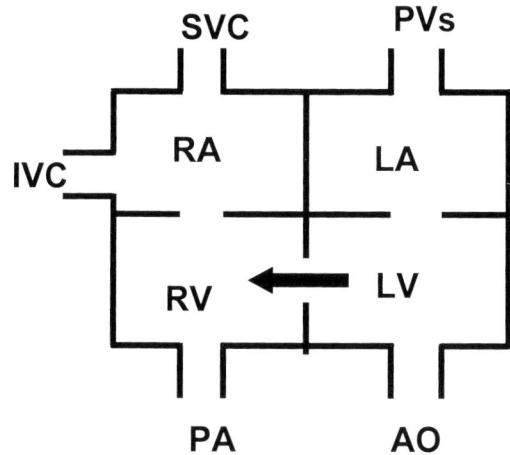

Fig. 2.4: Line diagram showing ventricular septal defect. Ao—Aorta, PA—Pulmonary artery, RA—Right atrium, RV—Right ventricle, SVC—Superior vena cava, IVC—Inferior vena cava, PVs—Pulmonary veins

Important Issues for Management

Spontaneous closure of VSD occurs in 15-50% of cases, in others the defect can become smaller. Even large defects at birth are known to become smaller by 6 months to one year of age. Development of aortic regurgitation or pulmonic stenosis in the course of a small VSD may also necessitate surgical correction.

Small Ventricular Septal Defect

The pulmonary artery pressure is normal, child is asymptomatic with no evidence of growth failure or congestive heart failure. There is no cardiomegaly and the second heart sound is normal. The diagnostic hallmark is the presence of a loud pansystolic murmur along the left sternal border which may be associated with a thrill.

ECG is normal and X-ray chest shows a normal sized heart with normal or slightly increased vascularity. Although the diagnosis of small VSD is obvious at the bedside, echo-Doppler helps to quantify the shunt and the pulmonary artery systolic pressure (PASP). By measuring the Doppler jet velocity across VSD, the gradient between left and right ventricular systolic pressure (RVSP) can be estimated. The RVSP equals the cuff systolic pressure minus the gradient across the VSD, RVSP is equal to PASP if there is no pulmonic stenosis. In small VSD, the PASP should be normal. The defect can be directly visualized on cross-sectional echocardiography. Color flow imaging shows turbulence across the defect and helps in diagnosis of multiple defects. If the defect is diagnosed to be small, patients should be followed medically. Parents must also be told about the need for prophylaxis against infective endocarditis. A large number of these defects may close spontaneously, mostly in the first two years of life.

Moderate Ventricular Septal Defect

The defect is usually less than half of the diameter of root of aorta with mild to moderate elevation of the pulmonary artery pressures. There may be some features of growth retardation, congestive heart failure is not usual. A flow related S3 or a short mid diastolic murmur is often heard at the apex. ECG is either normal or shows left ventricular volume overload pattern. There is mild to moderate cardiac enlargement on chest X-ray with evidence of increased vascularity. Echo-Doppler can quantify the shunt and show the septal defect. The degree of pulmonary hypertension can also be assessed by Doppler echo as described earlier.

Ventricular septal defects do not enlarge, they only get smaller. Some of these moderate VSD can close spontaneously or become smaller by one year of age and hence intervention during infancy is not required. However, if congestive heart failure, growth failure or pulmonary pressures show a rise, surgical closure may be performed even in infancy. In case moderate shunt with mild elevation of pulmonary pressure persist beyond one or two years of age, surgery is indicated.

Large Ventricular Septal Defects with Hyperkinetic Pulmonary Hypertension

A VSD is defined as large when it is equal to or more than the diameter of the aortic root. These defects are non-restrictive and therefore right ventricular systolic pressure is equal to the systolic pressure in the left ventricle.

The patient, usually an infant, has tachypnea, increased sweating, repeated chest infections, feeding difficulties and growth failure. Often there is congestive heart failure, precordium is hyperdynamic with cardiac enlargement. The systolic murmur of VSD is short, early systolic and S2 is widely split with a loud P2 component. There is mid-diastolic murmur at the apex. ECG shows biventricular hypertrophy, left atrial enlargement and q in V5,V6, due to left ventricular volume overload. Significant cardiomegaly with pulmonary plethora are seen on X-ray chest.

Echo-Doppler show enlarged left atrium and left ventricle. Large defects can be visualized (Fig. 2.5), but there is little turbulence across it as the right ventricular systolic pressure (RVSP) is nearly equal to the systolic pressure in the left ventricle.

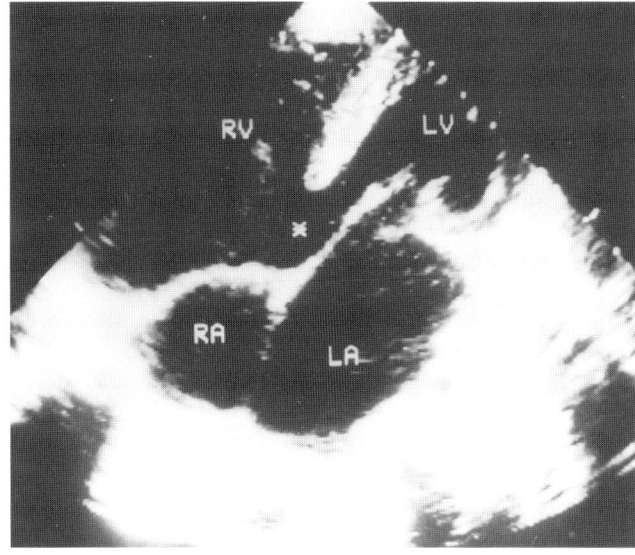

Fig. 2.5: Echocardiogram in four chamber view demonstrating a large ventricular septal defect (*). RA—Right atrium; LA—Left atrium; RV—Right ventricle; LV—Left ventricle

Cardiac catheterization and angiography may be needed for older children to estimate pulmonary vascular resistance. Left ventricular angiogram is able to show the defect as the contrast agent passes from left ventricle to right ventricle through the ventricular septal defect (Fig. 2.6).

Management and timing of surgery Infants with PASP more than 50% of the systemic systolic pressure (can be estimated by echo-Doppler) should have surgical closure by one year of age. Early surgery, even by 3 months of age, is indicated in infants with persistent congestive heart failure, recurrent chest infections and growth failure. Medical treatment includes correction of anemia, use of digoxin, diuretics and vasodilators for control of heart failure.

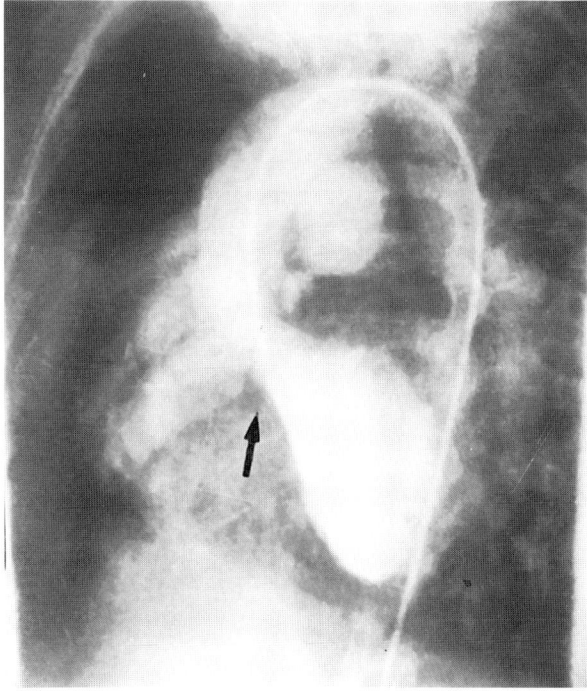

Fig. 2.6: Left ventricular angiography in left anterior oblique view, showing the ventricular septal defect through which contrast agent passes into the right ventricle (arrow)

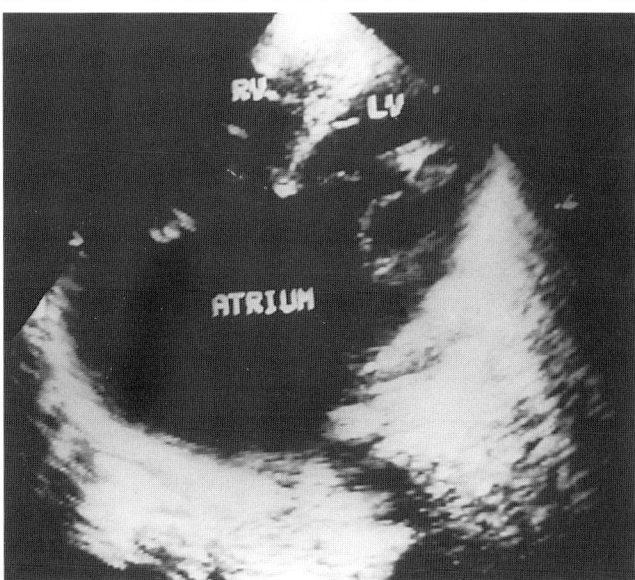

Fig. 2.7a: Echocardiography in four chamber view showing a common atrium, and a common atrioventricular valve

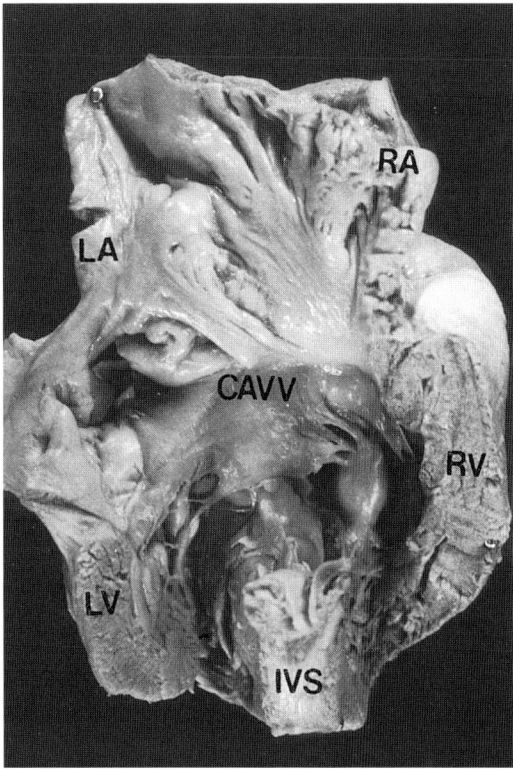

Fig. 2.7b: Gross specimen of heart showing common atrioventricular valve (CAVV). LA—Left atrium; RA—Right atrium, IVS—Interventricular septum, LV—Left ventricle, RV—Right ventricle

ATRIOVENTRICULAR SEPTAL DEFECT

This defect, also called endocardial cushion defect, is relatively uncommon form of CHD. Association of atrioventricular septal defect (AVSD) with Down's syndrome is well-established (40% of Down's syndrome with CHD have this defect).

Clinical Evaluation

The presentation is early, usually in infancy with congestive heart failure, growth failure and feeding difficulties. There may be mild cyanosis. The precordium is hyperdynamic with second sound widely split and intensity of P_2, elevated. A mid-diastolic murmur may be heard due to large flow across VSD. There is early development of pulmonary vascular obstructive disease especially in children with Down's syndrome.

ECG characteristically shows left axis deviation (mostly between –90 and –150). X-ray chest is suggestive of large intracardiac shunt as in VSD. Echo-Doppler is diagnostic of this anomaly (Figs 2.7a and b). It defines the anatomy of atrioventricular valves, ASD, VSD and quantifies the severity of valvular regurgitation. Early surgical correction by 6-9 months is advised. In untreated cases, the mortality is about 50% in the first year of life.

PATENT DUCTUS ARTERIOSUS

It is a tube that connects origin of left pulmonary artery to aorta just below left subclavian artery and is normally present in fetal life (Fig. 2.8). Functional closure occurs within 10-15 hours after birth in term babies, anatomical closure, however, occurs by 2-3 weeks leading to ligamentum arteriosum.

Incidence in term infants is about 1 in 2000 live births (5-10% of all CHD). Exposure to Rubella virus in the first trimester of pregnancy is associated with high incidence of patent ductus arteriosus (PDA) and other congenital malformations. The clinical picture depends on the size of the ductus.

Patients with large PDA are symptomatic in infancy with congestive heart failure, feeding difficulties, tachypnea, etc. The peripheral pulses are bounding and the precordium is hyperdynamic. The ductus murmur may be continuous or more often shorter due to high pressure in the pulmonary artery. ECG shows left ventricular hypertrophy with volume overload. There is cardiomegaly on X-ray chest with prominent aorta and pulmonary artery segment. Echo-Doppler reveals enlarged left atrium and left ventricle along with the ductal flow signal from which pulmonary artery pressure can be estimated. It is important to look for evidence of associated coarctation of aorta in all these cases. In

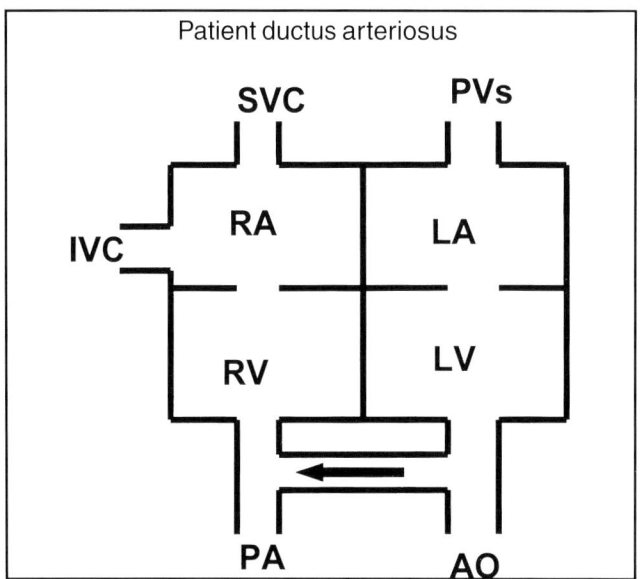

Fig. 2.8: Diagrammatic representation of patent ductus arteriosus. RA—Right atrium, LA—Left atrium, SVC—Superior vena cava, IVC—Inferior vena cava, PVs—Pulmonary veins, PA—Pulmonary artery, Ao—Aorta

cases with isolated PDA, surgical or device closure (Figs 2.9a and b) is performed without a prior cardiac catheterization. Since the operation is simple, early surgery in infancy is indicated in cases with large ductus. Those with smaller PDA can wait for closure.

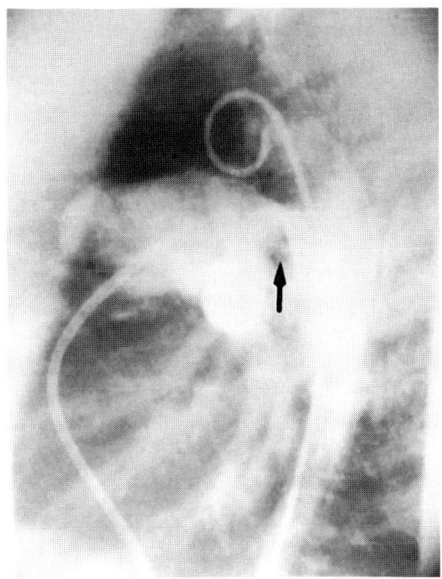
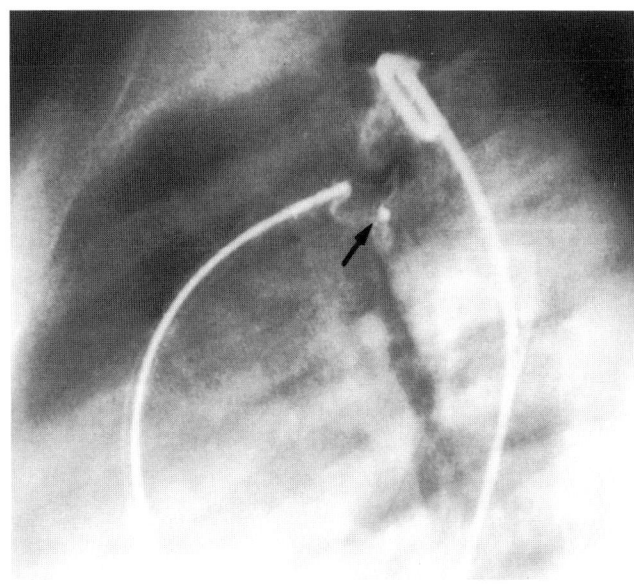

Figs 2.9a and b: Aortic angiography in left anterior oblique view showing a patent ductus arteriosus before (a) and after (b) device closure. The Amplatzer device is seen in place in Figure b (arrow)

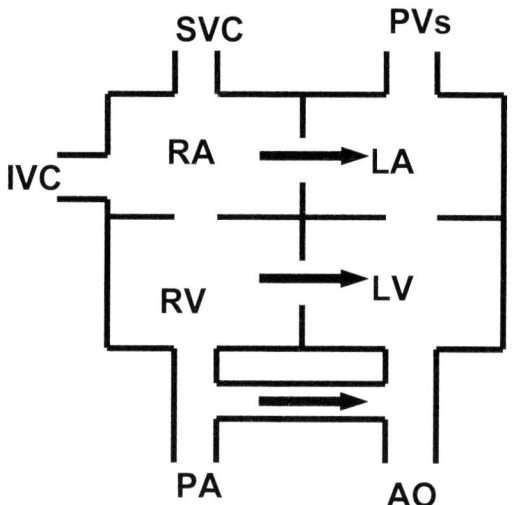

Fig. 2.10: Diagrammatic representation of Eisenmenger's syndrome. RA—Right atrium, LA—Left atrium, SVC—Superior vena cava, IVC—Inferior vena cava, PVs—Pulmonary veins, PA—Pulmonary artery, Ao—Aorta

EISENMENGER'S SYNDROME

Eisenmenger's syndrome can occur secondary to a large septal defect, which has resulted in severe pulmonary arterial hypertension (Fig. 2.10). It may occur as early as 3-4 years secondary to a large VSD or PDA, however, in patients with ASD, Eisenmenger syndrome is seen in 3rd or 4th decade. The pulmonary vascular resistance is elevated and it makes the shunt as bidirectional or predominantly right to left.

The patient, usually an older child, adolescent or adult appears well-compensated and is not in congestive heart failure. There may be mild cyanosis at rest or on exertion. There is mild left parasternal lift but no cardiomegaly. The second heart sound is closely split or single. There is no murmur of the defect as the degree of shunting is very small, a short ejection systolic murmur may originate from dilated pulmonary artery. Similarly there are no flow murmurs. Sometimes an early diastolic murmur of pulmonary regurgitation may be audible at the base. ECG reveals right ventricular hypertrophy, left ventricular forces may also be prominent in some cases. X-ray chest shows minimal cardiomegaly, prominent pulmonary artery segment and central plethora. The vascularity in the outer third of lung fields is reduced.

Echo-Doppler Large septal defect is visualized with little turbulence across it on color flow mapping. Usually there is no chamber enlargement. In late stages of Eisenmenger's syndrome, right atrium and right ventricle may dilate. Contrast echo performed by injecting agitated saline intravenously shows contrast going from right to left chamber across the defect.

Management Cardiac catheterisation and angiography is not needed to make a diagnosis of Eisenmenger's syndrome. However, in borderline cases especially in children below 5-6 years of age, a detailed hemodynamic study is required. Pulmonary vascular resistance (PVR) is determined from the heomdynamic data, first in the basal state and then its fall on inhalation of O_2 or nitric oxide is noted. Cases which show fall of PVR to 6 units or so, are still operable.

OBSTRUCTIVE LESIONS

The common lesions include pulmonic stenosis, aortic stenosis and coarctation of aorta. Obstructive lesions result in corresponding ventricular hypertrophy and hence no cardiomegaly or congestive heart failure occur till late stages of the disease. There is generally no history of frequent chest infections or failure to thrive. The obstruction results in a typical ejection systolic murmur due to the turbulence produced by obstruction.

Pulmonic Stenosis

Isolated pulmonic stenosis (PS) is generally valvular. Obstruction produces right ventricular hypertrophy and hence left parasternal impulse. Second heart sound is widely split due to delayed closure of pulmonic valve; however, normal respiratory variation of S_2 is maintained. In severe cases, pulmonary component of S_2 may become soft and a right sided S_4 may be audible. Valvular PS results in an inconstant click at 2nd left intercostal space (click accentuates in expiration), the S_1-click interval narrows as severity of PS increases. The characteristic murmur is ejection systolic which is loud and often associated with a thrill in cases with significant PS. The peak of murmur gets delayed as the severity of PS increases.

Electrocardiogram shows right axis deviation and right ventricular hypertrophy in moderate and severe cases. X-ray chest shows a normal sized heart with prominent pulmonary artery segment due to post-stenotic dilatation. Echocardiography not only diagnoses the condition but also helps in determining the severity of the obstruction by using Doppler echo. Right ventricular angiography (done usually prior to balloon dilatation) shows a thick and domed pulmonary valve with a thin jet of contrast agent through it.

Aortic Stenosis

Most often aortic stenosis (AS) is valvular due to a congenital bicuspid (rarely unicuspid) valve and results in left ventricular hypertrophy. Unlike PS, the S_2 in AS is narrow split and in severe cases, paradoxically split due to delayed A_2. The click is constant and localizes the obstruction to the valve. Ejection systolic murmur is best heard at 2nd right intracostal space and radiates to the carotids. Here also the peak of the murmur gets delayed as the severity of AS increases. Left sided S_4 is heard in severe cases. The carotid pulse in significant severe AS is typical with a slow upstroke. Rarely the AS may be supravalvular or subvalvular, click is absent in these cases.

Electrocardiogram may be completely normal even in severe cases, although it may show left ventricular hypertrophy at times with ST-T changes. X-ray chest shows normal sized heart with prominent ascending aorta. Here also echo-Doppler is diagnostic.

Coarctation of Aorta

Coarctation of aorta occurs due to narrowing at the junction of arch with descending thoracic aorta, most often just after the left subclavian artery origin (Fig. 2.11). This results in weak and delayed lower limb pulses, which is the hallmark physical sign of coarctation of aorta. It is therefore mandatory to palpate for femoral pulses in all cases suspected of CHD or hypertension. Blood pressure may not always be high in upper extremity. Left ventricle hypertrophies secondary to obstruction. There may not be any murmur over precordium, however, auscultation over the back of chest may reveal presence of soft continuous murmurs due to collaterals formation in older children. There may be associated bicuspid aortic valve resulting in a constant click. ECG is often normal and if ST-T changes along with left ventricular hypertrophy are present, one should suspect associated aortic stenosis. X-ray chest

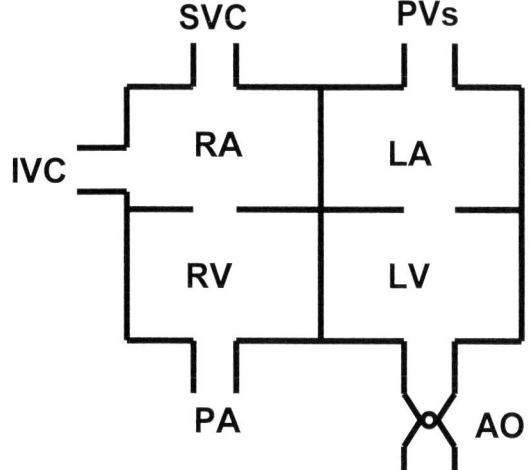

Fig. 2.11: Diagrammatic representation of coarctation of aorta. RA—Right atrium, LA—Left atrium, SVC—Superior vena cava, IVC—Inferior vena cava, PVs—Pulmonary veins, PA—Pulmonary artery, Ao—Aorta

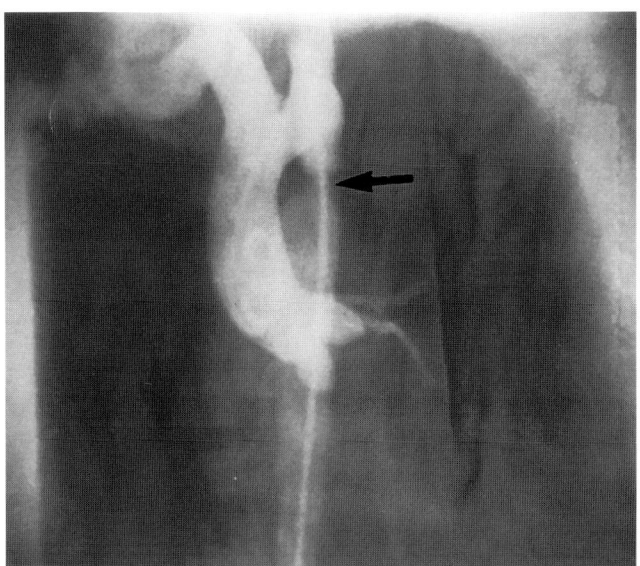

Fig. 2.12a: Aortic root angiogram in anteroposterior view showing a tight coarctation in the usual place (arrow)

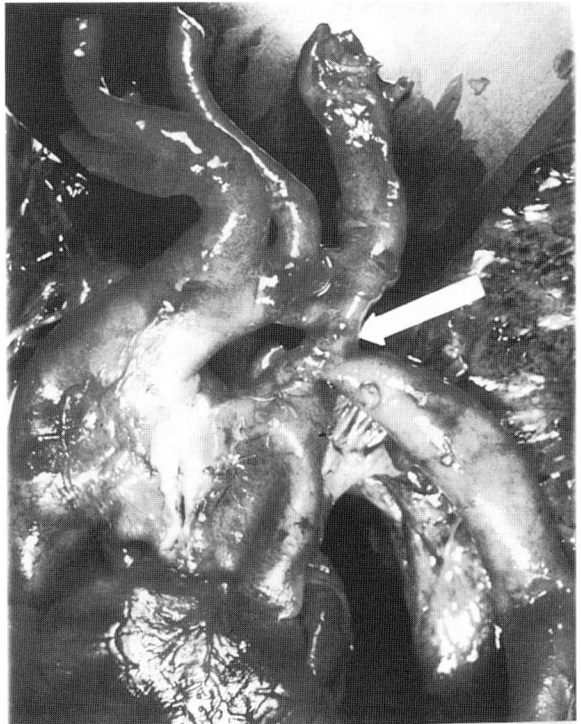

Fig. 2.12b: Gross specimen of heart and large vessels showing coarctation of aorta (arrow)

sometimes typically shows notching of undersurface of 3rd to 8th ribs due to large collaterals. The heart size is normal, but ascending and arch of aorta are prominent. Aortic angiogram further clarifies the diagnosis by showing narrowing of aorta just distal to left subclavian artery (Figs 2.12a and b).

Management of obstructive lesions Patients with mild and moderate lesions can be left on medical follow up alone. In those with severe obstructive lesions with ventricular dysfunction and congestive heart failure, an early relief of obstruction is necessary. Most of these obstructions can be successfully treated with balloon valvuloplasty/angioplasty. In a rare case unresponsive to balloon dilatation, surgery may be needed.

CYANOTIC HEART DISEASE

Cyanosis refers to the bluish coloration imparted to the skin when capillaries contain more than five grams of reduced hemoglobin. It is generally classified as peripheral and central, the latter can be due to abnormality of oxygen transport resulting from defects in the heart or respiratory tract.

In an infant with cyanotic heart disease, there has to be a right to left shunt, which results in unoxygenated blood bypassing the lungs. The degree of cyanosis also depends on the amount of pulmonary blood flow. Cyanosis is commonly accompanied by clubbing and polycythemia especially in older children. There are several congenital heart defects that result in cyanosis and these can be classified into the following groups.

1. Cyanosis with decreased pulmonary blood flow
   a. Tetralogy of Fallot and allied conditions
   b. Eisenmenger's syndrome secondary to a previous left to right shunt
2. Cyanosis with increased pulmonary blood flow
   a. Transposition of great arteries
   b. Unobstructed total anomalous pulmonary venous connection
3. Cyanosis with pulmonary venous hypertension
   a. Obstructed total anomalous pulmonary venous connection
   b. Hypoplastic left heart syndrome, aortic arch interruption
4. Others, e.g. single atrium, Ebstein's anomaly.

Diagnosis and management of some of the common cyanotic congenital heart defects seen in association with common extracardiac anomalies are described below:

Tetralogy of Fallot and Allied Conditions

The most frequently encountered lesion in this category is tetralogy of Fallot (Fig. 2.13). The other cardiac conditions with similar hemodynamics are called tetralogy variants. These include:
1. Double outlet right ventricle with pulmonary stenosis.
2. Atrioventricular septal defect and pulmonary stenosis.
3. Single ventricle and pulmonary stenosis.
4. Transposition of great arteries with ventricular septal defect and pulmonary stenosis.
5. Tricuspid atresia with restrictive ventricular septal defect and reduced pulmonary flow.

In tetralogy of Fallot (TOF), the large subaortic VSD results in equal pressures in right and left ventricle and hence right ventricular pressure cannot rise above systemic pressure. There is generally no congestive heart failure and no cardiomegaly unless complications develop. The most common cause of cardiomegaly in TOF is anemia in our country. A hemoglobin of 12.0 gm% may also be low in presence of deep cyanosis.

In addition to cyanosis and absence of cardiomegaly, these infants show mild left parasternal impulse, single second heart sound as P_2 is generally inaudible. There is an ejection systolic murmur of PS. The intensity of this murmur is inversely proportional to the severity of cyanosis and hence to the severity of PS. There is no right ventricular S_3 or S_4. An aortic ejection click may be heard in severe cases. X-ray chest shows normal sized heart with ischemic lung fields. The apex is right ventricular in type and there is concavity in the region of pulmonary artery segment resulting in the so-called "pulmonary bay" (Fig. 2.14). The aortic arch may be right sided. Electrocardiogram reveals right axis deviation upto + 135° or so and right ventricular hypertrophy. The transition starts early, sometimes in V_1 or V_2. Right ventricular strain does not occur in TOF.

It may be difficult to accurately diagnose the individual lesions of tetralogy variant clinically. Some of the helpful points are given below, absence of these, however, does not rule out the particular diagnosis.

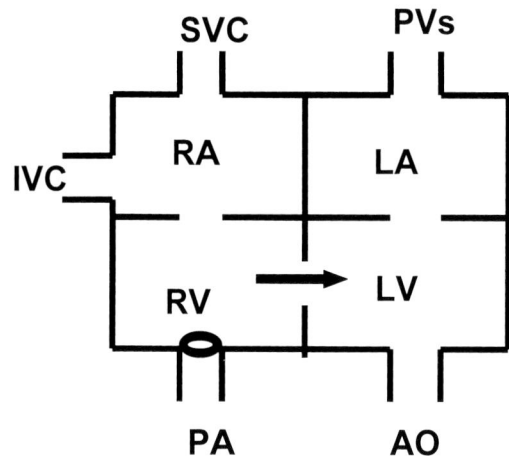

Fig. 2.13: Line diagram showing tetralogy of Fallot. RA—Right atrium, LA—Left atrium, SVC—Superior vena cava, IVC—Inferior vena cava, PVs—Pulmonary veins, PA—Pulmonary artery, Ao—Aorta

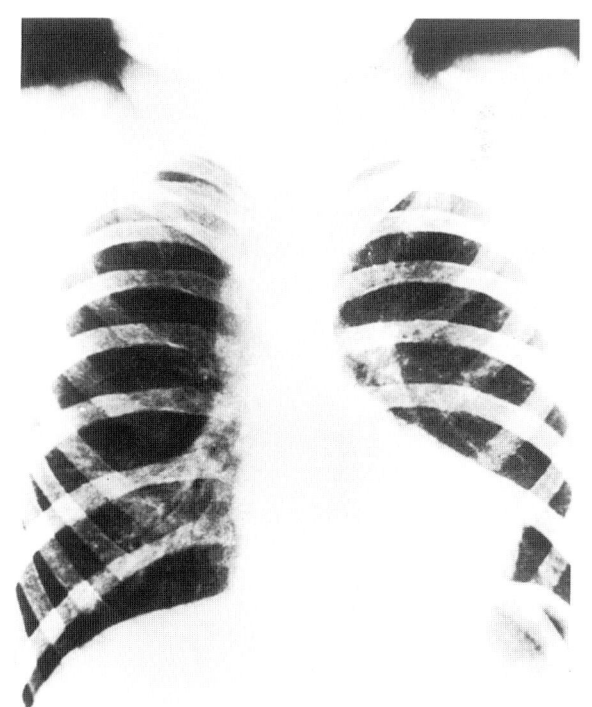

Fig. 2.14: X-ray chest from a patient with tetralogy of Fallot showing a normal sized, boot-shaped heart with pulmonary bay and oligemic lung fields

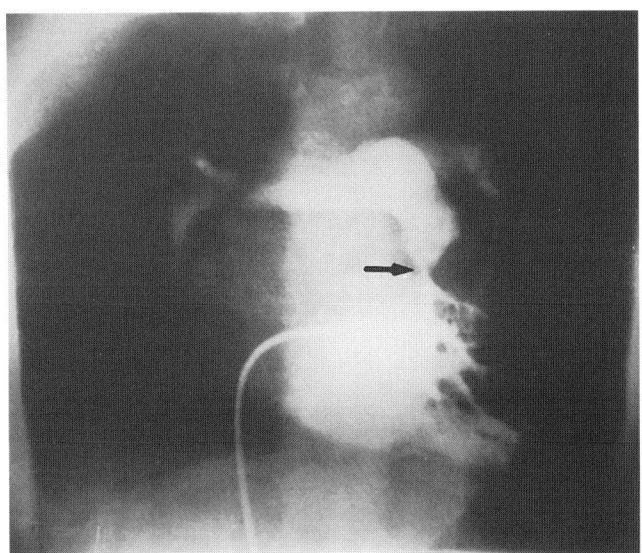

1. *Double outlet right ventricle with pulmonary stenosis* Clinical features and X-ray chest resemble those of TOF. ECG may reveal extreme right axis deviation along with right ventricular hypertrophy. In a rare case with restrictive VSD, left ventricular hypertrophy may also be present.
2. *Atrioventricular septal defect with pulmonary stenosis* Electrocardiogram is most helpful, demonstrating left axis deviation.
3. *Single ventricle with pulmonary stenosis* X-ray chest may show a prominent bulge along the upper left cardiac border, if the aorta is L-posed. ECG may show stereotyped complexes from V_1-V_6.

Echocardiography with color Doppler is diagnostic and can accurately define the various anatomic and hemodynamic features of TOF as well as its variants.

Cardiac catheterization and angiography demonstrates subvalvular obstruction of the pulmonary outflow, right ventricular hypertrophy and a large ventricular septal defect with overriding of the aorta (Figs 2.15a and b).

Management The urgency of treatment is determined by the degree of cyanosis and hypoxia. If a neonate is deeply blue and hypoxic, it may be best to do a palliative aortopulmonary shunt to relieve hypoxia. In older infants and children, a total surgical repair is advisable at about 9 months to a year of age.

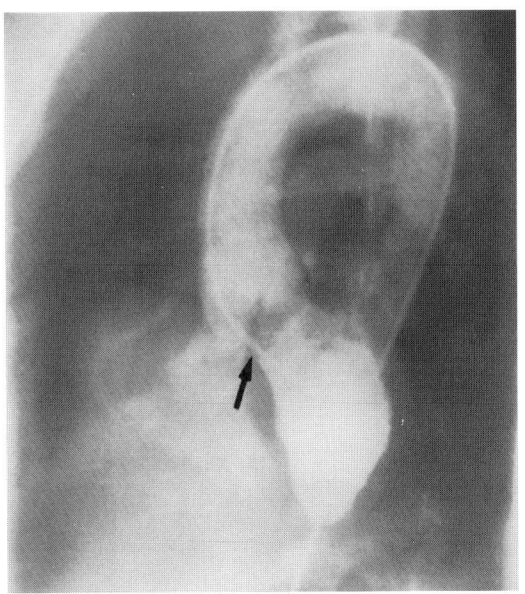

Figs 2.15a and b: Right ventricular angiogram (a) showing tight infundibular stenosis (arrow) and left ventricular angiogram (b) shows the large ventricular septal defect with overriding of aorta (arrow)

Complete Transposition of Great Arteries

In transposition (TGA) aorta arises from right ventricle and pulmonary artery from left ventricle (Fig. 2.16). The systemic and pulmonary circulations are therefore in parallel rather than in series and unless some communication exists between these two circulations, survival is unlikely. TGA is more common in males and almost always produces symptoms in neonatal period. In babies without a large VSD or ASD, intense cyanosis appears as the ductus arteriosus closes. Emergency balloon atrial septostomy to create an ASD is performed in these neonates with severe hypoxia. In infants with a sizable ASD/VSD or PDA, cyanosis is less severe, however, congestive heart failure is often seen resulting in tachypnea. The murmurs are generally soft or absent. ECG shows right axis deviation and right ventricular hypertrophy. X-ray chest demonstrates cardiomegaly and pulmonary plethora, in some cases a typical egg on side appearance of the heart may be appreciated. Echocardiography is diagnostic and clearly delineates the origin of pulmonary artery from left ventricle and aorta from right ventricle. Pulmonary artery can be differentiated from aorta by its bifurcation soon after origin (Fig. 2.17). Associated defects such as ASD, VSD, PDA, coarctation of aorta can be detected easily. Angiography shows origin of aorta from the right ventricle and pulmonary artery arises from the left ventricle.

Management As pointed out earlier, TGA without a sizable communication between the systemic and pulmonary circulations is an emergency and an urgent creation of an ASD should be performed in catheterization laboratory with Rashkind balloon catheter to relieve hypoxemia. In some cases, prostaglandin E1 infusion can be helpful in taking care of hypoxia by keeping the ductus arteriosus open.

The definitive treatment of babies with TGA and intact ventricular septum is surgery. An arterial switch operation which corrects physiology as well as anatomy should be performed in the first two to three weeks of life after which regression of left ventricular mass occurs as pulmonary vascular resistance falls and this regressed left ventricular mass may not remain suitable to take up systemic pressure after corrective operation. However, in

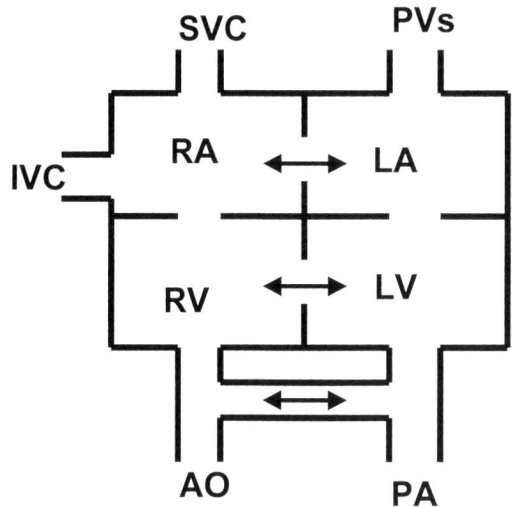

Fig. 2.16: Line diagram demonstrating transposition of great arteries. LA—Left atrium, SVC—Superior vena cava, IVC—Inferior vena cava, PVs—Pulmonary veins, PA—Pulmonary artery, Ao—Aorta

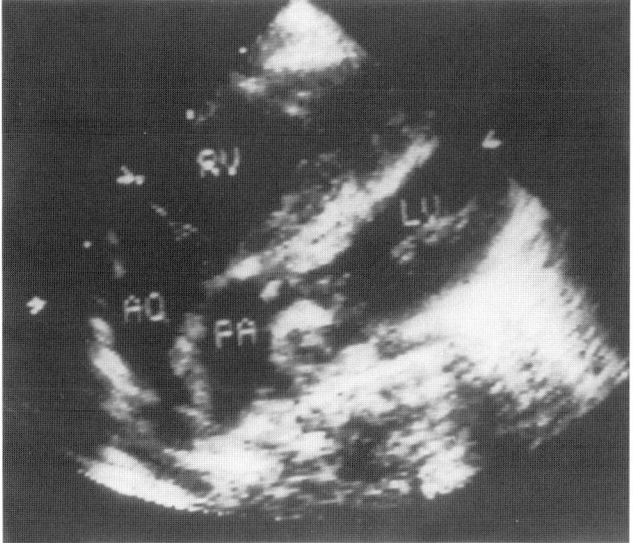

Fig. 2.17: Echocardiography in a patient with complete transposition showing origin of pulmonary artery (PA) from the left ventricle (LV) and origin of aorta (Ao) from the right ventricle (RV)

cases of TGA with large VSD, left ventricular pressure remains high due to VSD and in these an arterial switch operation can be performed even later, but preferably before 2-3 months to avoid irreversible pulmonary vascular obstructive changes in the lungs.

For infants with TGA and no VSD presenting beyond 2-3 weeks of life, a Senning operation is performed in which re-routing of circulation is done at atrial level. This operation makes right ventricle as systemic chamber and hence may not be ideal on long-term follow-up.

Total Anomalous Pulmonary Venous Connection (TAPVC)

In this condition, all pulmonary veins (mostly four) join anomalously to somewhere in systemic venous circulation mostly through a common chamber. There may be obstruction somewhere in their path resulting in obstructed variety. The anomalous connection may be as (a) *Supracardiac:* to left ventrical vein (most common) or right superior vena cava, (b) *Cardiac:* to right atrium or coronary sinus, (c) *Infracardiac:* to portal venous system or inferior vena cava, (d) *Mixed:* to more than one of the above mentioned sites. The infracardiac variety is almost always obstructive.

Unobstructed TAPVC

The presentation is usually in infancy with features of large left to right shunt, mild cyanosis and congestive heart failure. Examination reveals cardiomegaly, a wide fixed second heart sound, ejection systolic murmur at base and a tricuspid flow murmur. X-ray chest shows cardiomegaly, prominent pulmonary artery segment and pulmonary plethora. In supracardiac drainage, X-ray chest may show a classical figure of 8 appearance. Right axis deviation and right ventricular hypertrophy are seen on ECG. Again the exact diagnosis comes from echocardiography which localizes the site of drainage also. TAPVC may sometimes be a part of heterotaxy syndrome.

Management Unobstructed TAPVC, although not an emergency, must be corrected early at whatever age it is diagnosed. The correction is generally simple and safe except when it is a part of heterotaxy syndrome.

Obstructed TAPVC

The presentation is early in neonatal period mostly with cyanosis, congestive heart failure and absence of cardiomegaly and murmurs. In fact, the picture resembles that of pulmonary parenchymal disease like acute respiratory distress syndrome. X-ray chest typically shows a normal sized heart with severe pulmonary venous hypertension resulting in ground glass appearance of lungs due to severe pulmonary venous hypertension.

Management Obstructed TAPVC is medical emergency and these infants must be operated as early as possible, early demise is almost certain on medical treatment.

Persistent Truncus Arteriosus

In this condition, a single arterial vessel comes out of the heart overlying a VSD and supplies the systemic, coronary and pulmonary arterial system. Cyanosis is usually mild and pulse pressure may be wide. There is a constant ejection click and S2 is single. A systolic and sometimes an early diastolic murmur may be heard over the base, related to truncal valve insufficiency. An apical diastolic murmur due to increased flow may also be present. ECG shows right axis deviation and right or biventricular hypertrophy. X-ray chest typically shows cardiomegaly, absence of pulmonary artery segment, wide upper mediastinum and pulmonary plethora. Echocardiography can diagnose this condition accurately and quantify the severity of truncal valve stenosis and regurgitation if present.

Management Control of congestive heart failure followed by elective surgery at about 1-2 months of age is the desirable way of managing these infants.

Interruption of Aortic Arch

The aortic arch may be discontinuous with the rest of aorta, most often just after the left subclavian artery and the lower part of body is supplied by the right to left flow through PDA. Ductal constriction, results in decreased perfusion to lower part of the body with sudden deterioration and congestive heart failure. The presentation is within the first week or two of life. Differential cyanosis (cyanosis in lower limbs only) results due to right to left flow through PDA distal to the interruption. The femoral pulses may not be weak till ductus remains open. Echocardiography from suprasternal view clinches the diagnosis. These sick infants should be first stabilized by using Prostaglandin E_1 infusion to maintain ductal patency and then taken for early surgical correction of interruption.

Hypoplastic Left Heart Syndrome

The hypoplastic left ventricle may be associated with mitral valve atresia/stenosis, aortic valve atresia/stenosis and/or hypoplastic ascending and arch of aorta. Progressive congestive heart failure with mild to severe cyanosis sets in usually within the first week of life and leads to cardiogenic shock. X-ray chest shows cardiomegaly and pulmonary venous hypertension and echocardiography is diagnostic. Ductal patency is of vital importance and should be maintained by the use of Prostaglandin E_1 infusion in case surgery is being contemplated. There is no corrective surgery short of cardiac transplantation. Palliative surgery also has a high mortality and is done in stages. Most of the pediatric cardiologists are not very enthusiastic about treating this defect.

CONCLUSION

In congenital heart disease, a precise anatomic diagnosis at the bedside is not always possible. However, a good clinician, with the help of history, physical signs and ancillary investigations should be able to narrow down the diagnostic possibilities and categorise the child to a specific group of diseases. He should also be able to identify babies requiring immediate help, e.g. those suffering from ductus arteriosus dependent congenital heart diseases. Investigations like echocardiography may be necessary in arriving at a complete diagnosis of CHD.

SUGGESTED READING

1. Fyler DC: Atrial septal defect secundum. In Nadas' *Pediatric Cardiology*. Philadelphia: Hanely and Belfus. 513-24, 1992.
2. Garson A Jr, Bricker JT, Fisher DJ, Neish SR: *The Science and Practice of Pediatric Cardiology* (2nd ed), Williams and Wilkins, **1**: 1998.
3. Moller JH, Neal WA: *Heart Disease in Infancy*. Appleton-Century-Crofts, New York, 1981.
4. Moss and Admas' *Heart Disease in Infants, Children and Adolescents*. Emmanouilides GC *et al* (Eds): Baltimore: Williams and Wilkins, 1995.
5. Perloff JK: *The Clinical Recognition of Congenital Heart Disease* (4th ed). WB Saunders Company, 1994.

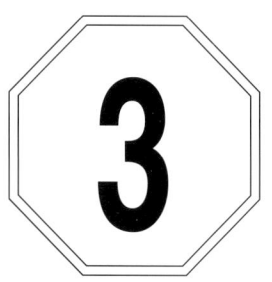

Rheumatic Heart Disease

Rheumatic heart disease (RHD) continues to be a cause of concern in the developing countries. In India it is a major public health challenge which contributes to high morbidity and mortality. The magnitude of the problem is well-appreciated by the prevalence figures ranging from 1/1000 to 5.5/1000 in school-going children (5-16 years age-Multicentre school survey by the Indian Council of Medical Research). Further, hospital based studies show that approximately a third of cardiac admissions are those of rheumatic heart disease. An evaluation of autopsy cases at the All India Institute of Medical Sciences, New Delhi revealed that cardiac autopsies accounted for 654 of 3157 total autopsies (20.7%) conducted in a period of 30 years. Rheumatic heart disease was the cause of death in 229 of the 654 cardiac autopsies (35%) thus making it the most common cardiac disease seen at autopsy.

Acute rheumatic fever (RF) is an inflammatory, recurrent, nonsuppurative disease which follows pharyngitis caused by group A beta-hemolytic streptococci. While a history of "sore" throat is obtained in some cases, in a substantial number it escapes notice by the patient. This generally affects children in the age range of 5-16 years. Following the pharyngitis there is a lag period of about 2-3 weeks after which clinical manifestations of rheumatic fever occur. It is believed that this period is a crucial one during which time the streptococcal antigens excite either an immune response and/or an autoimmune reaction to normal tissues in the body.

Diagnosis of rheumatic fever Presence of two major or, one major and two minor Jones criteria supported by laboratory evidence of preceding streptococcal infection is necessary for the clinical diagnosis of rheumatic fever (Table 3.1).

Table 3.1: Jones criteria (revised) for the diagnosis of rheumatic fever

Major criteria	*Minor criteria*
• Carditis	• Fever
• Polyarthritis	• Arthralgias
• Chorea	• Previous history of RF
• Subcutaneous nodules	• Elevated ESR, CRP, leucocytosis
• Erythema marginatum	• Prolonged P-R interval

Supporting evidence	Preceding streptococcal infection. History of recent scarlet fever. Positive throat culture for group A *Streptococcus*. Increased titres of streptococcal antibodies (streptokinase, streptolysin O and S, hyaluronidase and anti-DNAse B)
Clinical diagnosis of RF	Two major or, one major plus two minor criteria supported by antecedent streptococcal infection

RF—Rheumatic fever

Etiopathogenesis

Much evidence namely clinical, epidemiological, immunological and prophylactic exists to implicate Group A beta-hemolytic *Streptococcus* in the etiopathogenesis of rheumatic fever/rheumatic heart disease. It has been demonstrated that a number of proteins/enzymes in the cell wall and cell membrane of the *Streptococcus* reveal an identity and/or cross-reactivity with several mammalian tissues which are involved in the rheumatic process, e.g. the hyaluronate capsule of the group A *Streptococcus* bears identity to the human hyaluronate a substance which is present in the joints, valvular tissue, etc. Antibodies to group A cell wall polysaccharide cross-react with glycoprotein of heart valves while antibodies to membrane antigen of the group A *Streptococcus* exhibit reaction with sarcolemma of cardiac muscle, dermal fibroblast and caudate nucleus. In addition, M protein is one of the most important proteins of the *Streptococcus* which has antiphagocytic properties and is the major determinant of virulence. The molecular structure of M protein has revealed epitopes that exhibit cross-reactivity with cardiac myosin. Increased cellular immune response is evident by prominence of CD4+ lymphocytes in rheumatic heart lesions. It is believed that T cell mimicry between streptococcal antigens and heart proteins is responsible for autoimmunity in RHD. Pharyngitis caused by group A beta-hemolytic *Streptococcus* causes rheumatic fever after a latent period of 2-4 weeks. It is during this interval that hypersensitivity and/or autoimmunity to this bacterium develops to result in acute rheumatic fever. However, it is important to keep in mind that while pharyngitis caused by group A *Streptococcus* is so frequent, development of rheumatic fever varies from 1 to 3% only. How does then one explain this paradox? The reason for this observation is unexplained. However, it is likely that certain genetically predisposed individuals have an increased susceptibility to streptococcal antigens to develop the disease.

PATHOLOGY

Acute rheumatic carditis At autopsy the heart shows an involvement of all the three layers- **Pancarditis**.

Serofibrinous pericarditis It is most often observed in acute rheumatic carditis. Both layers of the pericardium are thickened and covered with varying amounts of fibrin that project between the two layers (Figs 11.11a and b). Healing produces fibrosis and adhesions between the two layers without any serious cardiac effects. Microscopically, fibrin covers the surface of the epicardium and an infiltrate comprising of lymphocytes, histiocytes and plasma cells is seen. Occasionally, fibrinoid necrosis with Aschoff bodies may be present (Figs 11.14a to d).

Endocarditis It involves either the valvular or the parietal (mural) endocardium but more commonly both sites are affected simultaneously. Rheumatic valvulitis has characteristic gross and microscopic features and is of extreme clinical importance as recurrent attacks of inflammation and healing produce valvular deformities which cause serious cardiac morbidity and mortality. All four cardiac valves may be involved in the following descending order of frequency—mitral, aortic, tricuspid and pulmonary. Mitral and aortic valves are more frequently affected than the tricuspid and the pulmonary valves. In the acute stage, the valve leaflets are edematous, opaque and lose their normal transparency. Tiny, firmly attached nodules 1 to 3 mm in diameter are present along the line of closure of the cusps. This lesion is commonly referred to as rheumatic vegetations (Fig. 3.1). The vegetations are present on the atrial surface of the mitral and tricuspid valves and on the ventricular surface of the semilunar cusps of the aortic and the pulmonary valves (Figs 3.2 and 3.3). Microscopically, the valve cusps show edema, increased vascularity and inflammatory cell infiltration of the valve substance by lymphocytes, histiocytes, few polymorphs and eosinophils. Rheumatic vegetations reveal fibrinoid necrosis of the valvular collagen on the surface of the valve which at its base is bordered by histiocytes in a palisading arrangement. Few aggregates of Aschoff cells may also be seen within the valve substance. Typical Aschoff nodules are not encountered in the valve (Figs 3.4 to 3.10).

Mechanism of formation of these vegetations is possibly related to injury to the endocardium and exposure of the subendocardial connective tissues caused by the hemodynamic stress and strain on

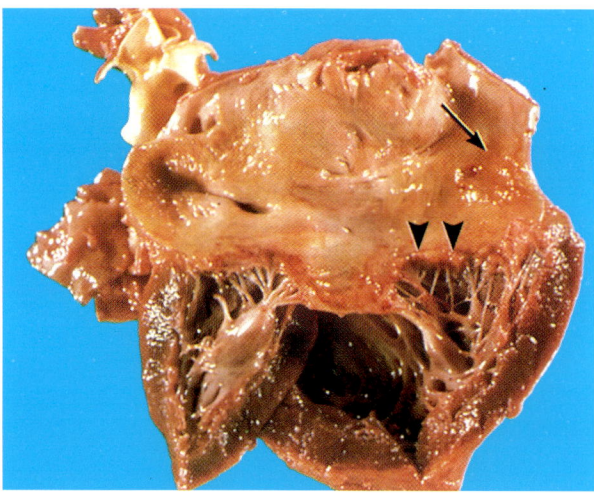

Fig. 3.1: Acute rheumatic carditis. Marked dilatation of left atrium and mitral valve ring is observed. The contact margins of both leaflets show tiny flat excrescences evident as congested foci (arrowheads). Left atrial endocardium above the posterior leaflet of the mitral valve (arrow) is irregular (MacCallum's patch)

Note: 15 years old male presented with fever for 2½ months, progressive effort intolerance and severe cough for 2 weeks. At autopsy heart weighed 350 gm. Aortic and mitral valves were affected.

the valves. The inflamed and exposed endocardial surface coupled with fibrinoid degeneration of the collagen favors the deposition of fibrin and platelets. Rheumatic vegetations on cardiac valves from autopsied cases of acute rheumatic carditis were evaluated by scanning electron microscopy. The

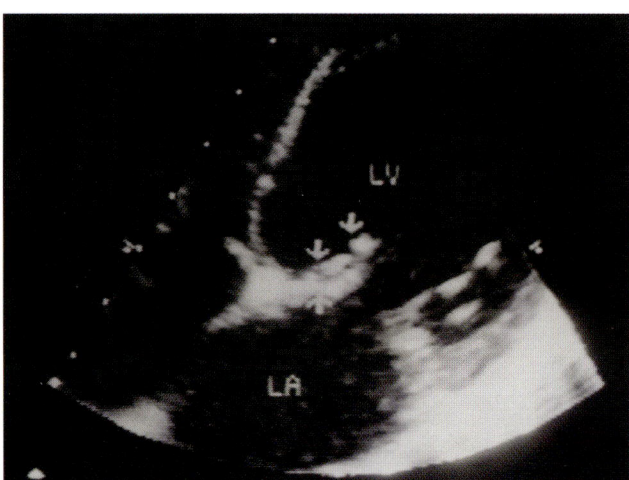

Fig. 3.2: Echocardiogram from a case of acute rheumatic fever with mitral regurgitation showing multiple small nodules (vegetations) (3-4 mm in size) on anterior mitral leaflet (arrows). LA—Left atrium, LV—Left ventricle

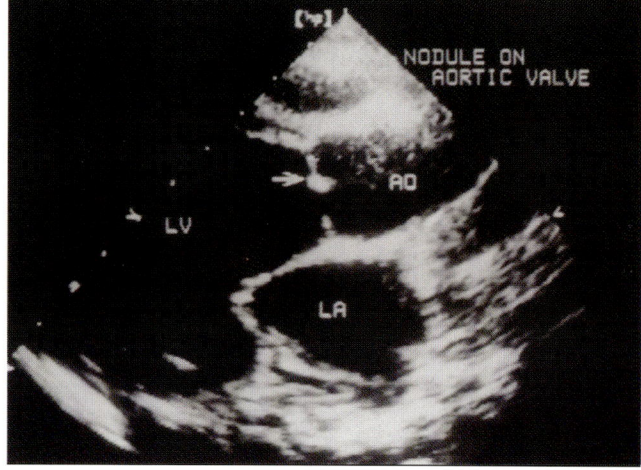

Fig. 3.3: Echocardiogram from a case of acute rheumatic fever with aortic regurgitation showing a small nodule (vegetation) (arrow) on aortic valve

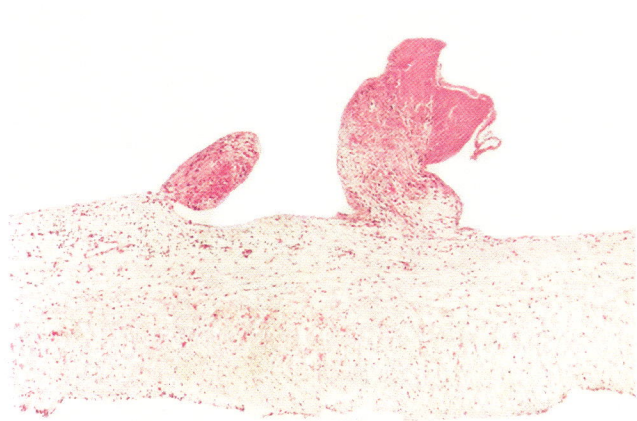

Fig. 3.4: Acute rheumatic carditis. The vegetation on the mitral valve is seen as an elevated projection from the surface of valve. Deep pink smudgy appearance represents fibrinoid degeneration of collagen. A few histiocytes and blood vessels are seen at the base. Valve substance does not show any inflammation

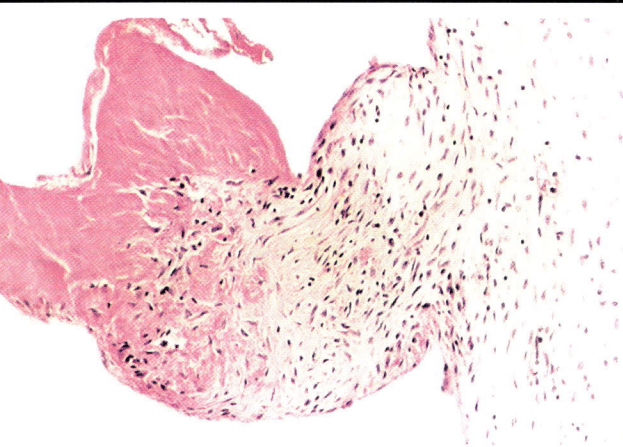

Fig. 3.5: Acute rheumatic carditis. Finger like projection from the valvular endocardium of the mitral valve (vegetation) is seen. Fibrinoid necrosis of the valvular collagen is well-appreciated. The base of the vegetation shows mesenchymal cells and few lymphocytes

normal mosaic arrangement of the endothelial cells was lost and the valvular collagen revealed marked architectural alterations (Figs 3.11 and 3.12). The collagen fibers were arranged irregularly forming large and small cavities between them. This arrangement served as a trap for circulating blood

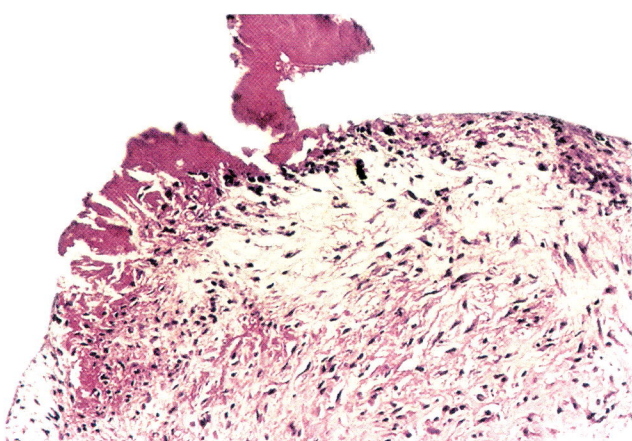

Fig. 3.6: Acute rheumatic carditis. Photomicrograph of vegetation on the mitral valve reveals deep pink smudgy appearance of surface valve collagen. The endocardium is discontinuous in this area. This change is bordered at its base by histiocytes. The subendocardial area shows edema and fibrinoid necrosis of the valve collagen and infiltration by few lymphocytes and histiocytes

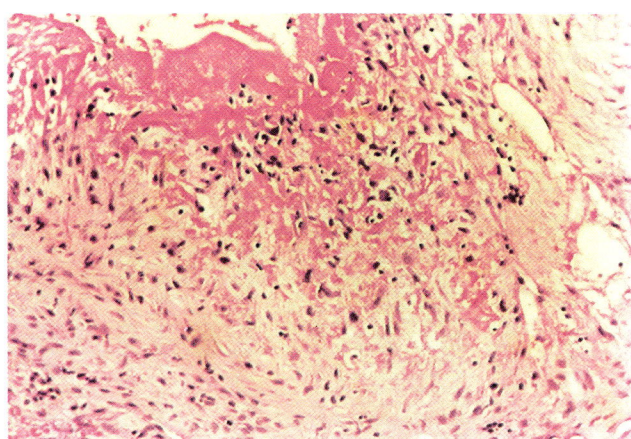

Fig. 3.7: Mitral valve from a case of acute rheumatic fever. Notice marked collagen degeneration on the surface of the valve. This is bordered by histiocytes and a few lymphocytes

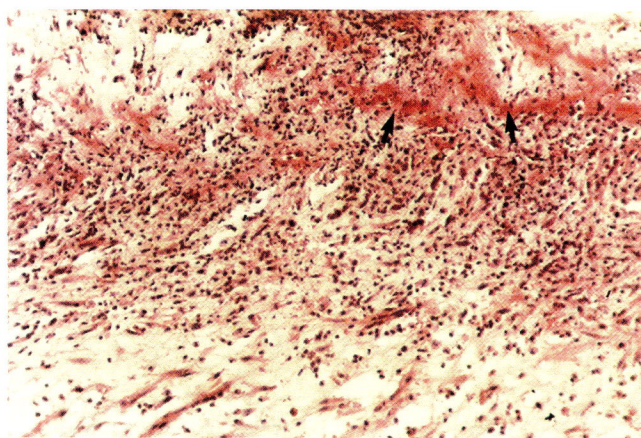

Fig. 3.8: Acute rheumatic mitral valvulitis. Valvular collagen shows edema, increased vascularity and dense infiltration by lymphocytes, histiocytes and few polymorphs. Additionally, necrosis of collagen is observed (arrows)

elements or infective organisms. Associated involvement of the mural (parietal) endocardium is often encountered in RF. The most common location is the endocardium lining the posterior wall of the left atrium above the posterior leaflet of the mitral valve. This lesion is commonly known as the **MacCallum's**

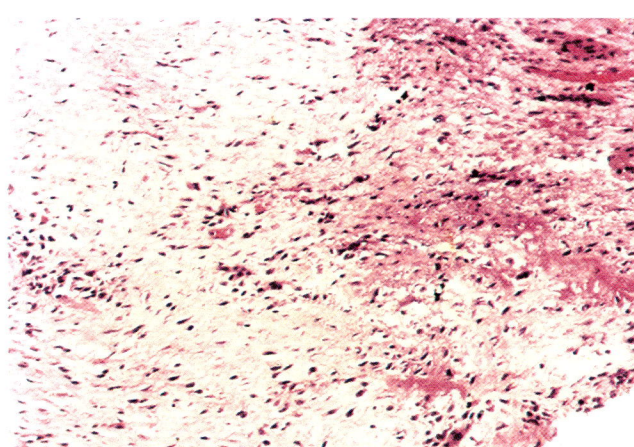

Fig. 3.9: Mitral valve from a case of acute rheumatic fever. Patchy fibrinoid necrosis of the valvular collagen is seen. This case had characteristic rheumatic vegetations

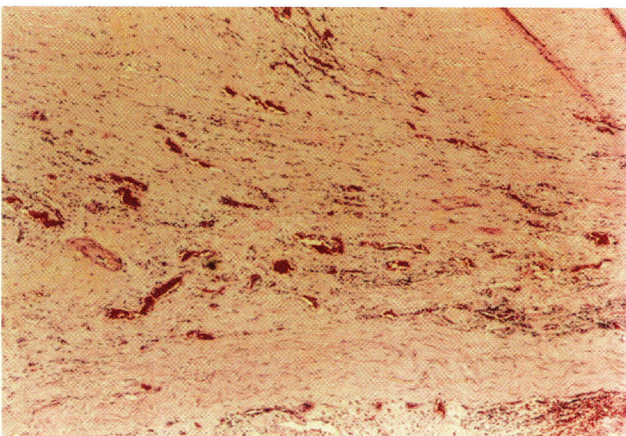

Fig. 3.10: Mitral valve from a case of acute rheumatic fever. Prominent neovascularization is noted along with infiltration by lymphocytes and other mononuclear cells

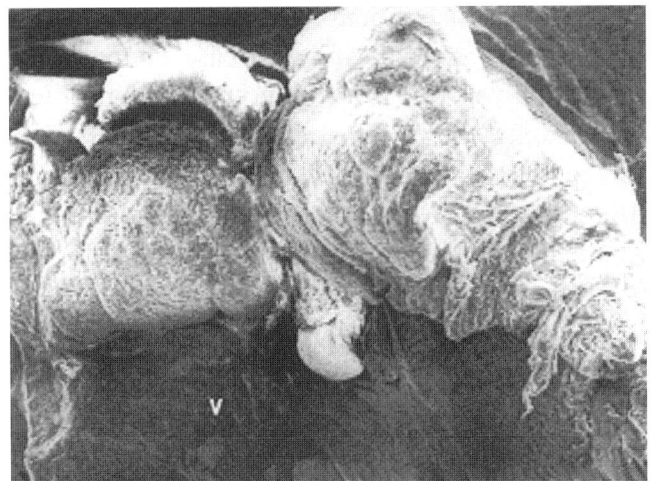

Fig. 3.11: Scanning electron micrograph of vegetations on the mitral valve in a case of acute rheumatic fever. These are seen as nodular bulbous projections over and undermining the valve surface (v). The surface of the vegetation is irregular and has a fine sieve-like appearance

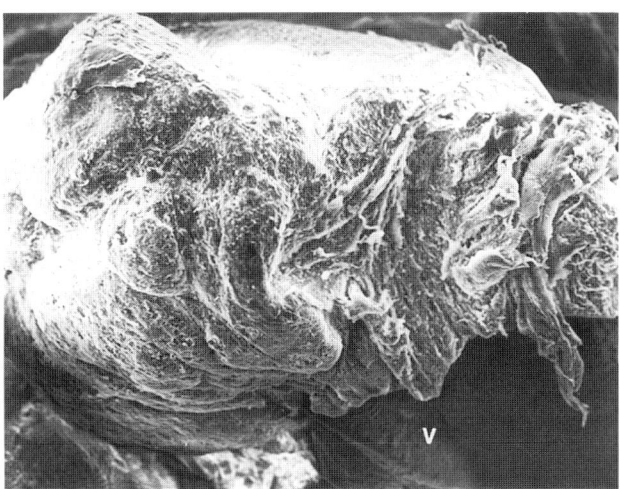

Fig. 3.12: Higher magnification of the scanning electron micrograph of rheumatic vegetation demonstrating the fine lattice-like arrangement that corresponds to the fibrinoid necrosis seen on light microscopy

patch which shows irregularly thickened endocardium (Fig. 3.1). Microscopically, edema and inflammation of the endocardium and subendocardial tissues is present. The infiltrate is composed of lymphocytes, histiocytes, few polymorphs and eosinophils. Antischkow and Aschoff cells may be seen. Classical Aschoff nodules are unusual although ill-formed Aschoff nodules have been observed (Figs 3.13 to 3.16).

Myocarditis It is a feature of acute carditis which is evident by an enlarged, soft and flabby heart with dilatation of all chambers especially the ventricles. Microscopically, rheumatic myocarditis is characterised by (i) presence of Aschoff bodies, (ii) non-specific interstitial myocarditis, and (iii) damage and destruction of the myofibers all of which result in a soft and dilated heart.

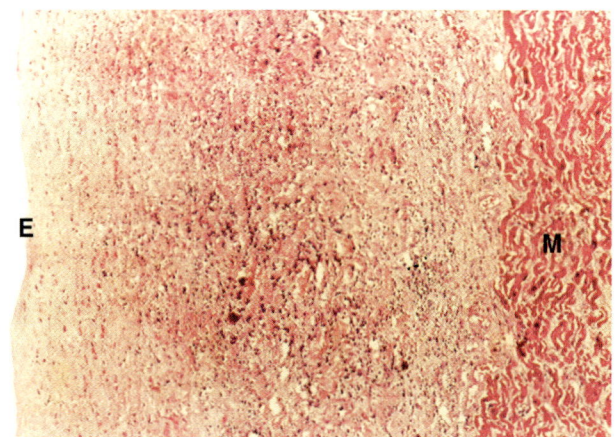

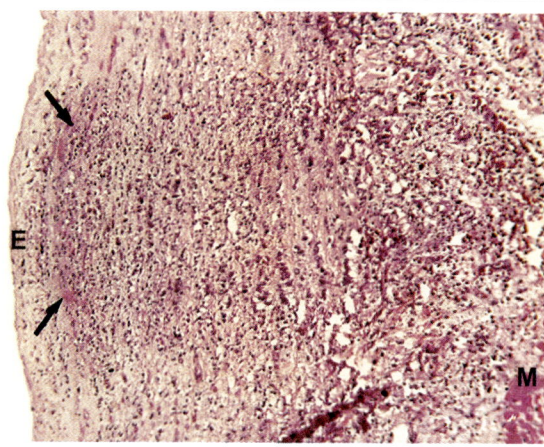

Fig. 3.13: Acute rheumatic carditis. Section from the MacCallum's patch reveals edema and increased cellularity of the left atrial endocardium. Focal fibrinoid degeneration of collagen, lymphocytic infiltration and histiocytes some of which are in aggregates reminiscent of Aschoff nodules are seen. E—Endocardium, M—Myocardium

Fig. 3.14: MacCallum's patch in a case of acute rheumatic fever. The endocardium is widened and cellular. Focal areas of necrosis of collagen (arrows) are seen. Aggregates of histiocytes (ill-formed Aschoff nodules) bordered by lymphocytic infiltration are present; E—Endocardium, M—Myocardium

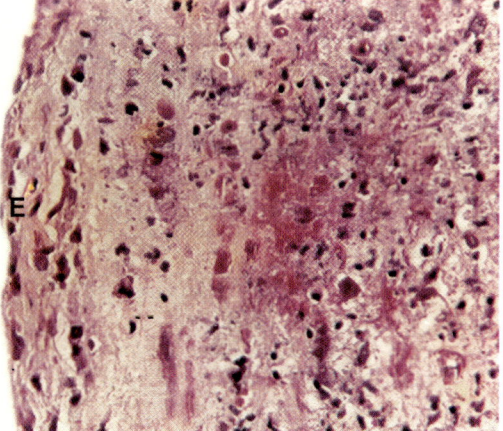

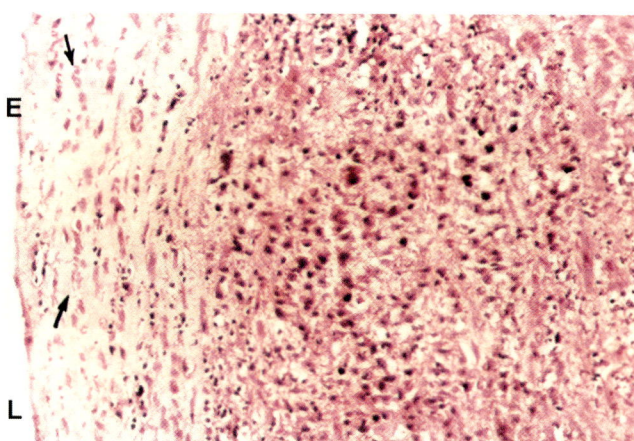

Fig. 3.15: MacCallum's patch (Fig. 3.14) from a case of acute rheumatic carditis. Higher magnification to demonstrate fibrinoid necrosis of collagen which appears smudgy. Infiltration by lymphocytes and histiocytes is observed; E—Endocardium

Fig. 3.16: Higher magnification of the MacCallum's patch from a case of acute rheumatic carditis. Clusters of cells having a appearance of an ill-defined Aschoff nodule are observed. Prominent myofibroblasts (arrows) are noted in the sub-endocardial region (E). L—Lumen

The most pathognomonic feature of rheumatic carditis is the **Aschoff body/nodule**. It may be present in various sites but is most commonly located in the interstices of the myocardium often adjacent to intramyocardial blood vessels and in the subendocardial tissue. It may occasionally be encountered in the pericardium, and adventitia of the aorta. Aschoff bodies are oval, elliptical or nodular structures which evolve through several stages. The earliest stage, is characterized by swelling, fragmentation and fibrinoid degeneration of the collagen which is surrounded by lymphocytes, macrophages and plasms cells (Figs 3.17 to 3.21). The appearance of the Aschoff body in the granulomatous stage is characteristic and comprizes of nodular aggregate of large, plump, mononuclear or multinuclear cells known as the Aschoff cells. Antischkow cells and lymphocytes are the other components of the Aschoff nodule (Figs 3.22 to 3.26). The Anitschkow cells are small elongated cells with single nucleus, scanty eosinophilic cytoplasm and indistinct cell borders. The Aschoff cells are large, ovoid in shape, have abundant to light basophilic cytoplasm and ill-defined, ragged cell borders. They may be uninucleate or multinucleated (Aschoff giant cells Fig. 3.19). The nuclei either have uniformly distributed chromatin or more often the chromatin is arranged as a bar with serrated edges, an appearance known as "caterpillar nuclei". In cross-sections the chromatin strand is surrounded by a halo and is commonly termed as "owl eyed" nuclei. Within three to four months the Aschoff bodies eventually heal by scarring. Myocarditis in RF is characterized by an interstitial infiltrate of lymphocytes, plasma cells and histiocytes. Occasionally polymorphs and eosinophils in variable numbers are also seen within the infiltrate. Focal and/or diffuse degeneration and necrosis of the myofibers is frequently encountered (Figs 3.20 and 3.21).

Aschoff nodules are present in a large number of left atrial appendages that are excised at the time of mitral valvotomy in cases of mitral stenosis (Figs 3.22 to 3.26). In a study of 325 excised left atrial appendages in rheumatic heart disease Aschoff nodules were detected in 106 cases (Table 3.2). These were located in the subendocardial tissue mostly

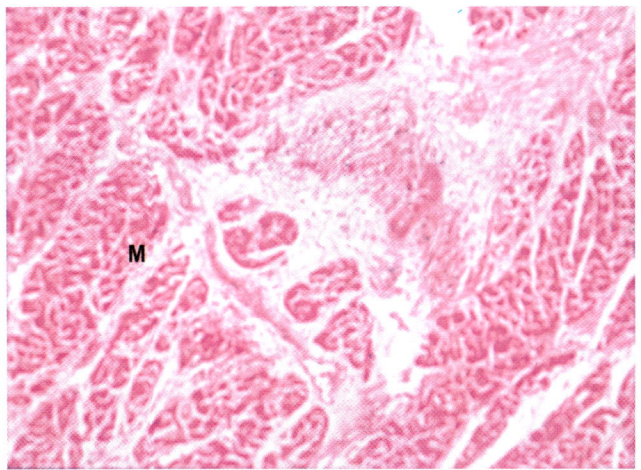

Fig. 3.17: Acute rheumatic carditis. An Aschoff nodule is seen in the interstitium of the myocardium in the paravascular location. Blood vessel wall shows fibrinoid necrosis. Myofibers (M) are unremarkable

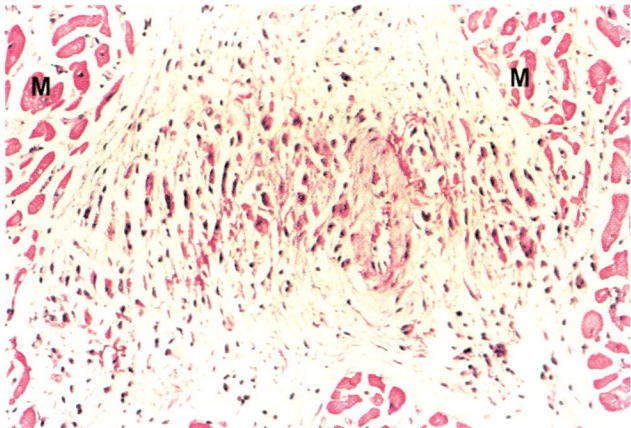

Fig. 3.18: Acute rheumatic carditis. A large area in the interstitium of myocardium is occupied by an ovoid, fairly well limited zone (Aschoff nodule) in which uninucleate and binucleate Aschoff cells are recognised. Myofibres (M) are unremarkable

Table 3.2: Aschoff nodules in excised left atrial appendage from cases rheumatic heart disease (N=325)

Age range (Years)	\textit{Aschoff nodules}					
	0	±	+	++	+++	Total
< 20	52	26	18	17	15	128 (39.4)
21-30	56	34	15	10	13	128 (39.4)
31-40	28	8	5	3	5	49 (15.07)
41-50	12	1	2	0	0	15 (4.61)
> 50	0	2	1	2	0	5 (1.53)
Total	**148**	**71**	**41**	**32**	**33**	**325**

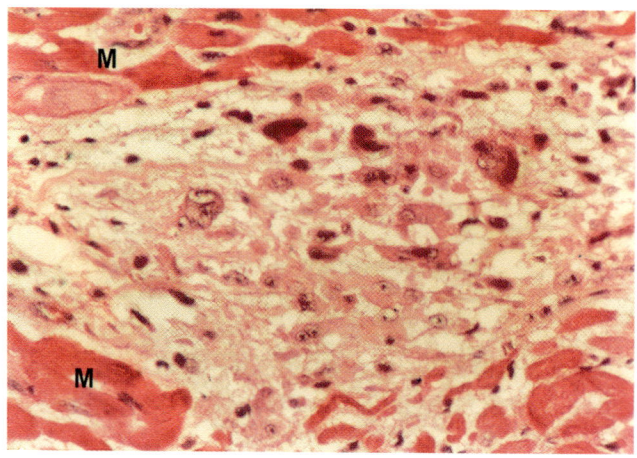

Fig. 3.19: Aschoff nodule. Uninucleate and binucleate Aschoff cells are seen. The cells are large and possess an ill-defined cell outline and abundant light eosinophilic cytoplasm. Nuclei are vesicular with prominent nucleoli. Myocardium (M) is seen at the periphery of the picture

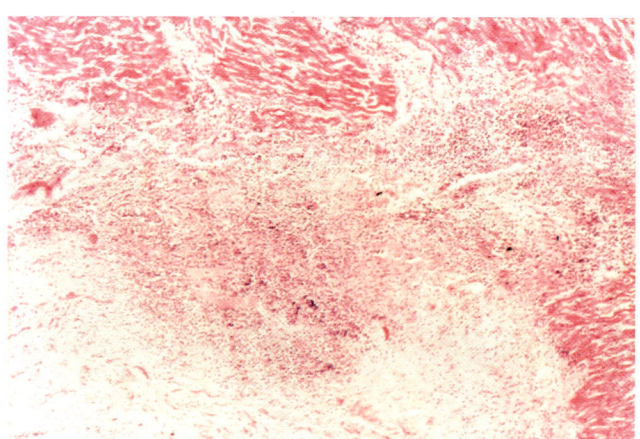

Fig. 3.20: Acute rheumatic carditis. The endocardium and interstitium of the myocardium reveal extensive myocarditis. Numerous Aschoff nodules were encountered in other sections

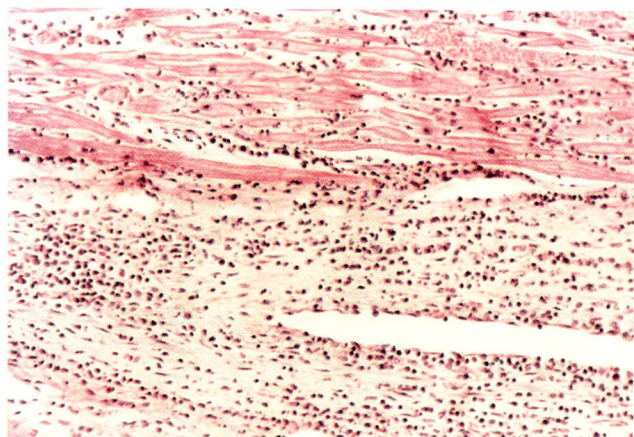

Fig. 3.21: Acute rheumatic carditis. Extensive inflammation is seen within the interstitium and endocardium. Predominant cell type is lymphocyte. Numerous eosinophils, polymorphs and nuclear debris is also present. Myofibers show marked degenerative changes and necrosis. Aschoff nodules were seen in other sections

Note: Besides the specific lesion of acute carditis (Aschoff nodules) it is not unusual to see acute necrotising carditis. This has also been observed occasionally in surgically excised left atrial appendages and mitral valves from cases of chronic rheumatic valve disease

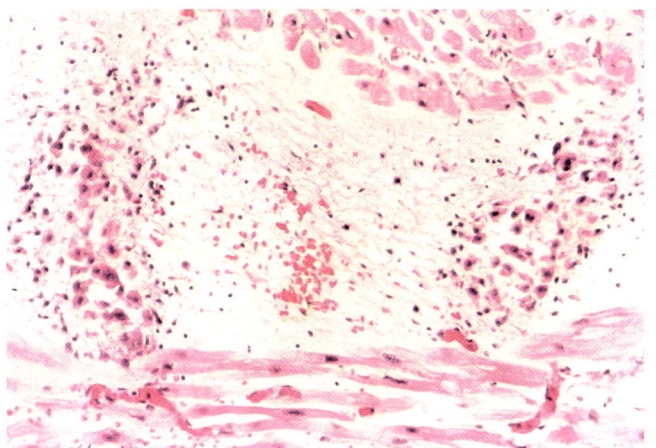

Fig. 3.22: Rheumatic heart disease. Excised left atrial appendage from a case of rheumatic mitral valve stenosis. Aschoff nodules (granulomatous phase) are seen within the interstitium of the myocardium

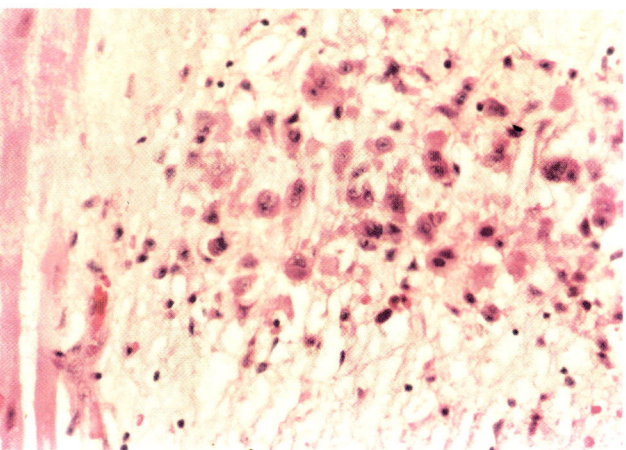

Fig. 3.23: Rheumatic heart disease. Excised left atrial appendage to demonstrate morphological features of Aschoff cells. Uninucleate and binucleate Aschoff cells are seen

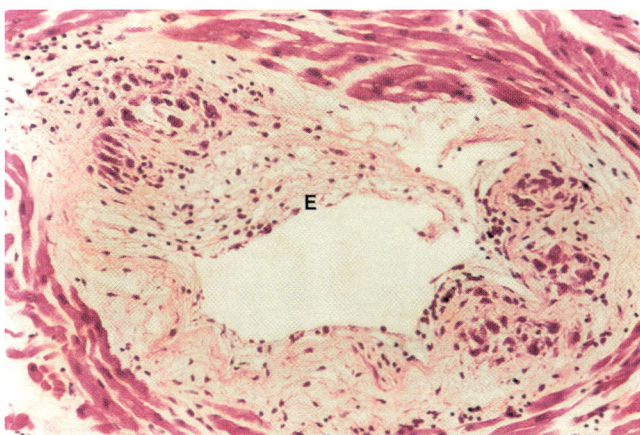

Fig. 3.24: Rheumatic heart disease. Excised left atrial appendage shows numerous Aschoff nodules in the subendocardium (E)

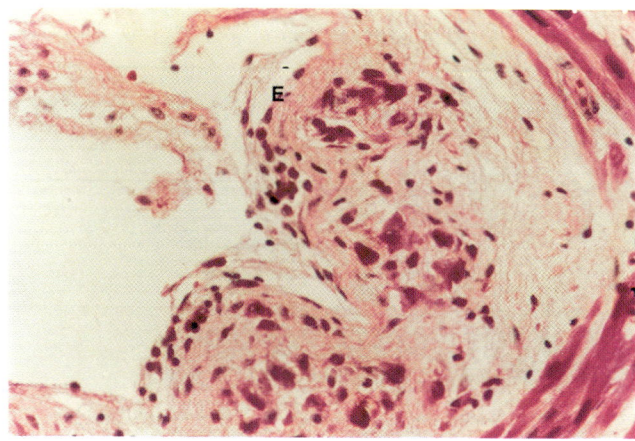

Fig. 3.25: Rheumatic heart disease. Excised left atrial appendage shows numerous Aschoff nodules in the subendocardium (E). Uninucleate and binucleate Aschoff cells are seen within the Aschoff nodule

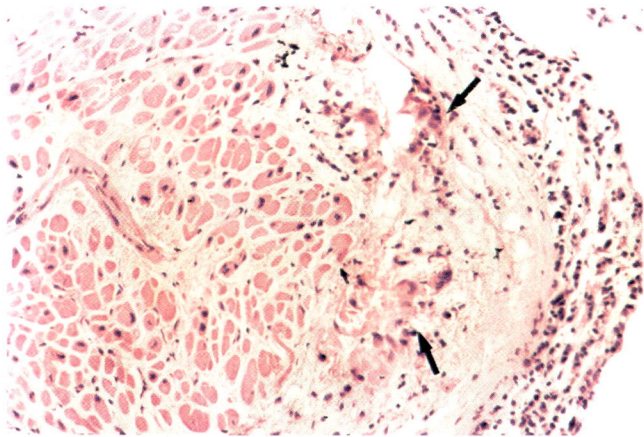

Fig. 3.26: Rheumatic heart disease. Excised left atrial appendage shows ill-formed Aschoff nodules (arrows) in the subendocardium. The endocardium reveals marked inflammation. The case was clinically quiescent and had no features of rheumatic activity

and at times in the interstitial tissue of the myocardium. As compared with surgically excised specimens, Aschoff nodules were infrequent or only sparsely distributed in autopsy cases of rheumatic heart disease. The number of Aschoff nodules were appreciably higher in active rheumatic heart disease as compared with inactive cases. Thus Aschoff nodules are encountered in the left atrial appendage in the "quiescent" phase of rheumatic heart disease. It has also been observed that variable degrees of lymphocytic infiltration is present within and surrounding the Aschoff nodules. A study of surgically excised left atrial appendages which were collected fresh to determine the phenotype of inflammatory cells using monoclonal reagents to T cells, T cell subsets, B cells and macrophages revealed that the endomyocardial infiltrates were comprized predominantly of T cells (predominantly CD4+ lymphocytes) and occasionally B cells. Frequent presence of Aschoff nodules and heavy mononuclear cell infiltrates in left atrial appendages from cases of chronic rheumatic heart disease suggest a possibility of subclinical/ongoing carditis.

Structure of the Aschoff nodules has been evaluated by both transmission and scanning electron microscopy. The Aschoff cell under the electron microscope reveals a ruffled cell membrane which is thrown into folds. Numerous profiles of rough endoplasmic reticulum many of which are distended to contain a light electron dense material are seen. Free ribosomes are increased. Few lipid droplets and dense bodies and an occasional Golgi apparatus are also present. The nuclei are large, round to ovoid with an irregular nuclear membrane showing occasional invaginations.

On scanning electron microscopy, Aschoff nodules are easily recognised as well-defined nodular aggregates sandwiched between the endocardium and myocardium. They are also present within the endocardium and interstitial tissue of the myocardium. The cells lie packed together and are oblong, elongated and often angulated. Surface of cells is either smooth or finely reticulated with a few blunt projections (Figs 3.27 and 3.28). Observations of electron microscopy suggest that Aschoff cells are of mesenchymal origin having characters of epithelioid cells and/or fibroblasts.

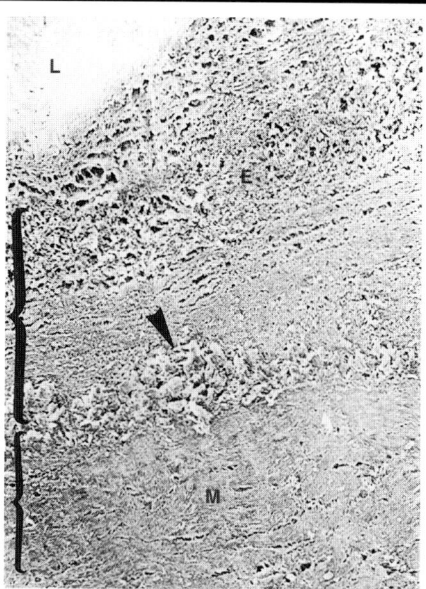

Fig. 3.27: Scanning electron micrograph (SEM) from a case of rheumatic heart disease (RHD). Numerous Aschoff nodules are observed in the excised left atrial appendage (LAA). The Aschoff nodules are seen as irregular, nodular cell groups (arrow head) sandwiched between the endocardium and myocardium. The endocardium is markedly thickened. L—Lumen; E—Endocardium; M—Myocardium. Larger bracket: Endocardium, smaller bracket: Myocardium

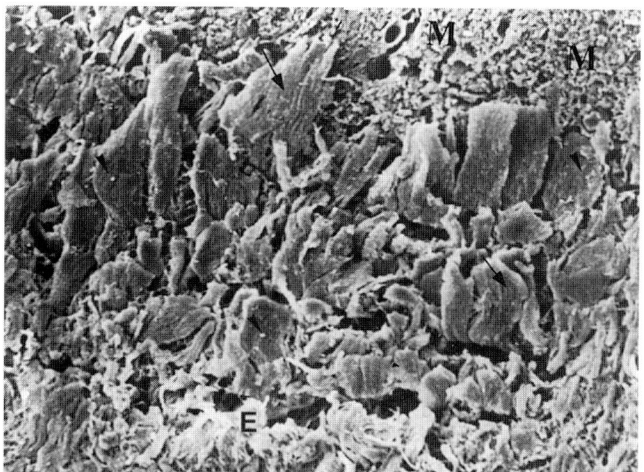

Fig. 3.28: Scanning electron micrograph of another case that had numerous Aschoff nodules in the excised LAA on conventional microscopy. Several cells have fine reticulations (small arrows) and blunt projections (small arrow heads) on their surface

Nature of Aschoff cells within Aschoff bodies seen in 35 excised left atrial appendages was evaluated using a panel of monoclonal and polyclonal antisera by the indirect immunoperoxidase staining for leucocyte common antigen, macrophage, desmin, vimentin, alpha-1-antitrypsin, alpha-1-antichymotrypsin, lysozyme, acid phosphatase and non-specific esterase. Aschoff cells revealed consistent and strong reactivity to several histiocytic markers which confirm the view that these cells derive from macrophages/histiocytes (Figs 3.29 to 3.31).

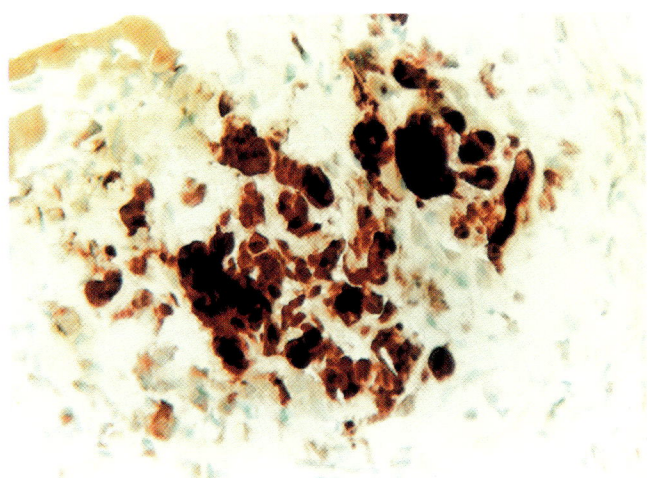

Fig. 3.29: Aschoff nodule in an excised left atrial appendage from a case of rheumatic mitral valve stenosis shows strong reactivity for non-specific esterase

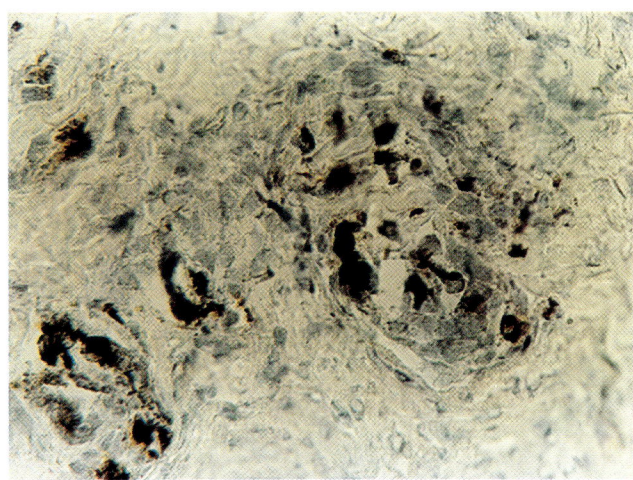

Fig. 3.30: Aschoff nodule in an excised left atrial appendage from a case of rheumatic mitral valve stenosis shows positive staining reaction for acid phosphatase

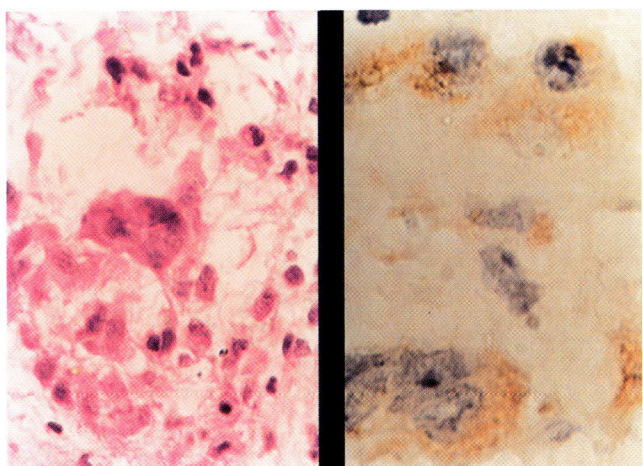

Fig. 3.31: Rheumatic mitral valve stenosis: Aschoff nodules in the excised left atrial appendage reveal strong reaction within cytoplasm when treated with antiserum to lysozyme. Peroxidase-antiperoxidase reaction

Note: Strong reactivity was also observed with α-1 antichymotrypsin, α-1 antitrypsin and CD68

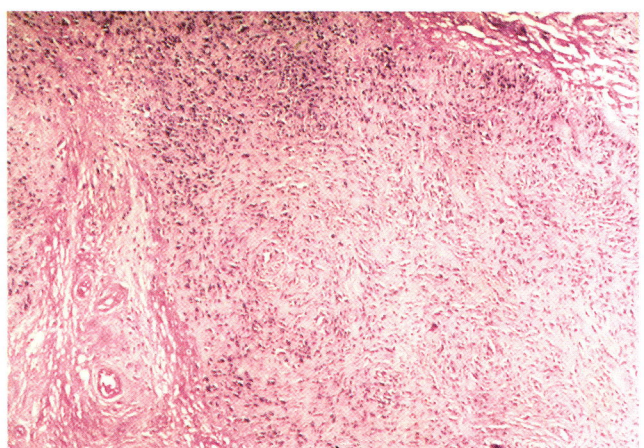

Fig. 3.32: Subcutaneous nodule from a case of rheumatic heart disease with suspected activity. Photomicrograph shows fibrinoid necrosis which is bordered by histiocytes. Blood vessels are also present

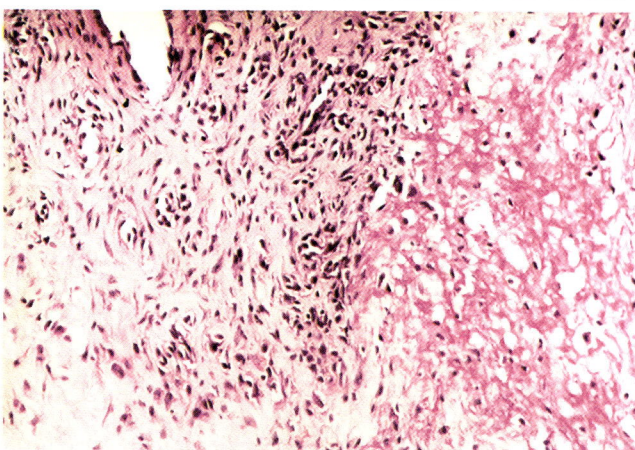

Fig. 3.33: Subcutaneous nodule from a case of rheumatic heart disease. The picture shows an area of fibrinoid necrosis of the collagen surrounded by histiocytes and blood vessels

Subcutaneous nodule It is one of the major clinical manifestation of acute rheumatic fever. It is located commonly on the extensor tendons of the wrists, elbows, knees and ankles of some patients of acute rheumatic fever. When present they are a good index of activity of the disease. Microscopically, subcutaneous nodules show fibrinoid necrosis of collagen which is bordered by histiocytes along with other mononuclear inflammatory cells (Figs 3.32 to 3.34). Induction of subcutaneous nodule has been carried out with an aim to make a diagnosis of rheumatic activity in patients with preexisting rheumatic heart disease. Twenty six patients with rheumatic fever and twenty with inactive rheumatic heart disease were studied. Following subcutaneous injection of autologous blood, 16/26 patients with rheumatic fever developed subcutaneous nodules while none of the 20 cases with inactive rheumatic heart disease developed them. The artificial subcutaneous nodule test in this study was 100% specific and predictive for rheumatic fever with an overall sensitivity of 62%. Histology of the artificial subcutaneous nodules was identical to the natural ones (Fig. 3.34). Thus artificial subcutaneous nodule induction is a simple and easy technique for the diagnosis of acute rheumatic fever when in doubt.

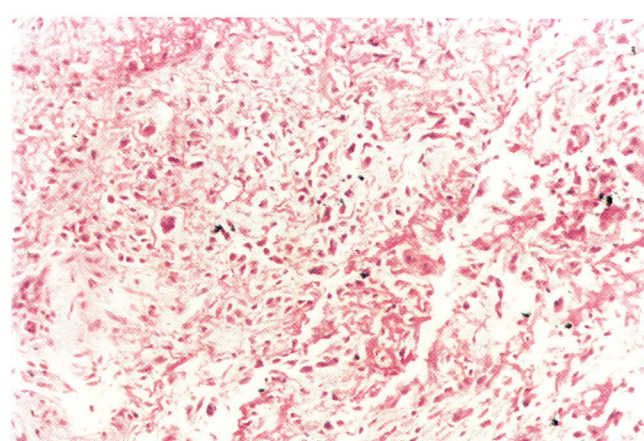

Fig. 3.34: Subcutaneous nodule from a case of rheumatic heart disease showing focal fibrinoid necrosis and aggregate of histiocytes. This was an artificially induced nodule (injection of autologous blood). Notice the resemblance to the naturally occurring subcutaneous nodule (Figs 3.32 and 3.33)

Ultrastructure evaluation of naturally occurring subcutaneous nodules in acute rheumatic fever shows an electron dense and smudgy material which has a distinct filamentous appearance in places. Latter is the collagen and corresponds to the fibrinoid necrosis seen under the light microscope. Several histiocytes and fibroblasts are seen at the edge of the smudgy material.

Central nervous system Chorea is another major criterion for the diagnosis of acute rheumatic fever. In chorea mild meningoencephalitis, small focal hemorrhages and perivascular cuffing by lymphocytes are seen in the cerebral cortex and basal ganglia. Neuron binding antibodies were evaluated in the sera of patients with acute rheumatic fever and chronic valvular rheumatic heart disease (both active and inactive) by the immunoperoxidase technique. It was observed that incidence of neuron-binding antibodies was highest in acute rheumatic fever (61%) in comparison with 54.2% in chronic rheumatic valvular disease with activity and 21% in inactive chronic valvular disease. Localization was observed in cytoplasm of caudate nucleus neurons. Various patterns of staining were noted.

Polyarthritis It affects multiple large joints. The pain is characteristically migratory in nature. Microscopically, in addition to infiltration of lymphocytes, macrophages and polymorphs, edema of the joint tissue and dilatation of blood vessels is present.

COMPLICATIONS AND SEQUELAE

Chronic rheumatic heart disease Recurrent rheumatic valvulitis results in **valvular deformities** which produce severe cardiac disability. Single or multiple valves in various combinations are affected by the rheumatic process. The mitral valve is most frequently affected either in isolation or in combination with other valves. In the developing countries the reported pattern of valvular involvement in descending order of frequency is as follows: Mitral valve alone; mitral, tricuspid and aortic; mitral and aortic; mitral and tricuspid; aortic alone and all four cardiac valves. Healing of the mural endocardium produces thickened endocardium in the posterior wall of the left atrium which is termed as **MacCallum's** patch. Healing of rheumatic myocarditis and pericarditis produces myocardial fibrosis and fibrous thickening of the pericardium respectively which is generally of little clinical consequence. **Congestive heart failure** in acute rheumatic carditis is due to the extensive myocardial involvement including myocarditis with necrosis. Valvular deformities consequent to the chronic rheumatic process is one of the most common causes of cardiac failure. Latter, in particular mitral valve stenosis produces pulmonary arterial and venous hypertension which leads to congestive heart failure. **Infective endocarditis** is another frequent complication of RHD. Valvular deformities and damage of the valves favor colonization of causative organisms. **Mural thrombi** in the cardiac chambers are a source of embolization commonly to brain, kidneys, spleen, lungs and other viscera. These form most commonly in the left atrium in cases of mitral stenosis and/or atrial fibrillation. **Sudden death** may occur due to obstruction of the mitral valve orifice by a large thrombus.

Rheumatic heart disease with such severe disabilities has simple methods of control. The means of promoting prevention of rheumatic fever/rheumatic heart disease is to provide education and create awareness in the public and community for recognition and management of cases of rheumatic fever through School and Community Health Education. Prevention of recurrent pharyngitis by group A *Streptococcus* through regular periodic administration of long acting penicillin injections or alternate antibiotics in itself has beneficial results. Besides strategies for primary and secondary prevention for rheumatic fever/rheumatic heart disease much interest has been generated for potentials of **vaccine** against rheumatic fever. Since M-protein in the streptococcal cell wall is the main virulence factor attempts are being made to prepare vaccine from this. Non-type specific M-protein vaccine from conserved regions of M-proteins have been prepared and tested in animals for protection. In addition to the M-protein vaccine, other vaccine candidates that are under scrutiny are cysteine protease, C5 peptidase, SFb-1 protein.

SUGGESTED READING

1. Bhatnagar A, Gover A, Ganguly NK: Superantigen-induced T cell responses in acute rheumatic fever and chronic rheumatic heart disease patients. *Clin Exp Immunol* **116(1)**: 100-06, 1999.
2. Brandt ER, Sriprakash KS, Hobb RI, Hayman WA, Zeng W, Batzloff MR, Jackson DC, Good MF: New Multi-determinant strategy for a group A streptococcal vaccine designed for the Australian Aboriginal population. *Nat Med* **6(4)**: 455-59, 2000.
3. Carpetis JR, Currie BJ: Rheumatic chorea in northern Australia: A clinical and epidemiological study. *Arch Dis Child* **80(4)**: 353-58, 1999.
4. Chopra P, Narula J, Sampath Kumar A, Sachdeva S, Bhatia ML: Immunohistochemical characterisation of Aschoff nodules and endomyocardial inflammatory infiltrates in left atrial appendages from patients with chronic rheumatic heart disease. *Int J Cardiol* **20**: 99-105, 1988.
5. Chopra P, Narula JPS, Tandon R: Ultrastructure of natural occurring subcutaneous nodule in acute rheumatic fever. *Int J Cardiol* **30**: 124-27, 1991.
6. Chopra P, Narula JPS: Scanning electron microscope feature of rheumatic vegetations in acute rheumatic carditis. *Int J Cardiol* **30**: 109-12, 1991.
7. Chopra P, Tandon HD, Raizada V, Gopinath N, Butler C, William RC Jr: Comparative studies of mitral valves in rheumatic heart disease. *Arch Int Med* **143**: 661-66, 1983.
8. Chopra P, Tandon HD: Pathology of rheumatic heart disease with particular reference to tricuspid valve involvement. *Acta Cardiologica* **32**: 423-33, 1977.
9. Chopra P, Wanniang J, Sampath Kumar: Immunohistochemical and histochemical profile of Aschoff bodies of rheumatic carditis in excised left atrial appendages-An immunoperoxide study in fresh and paraffinembedded tissue. *Int J Cardiol* **32**: 199-207, 1992.
10. Chopra P: Application of scanning electron microscopy in the characterisation of Aschoff nodules in rheumatic heart disease. *Jap Heart J* **26(4)**: 531-38, 1985.
11. Chopra P: Origin of Aschoff nodule: An ultrastructural light microscopic and histochemical evaluation. *Jap Heart J* **24(2)**: 227-35, 1985.
12. El Demellawy M, El Ridi R, Guirguis NI, Abdel Alim M, Kotby A, Kotb M: Preferential recognition of human myocardial antigens by T lymphocytes from rheumatic heart disease patients. *Infect Immun* **65(6)**: 2197-205, 1997.
13. Fischetti VA: The *Streptococcus* and the host: Present and future challenges. *Amer Soc Microbiol News* **63(10)**: 541-45, 1997.
14. Fraser WJ, Haffejee Z, Jankelow D, Wadee A, Cooper K: Rheumatic Aschoff nodules revisited II: Cytokine expression corroborates recently proposed sequential stages. *Histopathology* **31**: 460-64, 1997.
15. Galvin JE, Hemric ME, Kosanke SD, Factor SM, Quinn A, Cunningham MW: Induction of myocarditis and valvulitis in Lewis rats by different epitopes of cardiac myosin and its implications in rheumatic carditis. *Am J Pathol* **160**: 297-306, 2002.
16. Guilherme L, Cunha-Neto E, Coelho V, Snitcowsky R et al: Human heart-infiltrating T-cell clones from rheumatic heart disease patients recognize both streptococcal and cardiac proteins. *Circulation* **92**: 415-20, 1995.
17. Narin N, Kutukculer N, Ozyurek R, Bakiler AR et al: Lymphocyte subsets and plasma IL-1, IL-2 and TNF-concentrations in acute rheumatic fever and chronic rheumatic heart disease. *Clin Immunol Immunopathol* **77**: 172-76, 1995.
18. Raizada V, Williams JC Jr, Chopra P, Gopinath N, Prakash K, Sharma KB, Cherian KM, Aurora R, Nigam M, Zabriskie JB: Tissue distribution of lymphocytes in rheumatic heart valves as defined by monoclonal T cell antibodies. *Amer J Med* **74**: 90-96, 1983.
19. Roberts S, Kosanke S, Dunn ST, Jankelow D, Duran CMG, Cunningham MW: Pathogenic mechanisms in rheumatic carditis: focus on valvular endothelium *J Inf Dis* **183**: 507-11, 2001.
20. Veasy LG, Hill HR: Immunologic and clinical correlations in rheumatic fever and rheumatic heart disease. *Pediatri Infect Dis J* **16(4)**: 400-07, 1997.

4 Valvular Heart Disease

Not only does the prevalence of rheumatic fever continue to be high but recurrent streptococcal infections lead to severe and crippling valvular deformities which are a common cause of cardiac disability and high mortality. Additionally, in the Indian subcontinent, rheumatic heart disease affects the pediatric and juvenile age groups resulting in **juvenile mitral stenosis** in a high proportion of cases. This subgroup is associated with a fulminant disease, severe pulmonary hypertension, rapidly progressive clinical course and high morbidity and mortality.

For the **normal functioning** of a valve, the entire valve apparatus, i.e. the valve ring, valve cusps, commissures, chordae tendinea, papillary and ventricular muscle play an important role. Involvement of one or more of these components result in malfunction of the valve. **Atrioventricular valves** are comprized by the mitral and the tricuspid valve. The **mitral valve apparatus** includes the **annulus**; two **valve leaflets**—a tongue-shaped anterior leaflet and a narrower spread out posterior leaflet; junction of the leaflets-**commissures; chordae tendinea** and the **papillary muscles**. Components of tricuspid valve apparatus are identical except that it has three valve leaflets: the anterior, septal and posterior. The **semilunar valves** consist of the pulmonary and the aortic valve. Both semilunar valves consist of 3 **semicircular cusps** each. They are the anterior, right and left in the pulmonary valve and right and left coronary cusps and noncoronary cusp in the aortic valve. The vessel wall behind each cusp forms a pouch like dilatation known as the **sinus of Valsalva**. Junction of the adjacent cusps is termed **commissures**. The ostia of the left and right coronary arteries are located in the center of their respective sinuses and thus normally covered by the valve cusps.

Rheumatic Valve Disease

Though a number of congenital and acquired conditions cause valvular heart disease, rheumatic heart disease remains the most common cause in India and other developing countries. Rheumatic heart disease (RHD) can affect all four valves but the most common to be involved are mitral and aortic valve combined. In an evaluation of 229 autopsied cases of rheumatic heart disease various combination of valvular involvement were encountered (Table 4.1). Rheumatic process in terms of both extent and severity is most marked in the mitral valve. Valve leaflets, commissures and chordae tendinea show variable degrees of fibrosis.

Pathogenesis of rheumatic valve disease An observation of inflammatory cells in excised tissues (left atrial appendages and valves) made on conventially processed hematoxylin and eosin stained sections have provided an important basis for study of pathogenesis of rheumatic heart disease. Latter seems to be related to production of hyperimmune responses in a susceptible host against group A streptococci. In a study conducted by us, analysis

Table 4.1: Frequency of valvular involvement in chronic rheumatic heart disease (N=229)

Valves affected	Number of cases	Percent
Mitral, aortic	60	26.2
Mitral, tricuspid	25	10.9
Mitral, aortic, tricuspid	61	26.6
Mitral, aortic, tricuspid, pulmonary	7	3.05
Mitral alone	74	32.3
Aortic alone	2	0.87
Tricuspid alone	–	
Pulmonary alone	–	

of the phenotypic profile in freshly excised cardiac valves revealed that 45% of the cell population was made up of macrophages and rest were lymphocytes. The T-helper/inducer population of lymphocytes was predominant (Table 4.2). Similar phenotypic profile was observed in excised left atrial appendages (LAA) from cases of rheumatic mitral valve stenosis. In many cases T4 cells were closely juxtaposed to fibroblast and collagen fibers. Aschoff bodies and inflammatory cell infiltration in absence of rheumatic activity observed in excised LAA and valves from cases of rheumatic heart disease suggests that there is recurrent and smouldering inflammation due to an ongoing insult/injury by some persistent antigenic stimulus initiated by group A beta-hemolytic *Streptococcus* that have primed the various target tissues to culminate in chronic fibrosing rheumatic valvular heart disease. Indeed, investigations in this direction have provided insight into the pathogenesis of this disease. In one study, the phenotypic profile revealed predominance of CD4 positive T cells. Increased expression of IL-1, IL-2 and TNF has also been demonstrated in cardiac tissues in acute rheumatic fever. Additionally, T-cell clones obtained from surgical tissues of RHD simultaneously recognized streptococcal M and heart proteins. Cross-reactive T cell clones suggest their involvement in the pathogenesis of RHD. The progressive fibrotic process leading to crippling valvular deformity may be a result of continued, low grade inflammation, and elaboration of cytokines and other factors by CD4 + T lymphocytes.

Mitral Valve Disease

Mitral stenosis with or without incompetence is the most common acquired valvular disease. This valve is affected either in isolation or more commonly in combination with the other cardiac valves.

Mitral stenosis (MS) The most common cause of mitral valve stenosis in developing countries remains **rheumatic heart disease**. Rarely, infective endocarditis and congenital defects cause MS. Recurrent attacks of rheumatic valvulitis cause healing with fibrosis resulting in valvular deformities. The mitral valve leaflets, including the valve ring, the commissures and the chordae tendinea undergo scarring of one or more of the various valve components. The fibrotic leaflets become fused and retracted such that the papillary muscles are pulled up closer to the leaflets (Figs 4.1 to 4.7). At times the fibrotic process may be severe enough to transform the valve into a **funnel-shaped** structure (Figs 4.19 and 4.22). Fusion of the leaflets at the free margins may result in a diphragm with a tiny hole or a slit giving the appearance of **"button hole"** or **"fish mouth"** types of MS respectively (Figs 4.8 to 4.10). This type of deformity of the mitral valve is commonly encountered in childhood and has been termed as **juvenile mitral stenosis**. The latter subset of patients appears to be unique to the Indian subcontinent and is characterized by an aggressive clinical course, cardiomegaly, markedly elevated pulmonary arterial and venous pressure, heart failure and a high mortality.

The normal mitral valve area is 4-6 sq cm. Mitral valve area less than 1 sq cm qualifies for severe MS. Clinical effects of MS are a result of obstruction to the flow of blood from the left atrium and the pressure that builds up in this chamber. Dilatation and hypertrophy of the left atrium occur due to the accumulation and stasis of blood (Figs 4.4 and 4.8 to 4.10). Occasionally the atrium may assume a large size (Figs 4.4 and 4.8). Fibrous thickening of the atrial endocardium particularly of the posterior wall of the left atrium is present. The elevated pressure in the left atrium reflects into the pulmonary veins producing **chronic pulmonary venous congestion**. Latter, eventually leads to pulmonary capillary,

Table 4.2: Lymphomononuclear cells in excised mitral valves and left atrial appendages (LAA) from cases of rheumatic heart disease

Tissue	T helper/Inducer	T Suppressor/Cytotoxic	Macrophages	B Cells
Mitral valves (n-50)	30.16 ± 7.2	19.2 ± 7.2	44.54 ± 10.9	4.96 ± 2.46
LAA (n=50)	44.1 ± 7.6	23.5 ± 4.8	29.3 ± 9.6	2.6 ± 0.5

Valvular Heart Disease

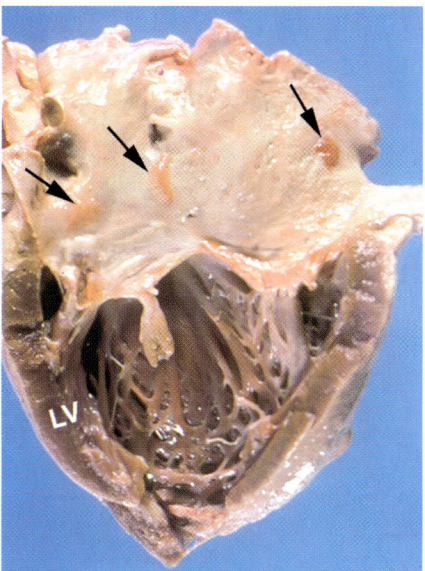

Fig. 4.1: Rheumatic heart disease. The normal morphology of the anterior and posterior leaflets of the mitral valve is lost. The leaflets of mitral valve are thickened and appear as elevated ridges. The chordae tendinea are fused and appear as cords. MacCallum's patch is observed in the posterior wall of the left atrium. Multiple mural thrombi are also seen (arrows). Left ventricle (LV) is both dilated and hypertophic

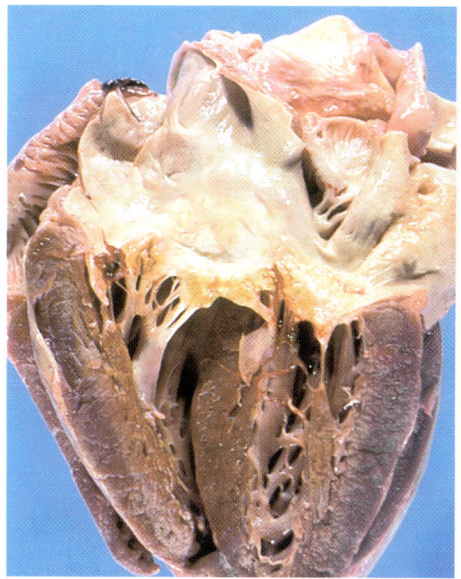

Fig. 4.2: Rheumatic heart disease. Mitral valve ring diameter is reduced. Fibrosis and contracture of both mitral valve leaflets, commissures and chordae tendinea are observed. Focal calcification is also present. Valve was gritty on cutting. Marked left ventricle hypertrophy consequent to incompetence of the valve is seen

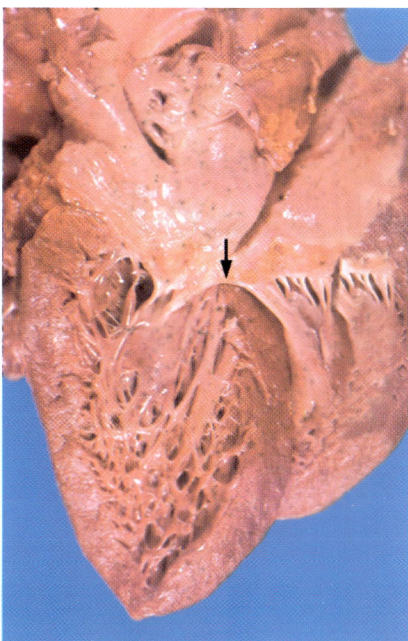

Fig. 4.3: Rheumatic heart disease. This photograph demonstrates thickening and distortion of the normal structure of the leaflets of the mitral valve. The leaflets are thickened and retracted and commissural fusion (arrow) is present. The chordae tendinea are also thickened and shortened. Left ventricular hypertrophy is seen

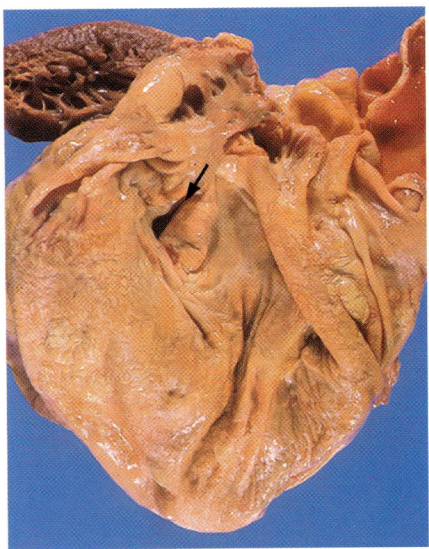

Fig. 4.4: Rheumatic heart disease. Left atrium is hugely dilated and the wall is very thin. Distributed throughout the endocardial surface of the atria which is numerous opaque, firm, grey white areas 0.1 to 0.2 cm in diameter (organised thrombi). Mitral valve is severly stenosed allowing only tip of a finger to pass through (arrow). Leaflets are thickened but not calcified, commissures are fused and the chordae tendinea are thickened and shortened

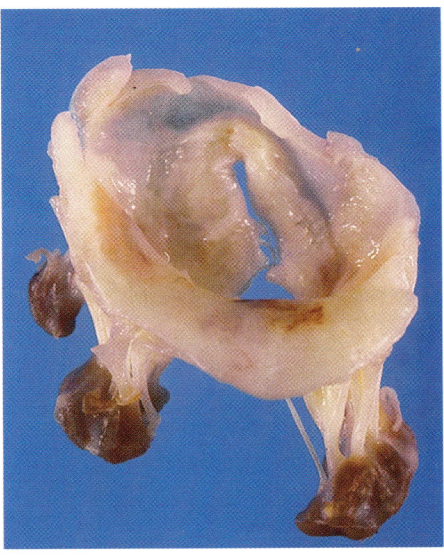

Fig. 4.5: Rheumatic heart disease. Surgically excised incompetent mitral valve. The leaflets of mitral valve are thickened and fibrosed. The valve orifice is narrowed. Chordae tendinea are thickened and shortened

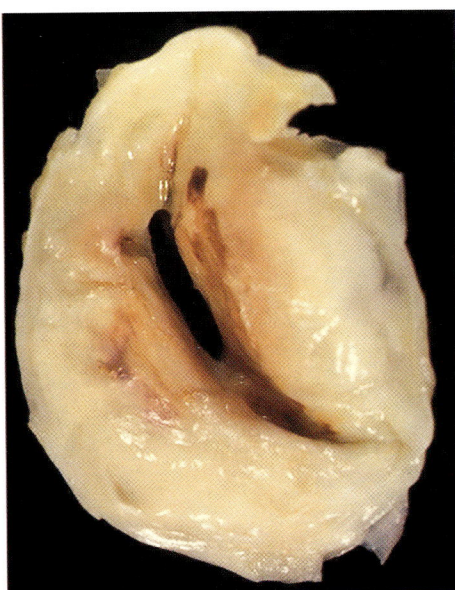

Fig. 4.6: Rheumatic heart disease. Atrial view of the excised mitral valve shows marked thickening and distortion of valve leaflets. Congestion and focal irregularities of the endocardium are seen at the contact margins

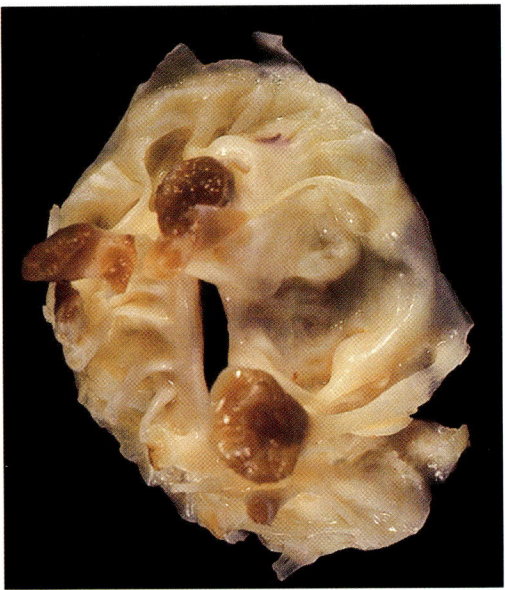

Fig. 4.7: Rheumatic heart disease. Ventricular aspect of the excised incompetent mitral valve. The chordae tendinea are thickened, fused and plastered. Cut edges of papillary muscles are seen almost embedded in the fibrous tissue

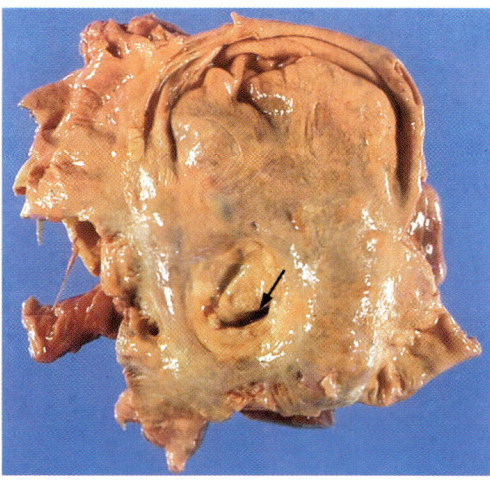

Fig. 4.8: Rheumatic heart disease. Atrial view of the left atrium reveals stenotic mitral valve (arrow). The valve leaflets are thickened along with commissural fusion. Left atrium is markedly dilated

arteriolar and arterial hypertension which in turn causes **right ventricular hypertrophy** and finally **right heart failure** develops. In predominant MS, the left ventricle is either normal or atrophic. Atrial dilatation in MS is often accompanied by **atrial fibrillation** which in turn favors blood stasis and **thrombus** formation both within the atrium (Fig. 4.9) and the left atrial appendage. **Systemic**

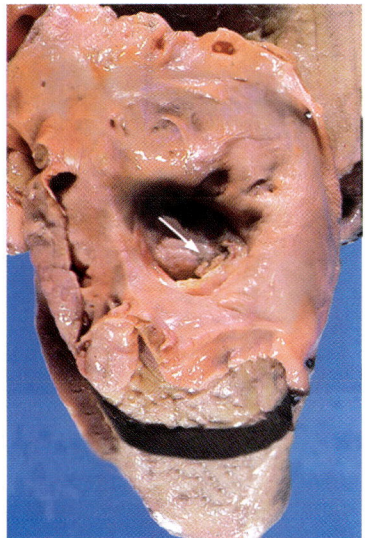

Fig. 4.9: Rheumatic heart disease. Close up of atrial view of the stenotic mitral valve. Thrombus is seen to occlude the lumen (arrow). Multiple tiny mural thrombi are seen in the dilated left atrium

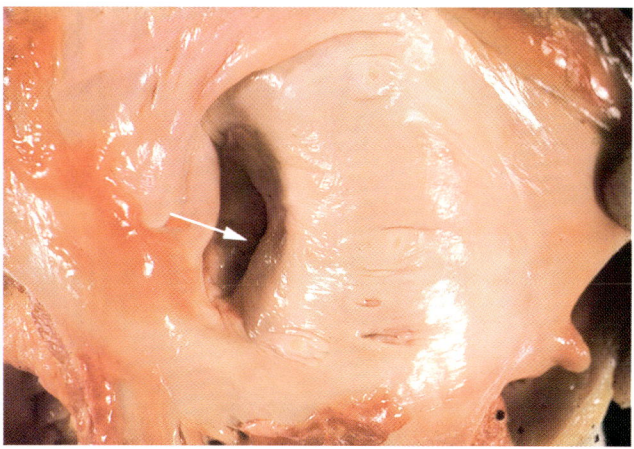

Fig. 4.10: Rheumatic heart disease. Close up of atrial view of the stenotic mitral valve which appears as a slit (arrow). Mural thrombi are present on the left atrial endocardium

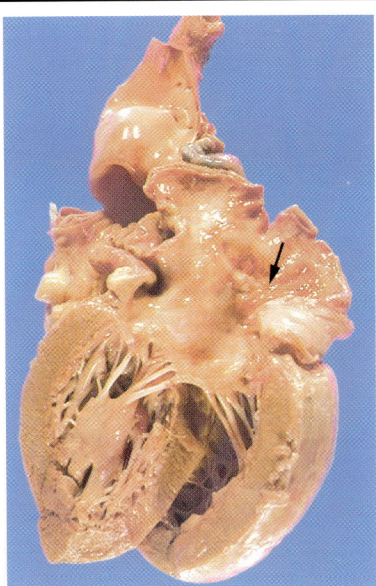

Fig. 4.11: Rheumatic heart disease. The valve leaflets particularly the posterior leaflet of the mitral valve is thickened and shortened as are the chordae tendinea. Left atrial endocardium shows tiny mural thrombi well-marked in the posterior wall (arrow). Marked left ventricular hypertrophy is observed. This is consequent to incompetence of the mitral valve

embolization therefore is a common complication of left atrial thrombosis producing clinical effects related to the organ which suffers ischemia.

Mitral incompetence/regurgitation (MR) Incompetence or insufficiency of the mitral valve may result from **structural abnormalities** of the **valvular leaflets, dilatation of the valve ring** and conditions causing **dysfunction** of the **papillary muscles**. In developing countries, the most common cause of MR is **rheumatic heart disease**. It is invariably associated with aortic valve disease. Fibrous thickening and scarring of the valve leaflets cause them to become rigid and there is retraction of the free edges of the valve leaflets (Figs 4.1 to 4.3, 4.5 to 4.7 and 4.11). Associated fusion of the commissures and thickening and fusion of the chordae tendinea is usually present. Insufficiency of the mitral valve is invariably accompanied with some degree of stenosis. Pure MR is unusual although it may occur in isolation. **Microscopic** examination of valves in chronic RHD shows marked distortion of architecture with dense fibrocollagen deposition. Prominent thick-walled blood vessels are present. The degree of inflammation is variable and in some cases significant amount of inflammatory cell infiltration is noted. The inflammatory cell infiltrate seems to be directly proportion to the severity of calcification. Inflammatory cells are comprised of lymphocytes, plasma cells and histiocytes. They occur either in small groups particularly around areas of calcification or are dispersed within the valve substance (Figs 4.12 to 4.14).

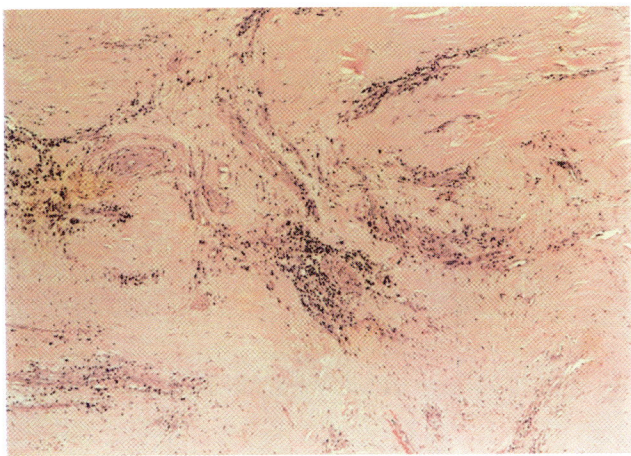

Fig. 4.12: Excised mitral valve from a case of rheumatic heart disease. Numerous thick-walled blood vessels are present in the valve substance. Infiltration by lymphocytes is striking. Hyalinisation of the valve collagen is also observed

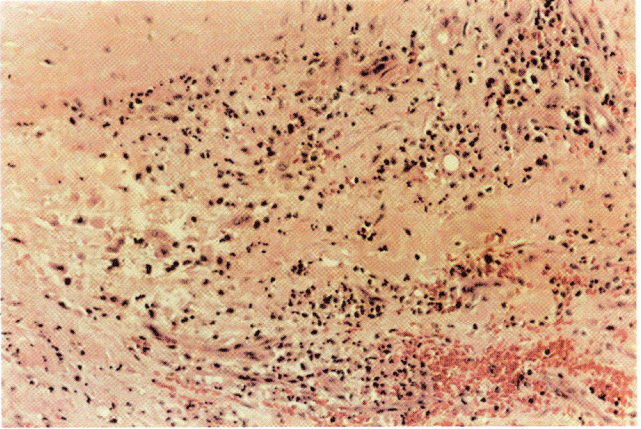

Fig. 4.13: Rheumatic mitral valvulitis. Section from another area of the valve demonstrated in Figure 4.12. Edema of collagen, extravasation of red blood cells and infiltration by histiocytes resembling Aschoff cells and lymphocytes are seen. These features suggest recurrent acute rheumatic valvulitis

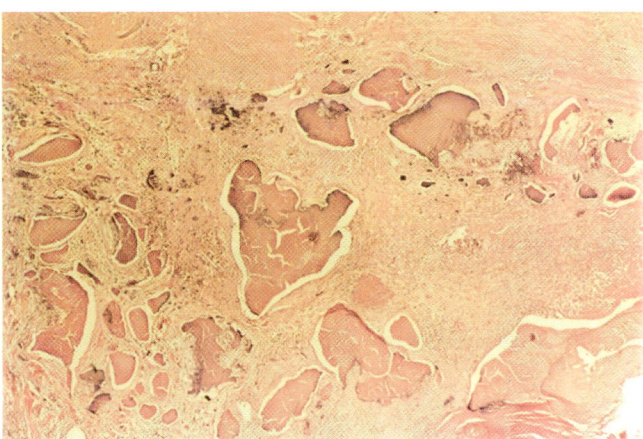

Fig. 4.14: Excised incompetent mitral valve from a case of rheumatic heart disease. Sections from the valve show marked inflammatory cell infiltration around areas of calcification. Besides lymphocytes a large number of plasma cells are also noted

It has been out experience that features of acute rheumatic valvulitis are not infrequent in excised diseased and distorted valves from cases of RHD (Figs 4.15 to 4.17).

Besides RHD, **floppy mitral valve** or **mitral valve prolapse** syndrome is an important cause of mitral incompetence. In this condition the valve leaflets are large and bulky and appear mucoid and gelatinous. The chordae tendinea also show identical changes (Fig. 4.18). Microscopically, loss of valvular collagen along with an increase in the ground substance in the cusps and the chordae tendinea is characteristically observed. The myxomatous material is rich in mucopolysaccharides. These abnormal cusps buldge into the atrium during ventricular systole resulting in incompetence of the

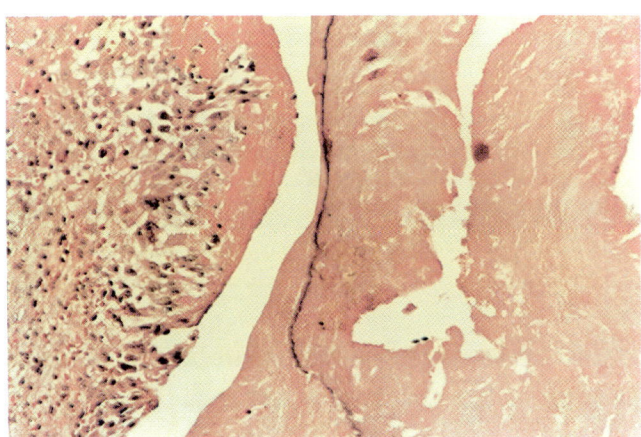

Fig. 4.15: Rheumatic heart disease. Mitral valve replacement was done. The excised valve in addition to showing areas of hyalinization, calcification, neovascularization and inflammation showed changes of acute rheumatic valvulitis. Notice fibrinoid necrosis on the surface bordered by histiocytes. This case demonstrates acute on chronic rheumatic valvulitis

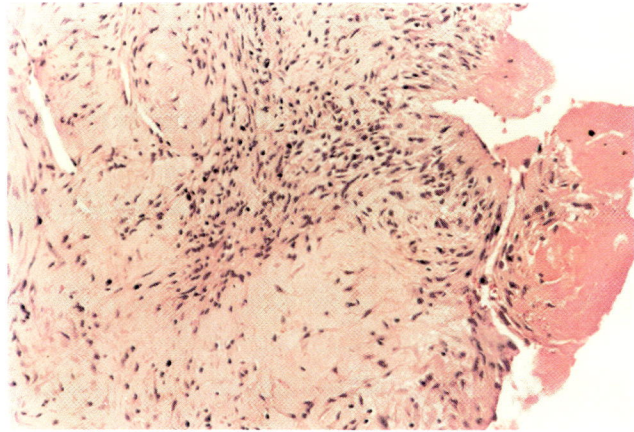

Fig. 4.16: Excised incompetent mitral valve from a case of chronic rheumatic heart disease. The valve shows rheumatic vegetation-fibrinoid necrosis of valvular collagen which is bordered by a palisade arrangement of histiocytes. Prominent lymphocyte infiltration is also present. Clinically no features of rheumatic activity were detected

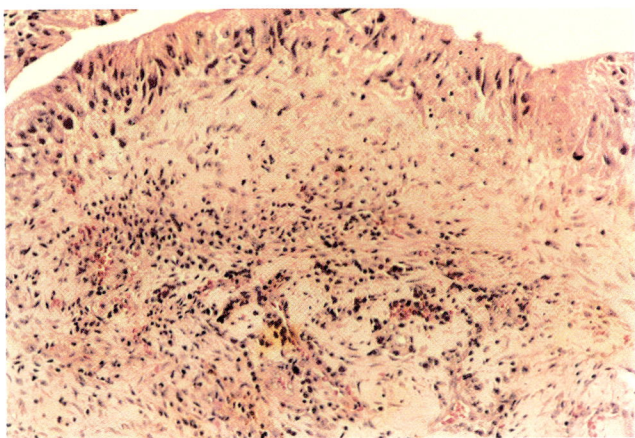

Fig. 4.17: Rheumatic heart disease. Mitral valve replacement was done for mitral incompetence. In addition to changes of chronic rheumatic mitral valvulitis, in foci changes of acute valvulitis were noted. Photomicrograph shows necrosis of collagen on the valve surface with a palisade arrangement of histiocytes. Valve substance shows neovascularization and infiltration by lymphocytes. Clinically no features of rheumatic activity were detected

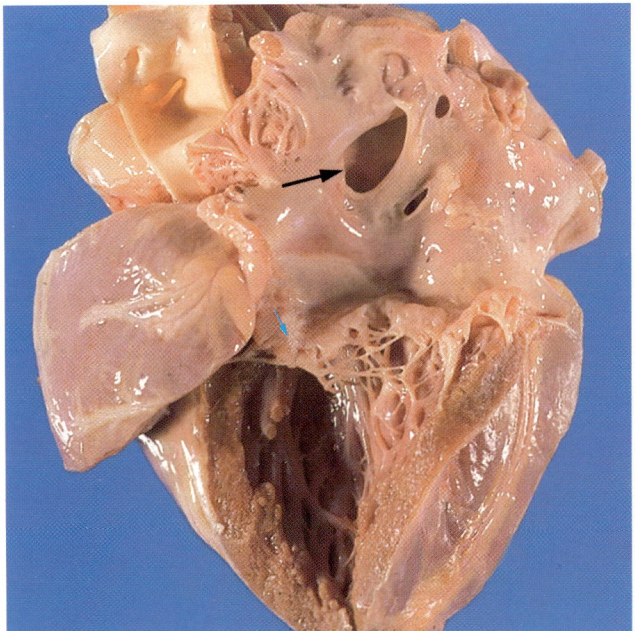

Fig. 4.18: Ostium secundum variety of atrial septal defect (Black arrow). Mitral valve leaflets show myxomatous degeneration. Tiny mucoid elevations are seen on the atrial aspect of the leaflet especially the posterior leaflet of mitral valve (Blue arrow)

valve. Mitral valve prolapse may either be completely asymptomatic, or may present as MR which may be severe enough to warrant medical and/or surgical treatment. Rupture of chordae tendinea and increased risk of developing infective endocarditis and embolic complications are the other associated events with the floppy mitral valve. Etiology is unknown and possibly represents a hereditary connective tissue abnormality as is observed in some cases of Marfan's syndrome and other connective tissue disorders like Ehlers-Danlos syndrome and pseudoxanthoma elasticum.

Sudden mitral valve incompetence may result from rupture of the chordae tendinea, the common underlying causes being mitral valve prolapse, infective endocarditis and ischemic necrosis. This may lead to fatal left ventricular failure.

Aortic Valve Disease

This may present either as stenosis or incompetence of the valve. Involvement of both aortic and mitral valves together is a feature of rheumatic heart disease. On the other hand, **isolated aortic valve involvement** causing aortic stenosis and/or regurgitation is most commonly due to a **congenital deformity** of the valve.

Aortic valve stenosis (AS) may be either acquired or congenital in nature. **Acquired AS** when present along with mitral valve disease is most commonly due to **rheumatic heart disease**. RHD only very infrequently causes isolated AS. **Congenital bicuspid** aortic valve is believed to be the underlying abnormality in over half the cases of isolated AS. **Calcific AS** occurs commonly in congenitally bicuspid or unicuspid valves. In individuals over 70 years of age tricuspid aortic valve may undergo calcification. This is known as **senile calcific aortic stenosis**. Calcific deposits are usually present in the sinuses of Valsalva and the free margins of the cusps. Understandably, AS causes an increased work load and results in left ventricular hypertrophy. The coronary perfusion may be impaired due to low pressures in the aorta during ventricular diastole. Left ventricular hypertrophy combined with low coronary perfusion may predispose to angina pectoris, syncope and sudden death. Left ventricle failure develops eventually.

Aortic valve incompetence/regurgitation (AR) It occurs as a result of thickening and distortion of the cusps, commissural fusion, calcification of valves, destruction and/or perforation of the cusps and in conditions associated with aortic root dilatation (Figs 4.19 to 4.24). **RHD** remains an important cause of thickening and distortion of the aortic valve apparatus which may manifest as stenosis and/or incompetence of the valve and is commonly associated with involvement of the mitral valve. Isolated aortic valve disease of rheumatic etiology is extremely uncommon. **Infective endocarditis** of the aortic valve may either lead to distortion of the cusps or in some cases may produce erosion, perforation and destruction of the cusps causing sudden and significant incompetence of the aortic valve. Dilatation of the aortic valve ring occurs consequent to certain diseases affecting the aorta. In **Marfan's syndrome** a genetic disorder of connective tissues, AR is common. The wall of the aorta shows loss of elastic tissue of the media in addition to accumulations of increased amounts of mucoid or myxoid material which produces weakening of the tissues of the aorta. **Syphilitic aortitis** also causes stretching and dilatation of the aortic root along with widening of the commissures. Similar structural changes have been noted in AR associated with **ankylosing spondylitis** and **rheumatoid arthritis**. AR may also result from **dissecting aortic aneurysm** which may extend towards the aortic valve, **myxomatous degeneration** of aortic valve cusps, **atherosclerosis** and **Takayasu aortitis**.

Incompetence of the aortic valve results in marked cardiac enlargement due to both hypertrophy and dilatation. Due to the low diastolic blood pressure consequent to regurgitation of blood, the coronary blood flow is impaired. Latter combined with the increased oxygen demands of the hypertrophied heart, manifest as angina pectoris. The continuous volume overload of the left ventricle results in left ventricular failure.

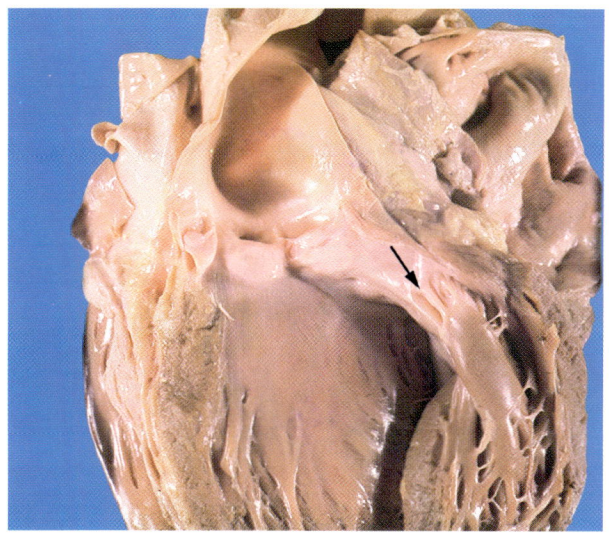

Fig. 4.19: Rheumatic heart disease with involvement of the mitral and aortic valves. Commissural fusion of aortic valve cusps is seen. Mitral valve was also involved. Picture shows the aortic aspect of the mitral valve which appears as a funnel (arrow) due to fibrosis and fusion of the leaflets and chordae tendinea. Left ventricle shows hypertrophy and dilatation due to incompetence of the aortic valve

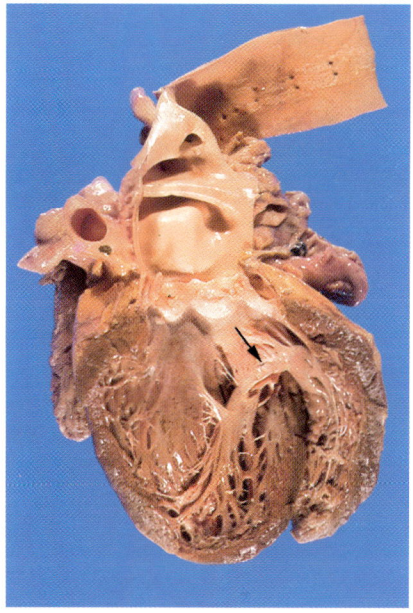

Fig. 4.20: Rheumatic heart disease. Picture shows involvement of the aortic and mitral valves. The normal architecture of the aortic valve cusps is lost. The cusps are thickened and commissures are fused. In addition, the free margins of the aortic valve cusps are covered by irregular nodular elevations (non-bacterial thrombotic endocarditis). Mitral valve is distorted and thickened due to fibrosis of the valve apparatus (arrow). Left ventricular dilatation is observed. Tricuspid was also involved in this case

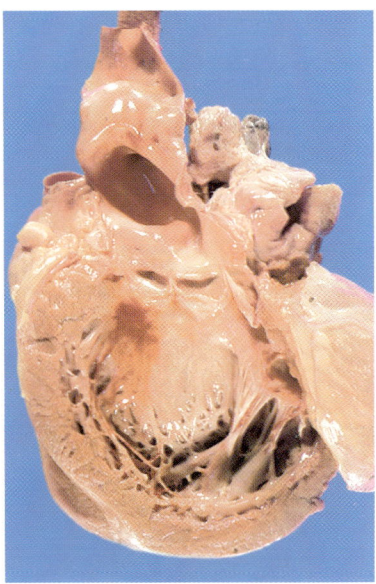

Fig. 4.21: Rheumatic heart disease. Prominent commissural fusion of the aortic valve cusps is observed. Marked left ventricular hypertrophy and dilatation ("cor bovinum") consequent to aortic valve incompetence is seen. Mitral valve was also involved in the rheumatic process. Its valve leaflets and chordae tendinea are thickened. Fresh hemorrhage is seen in the posterior wall of left ventricle

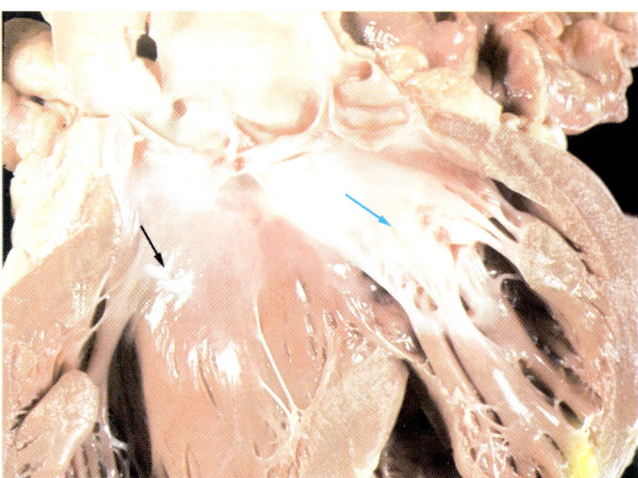

Fig. 4.22: Rheumatic heart disease. Aortic valve ring is dilated. The valve cusps are thickened and everted and commissural fusion is present. The aortic valve sinuses incuding coronary artery ostia are exposed. The mitral valve and its chordae tendinea are thickened and appear as a funnel (blue arrow). Left ventricle is markedly dilated due to long-standing incompetence of the aortic valve. Latter is also evident by focal thickening of endocardium and formation of "pockets of Zahn" in the left ventricular outflow tract (black arrow)

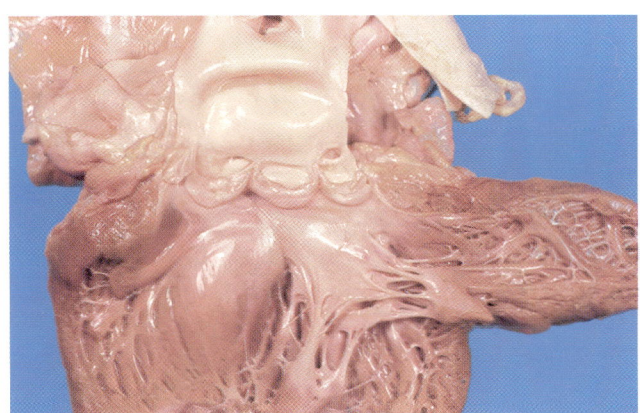

Fig. 4.23: Rheumatic heart disease. All three cusps of the aortic valve are thickened especially the free margins which are everted thus exposing the sinuses. The commissures of the valve cusps are fused. Diseased mitral valve can also be seen in this picture. Chordae tendinea of mitral valve are thickened and fused. Left ventricle dilatation is striking indicating incompetence of the aortic valve

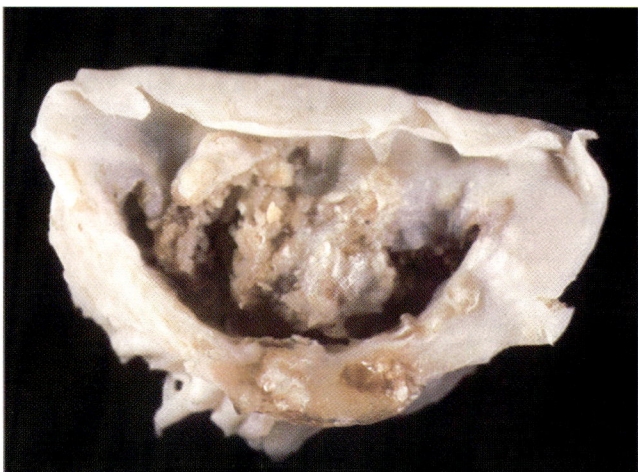

Fig. 4.24: Excised calcified aortic valve. The commissures are fused and the cusps are markedly fibrosed. Large aggregates of calcium are seen covering the cusps and occupying the narrowed lumen

Valvular Heart Disease

Tricuspid valve insufficiency This may be either **functional** resulting from failure and dilatation of the right ventricle and the valve ring (Fig. 4.25) or due to an **organic** involvement of the valve (Figs 4.26 and 4.27). Latter is most often caused by rheumatic valvulitis. Involvement by the rheumatic process is much milder in severity and intensity as compared with the mitral valve.

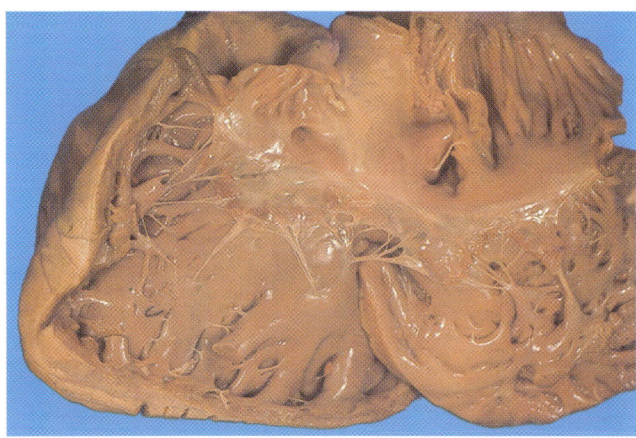

Fig. 4.25: Photograph shows marked dilatation of tricuspid valve ring and the right ventricle. This was a case of rheumatic heart disease with involvement of the aortic and mitral valves. Signs of tricuspid valve regurgitation were present. Latter is of a functional nature as the valve apparatus is normal

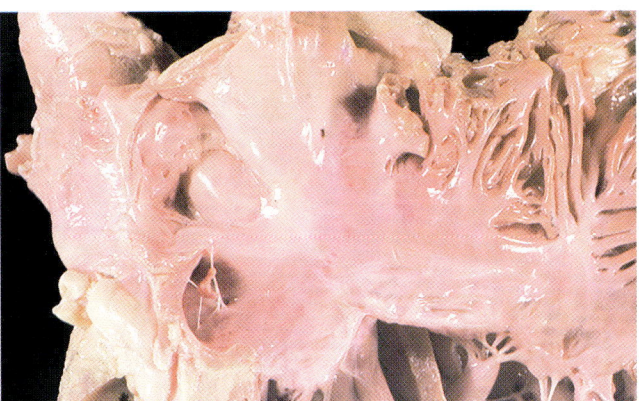

Fig. 4.26: Rheumatic heart disease. Tricuspid valve leaflets are thickened. The chordae tendinea are thickened, fused and reduced in length. Mitral and aortic valves were also involved in this case
Note: Tricuspid regurgitation was present. This is organic in nature as opposed to functional incompetence illustrated in Fig. 4.25

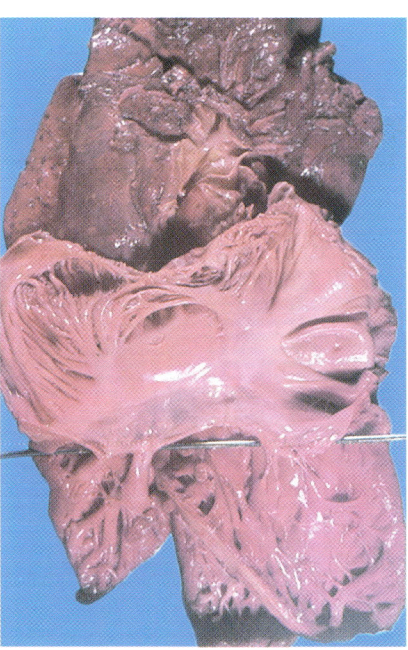

Fig. 4.27: Rheumatic heart disease. Photograph of tricuspid valve shows involvement of the leaflets and the chordae tendinea. The leaflets are fibrosed and thickened. The chordae tendinea are severaly affected and show marked fibrosis, thickening, shortening and fusion: A probe highlights these changes. The mitral and aortic valves were also diseased

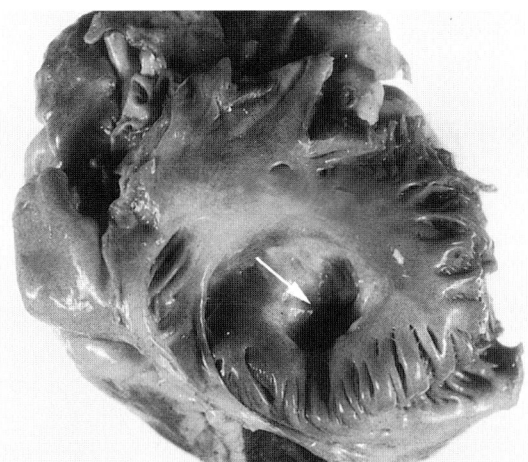

Fig. 4.28: Rheumatic heart disease. Tricuspid stenosis is observed (arrow). The mitral and aortic valves were also stenosed in this case
Note: Tricuspid involvement by the rheumatic process is milder as compared with the left sided valves. It is involved along with disease of the aortic and mitral valves. Tricuspid stenosis of rheumatic origin though documented is uncommon

Tricuspid valve stenosis RHD is the most common cause of acquired tricuspid valve stenosis which is associated with involvement of other heart valves (Fig. 4.28). Rarely it may occur consequent to infective endocarditis, carcinoid syndrome or exist as a congenital anomaly.

Both tricuspid valve stenosis and incompetence cause dilatation of the right atrium with elevated right atrial pressures, systemic venous congestion and right heart failure.

Pulmonary valve stenosis It is almost always congenital in nature. Involvement of this valve has also been reported in carcinoid syndrome, rheumatic heart disease and infective endocarditis. Clinically, effects of right ventricular hypertrophy result.

Pulmonary valve insufficiency It may result from dilatation of the pulmonary artery and the valve ring secondary to pulmonary hypertension and right ventricular failure. Rarely, rheumatic valvulitis, infective endocarditis, carcinoid syndrome and congenital malformations may cause insufficiency of the pulmonary valve.

Prosthetic Heart Valves

Valvular heart disease can be successfully treated by surgical means. The diseased valve can be replaced by prosthetic valve or tissue valves. Valve prostheses are of two types: (i) mechanical and (ii) bioprostheses.

Mechanical prostheses Several types of mechanical prostheses have been designed and marketed. Essentially, these are comprised of a metal or pyrophytic carbon-coated graphite frame, silicon ball or tilting disc, and teflon sewing ring. The prototype of the ball and cage mechanical prostheses is the Starr-Edwards valve and that of the tilting disc group is the Björk-Shiley valve and hinged bileaflet prostheses is the St. Jude prosthetic valve. Prosthetic valves have potentials for various complications. Patients with this device have to be maintained on **life-long anticoagulation** and therefore they suffer an increased risk of **hemolysis**. The incidence of this has lessened considerably due to better designing. **Dehiscence** of sutures may result in **paravalvular leak**. Ring and surface of the valve can be covered by overgrowth of fibrous tissue (**pannus formation**) This overgrowth may impede effective functioning or the mechanical prostheses. **Infective endocarditis** of mechanical prosthesis is of considerable concern. Sutures give way in most cases of infective endocarditis resulting in **paravalvular leak** and **regurgitation** of valve. The vegetations may grow and extend to cover/block the valve. Mortality in such instances is high. **Thromboembolism** is another consequence. Other complications include fracture of the ball within the cage fragments of which may embolise.

Bioprostheses The major risk of mechanical prosthetic valves is thromboembolism and effects of anticoagulation. Tissue valves were developed with an aim to have nonthrombogenic valves. Bioprosthesis also known as tissue valves are made of various types of biological material such as fascia lata, dura mater, bovine or porcine pericardium, porcine aortic valve or human aortic valve (homograft). These are then mounted on to prosthetic frames. Fascia lata and dura mater bioprostheses are discontinued and are not used presently due to high failure rate. The biological tissues before being constructed as valves are treated with glutaraldehyde. This treatment provides for strengthening of valve structure and flexibility and renders the tissue nonviable thus preventing any immune response to the valve. Valves constructed from bovine pericardium or procine aortic valves after treatment with glutaraldehyde are mounted on metallic stents. These are commercially available as Ionescu-Shiley bioprostheses. Those used from the procine aortic valve is better known as Hancock or Carpentier-Edwards bioprostheses. Eventually these tissue valves also suffer two major problems namely **degeneration** and **tearing of valve** and frequent occurrence of **dystrophic calcification**. Though these showed encouraging early results high degree of failure was reported and therefore they had to be removed from the patients. Additionally, since bioprostheses have a cloth-covered ring, potential for overgrowth of fibrous tissue on the ring exists which may cause hemodynamic changes. The common complications associated with bioprostheses are **tears of valve leaflets, calcification, paravalvular leak** and **infective endocarditis. Thrombosis** and **thromboembolism** causing obstruction of the valve may also occur in some cases.

Biologic Valves

In this group homografts and autografts are included. To overcome the serious problem of thromboembolism associated with prosthetic valves and rapid degenerative changes and consequently failure of bioprostheses there was a constant search for natural tissues to serve as valve replacement material. Biologic valves were thus devised by using homograft or autograft valves.

Homografts The mitral, aortic and pulmonary valves are removed from cadavers and collected and stored in appropriate conditions. Over the years with improvement in the techniques of collection and preservation of the valve and sterilization with antibiotics in place of chemical sterilization or irradiation, homografts have produced good results. Stent mounted allografts have been used for mitral valve replacement.

Autografts The use of biologic tissue has been further defined by replacement of the diseased valve by the patient's own valve. For example, patient's pulmonary valve can be used to replace the aortic valve while the patients tricuspid valve can be remodelled to replace the diseased mitral valve. The normal valve that is removed for use can be replaced by homograft.

Tissue engineering techniques and genetic engineering are being surveyed to develop tissue valve substitutes.

SUGGESTED READING

1. Chopra P, Bhatia ML: Chronic rheumatic valvular heart disease in India: A reappraisal of pathologic changes. *J Heart Valve Disease* **1**: 92-101, 1992.
2. Choudhary SK, Mathur A, Sharma R, Saxena A, Chopra P, Ray R, Kumar AS: Pulmonary autograft: Should it be used in young patients with rheumatic heart disease. *J Thoracic C Cardiovasc Surg* **118**: 483-90, 1999.
3. Goswami KC, Rao MB, Dev V, Shrivastava S: Juvenile tricuspid stenosis and rheumatic tricuspid valve disease: An echocardiographic study. *Int J Cardiol* **15**: **72(1)**: 83-86, 1999.
4. Hara JH: Valvular heart disease. *Prim Care* **27(3)**: 725-40; vii, 2000.
5. Kumar AS: Valvular heart disease—repair or replacement? *J Indian Med Assoc* **97(7)**: 282-86, 1999.
6. Kumar SA, Iyer KS, Chopra P: Quadrivalvular heart disease. *Int J Cardiol* **7**: 66-69, 1985.
7. Pauperio HM, Azevedo AC, Ferreira CS: The aortic valve with two leaflets–a study in 2,000 autopsies. *Cardiol Young* **9(5)**: 488-98, 1999.
8. Roldan CA: Valvular disease associated with systemic illness. *Cardiol Clin* **16(3)**: 531-50, 1998.
9. Rose AG: Etiology of valvular heart disease. *Curr Opin Cardiol* **11(2)**: 98-113, 1996.
10. Sabet HY, Edwards WD, Tazelaar HD, Daly RC: Congenitally bicuspid aortic valves: A surgical pathology study additional cases. *Mayo Clin Proc* **74(1)**: 14-26, 1999.

Infective Endocarditis

Infective endocarditis (IE) is infection of both valvular and parietal endocardium. It is characterized by masses (vegetations) on the valve surface. Traditionally, depending upon the clinical course IE is categorized as **acute** and **subacute**. **Acute IE** is generally caused by organisms of high virulence, has an aggressive clinical course with high mortality and is associated with serious cardiac and extracardiac complications. In immunocompromised hosts, however, even organisms of low virulence may cause a fulminant disease. **Subacute IE** is caused by organisms of low virulence commonly affecting a previously diseased valve. The infection caused is less invasive and destructive as compared with acute IE. Clinical course is generally prolonged with more morbidity than mortality.

Changed trends of infective endocarditis The availability and wide practice of cardiac surgery involving open heart surgery for valvular and congenital heart disease, cardiac interventions, pacemakers, etc. have provided potential sources of infection. Despite the availability of a wide range of antibiotics, infective endocarditis has emerged as a major problem and its management has given a major challenge. The types of infective organisms isolated in various clinical situations have undergone a change in the postantibiotic era. Organisms of low virulence may be highly virulent in certain situations, e.g. in the preantibiotic era *Streptococcus viridans* was the most common pathogen while in the postantibiotic era *Staphylococcus aureus* has emerged as an important organism in infective endocarditis that causes fulminant disease. Other organisms include Pseudomonas, Klebsiella, Enterococci, etc.

Predisposing factors Bacteremia/septicemia due to various causes is a prerequisite for development of IE. Damaged and scarred valves, e.g. consequent to rheumatic heart disease (RHD) and congenital heart defects are at risk to develop IE. In developing countries RHD still remains the underlying pathologic process in a vast majority of cases. Congenital heart disease such as tight stenoses, ventricular septal defects, tetralogy of Fallot, patent ductus arteriosus, etc. are predisposed to IE. Various types of **intervention** procedures, **indwelling catheters** and **intracardiac devices** increase the risk of introducing infection. **Immunocompromised hosts, intravenous drug abusers** and **prosthetic valves** are also a high-risk group. Infection by a virulent organism may affect a damaged and even normal valve.

Bacteremia consequent to fulminant infections of skin, respiratory tract, genitourinary tract may cause endocarditis. Normal valves may also get involved in bacteremia due to highly virulent organisms. Bacteremia has been documented even in procedures like dental extractions, catheterization of genitourinary tract, cystoscopy and during normal delivery.

Infective organisms A variety of organisms including bacteria, fungi, chlamydia, rickettsia, viruses, etc. may cause infection. Bacterial species, however, is the commonest cause of IE. Streptococci (50-70%), Staphylococci (25%) and Enterococci (10%) account for the vast majority of cases of IE. In Streptococcal caused endocarditis *S. viridans* is isolated in about 75% of the cases *S. bovis* and other streptococci cause IE in 20% and 5% cases respectively. *Staphylococcus aureus* is about 10 times commoner than *S. epidermidis*. Amongst **other organisms** almost all bacteria and organisms can cause endocarditis. **HACEK organisms** (Haemophilus, Actinobacillus, Cardiobacterium, Eikenella and Kingella) are a group of gram-negative organisms which produce a less virulent, indolent (subacute) form of the disease in about 2-3% cases. These organisms are difficult to isolate and therefore awareness of these agents and special appropriate steps have to be taken for their recovery. **Fungi** rarely cause IE in native valves. They occur particularly in **immunosuppressed** individuals, in **intravenous drug abusers** and in patients with **prosthetic valves**. Candida, Aspergillus are of commoner occurrence than *Cryptococcus neoformans, Histoplasma capsulatum* and *mucormycosis*. Rarely, spirochetes, *Rickettsiae*, *Chlamydia pneumoniae,* etc. can also cause endocarditis.

Pathology

Mitral and aortic valve involvement is commoner than the involvement of right sided valves. On naked eye examination, acute infective endocarditis is characterized by large friable vegetations. The color varies from dark red to pale or yellow. Their size may range from 5 mm to 2 cm (Figs 5.1 to 5.11a, 5.12 and 5.13). Vegetations caused by fungi are

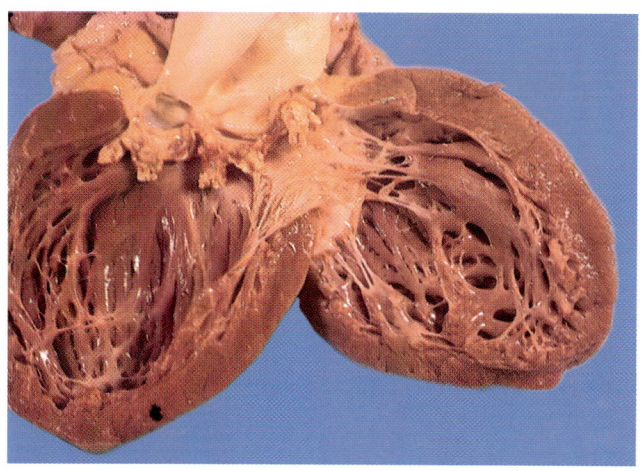

Fig. 5.1a: Infective endocarditis of aortic valve. Large vegetations cover the three cusps of the aortic valve and project into the left ventricle outflow tract. Left ventricle shows both hypertrophy and dilatation

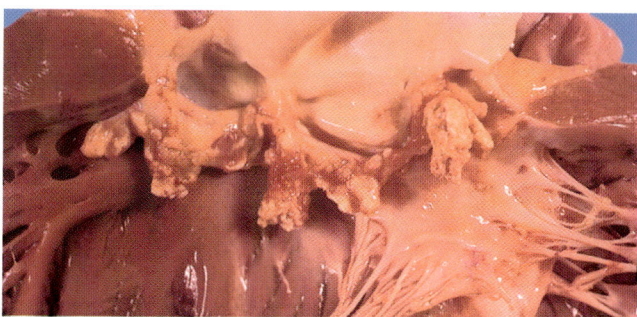

Fig. 5.1b: Infective endocarditis of aortic valve. This photograph shows a closer view of the vegetations illustrated in Figure 5.1a. They are polypoidal, congested and have an irregular surface
Note: This 18 years male was a case of rheumatic heart disease with involvement of the mitral and aortic valves. Gram-positive cocci were demonstrated within the vegetations

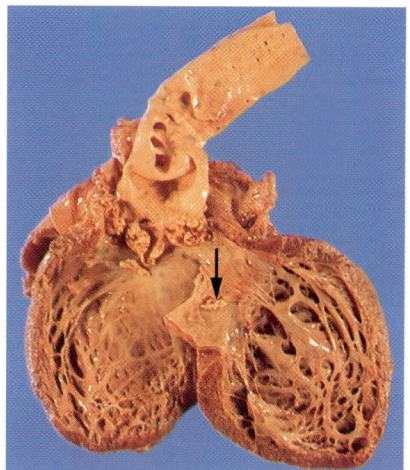

Fig. 5.2: Infective endocarditis of aortic valve to demonstrate the destructive nature of vegetations which are polypoidal, irregular and have infiltrated and destroyed the aortic valve cusps. Vegetations are seen to extend on to the aortic aspect of the anterior leaflet of the mitral valve (arrow). Left ventricle reveals marked dilatation of the chamber

Infective Endocarditis

generally larger and pale in color. Suppuration, destruction of valve structures with perforation and/or rupture of cusps is not uncommon (Figs 5.1 to 5.7 and 5.13). The vegetations can extend from the valve to the adjacent mural endocardium, to the intima, from aortic to mitral valve and *vice versa* (Figs 5.2 and 5.6). Vegetations can extend into the ostia of coronary arteries. The extension of vegetations may

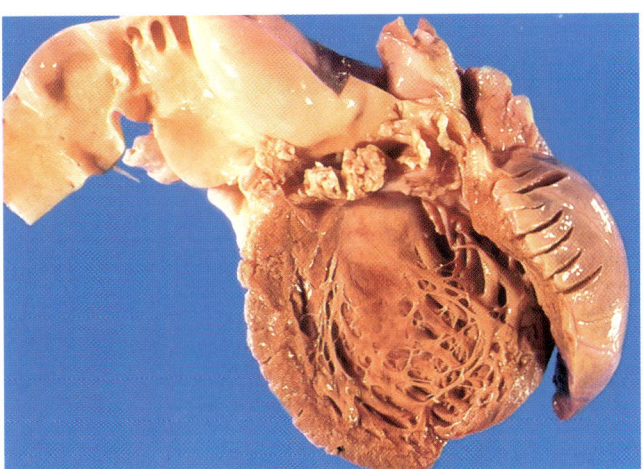

Fig. 5.3: Infective endocarditis of aortic valve. The valve cusps are totally eroded and destroyed and replaced by large, irregular grey white masses (vegetations). Left ventricle shows marked hypertrophy and dilatation

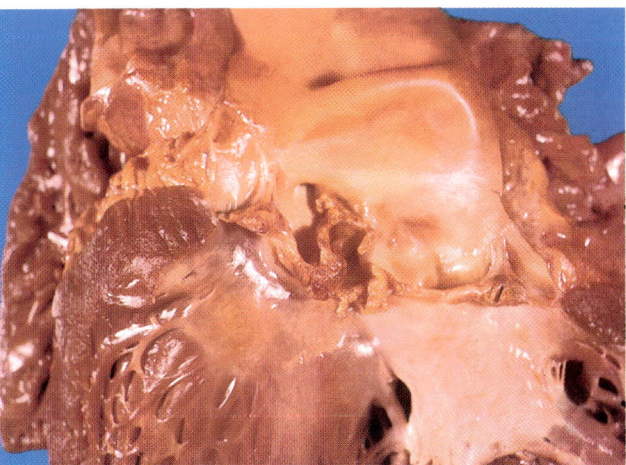

Fig. 5.4: Infective endocarditis of aortic valve. The cusps are destroyed and markedly distorted. The thickened cusps show polypoid, fragile vegetations mainly on the ventricular surface

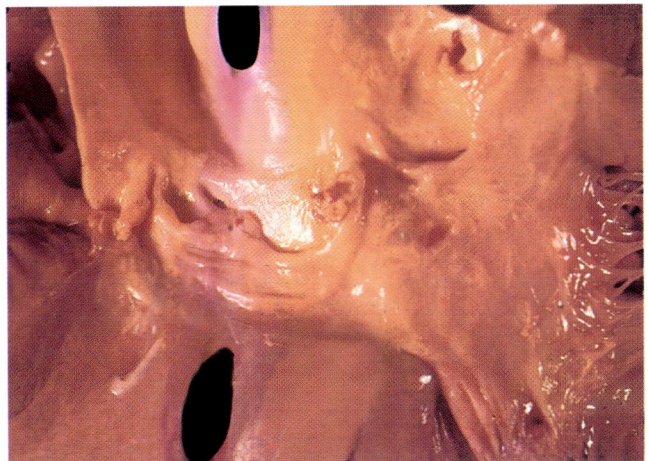

Fig. 5.5a: Congenital bicuspid aortic valve. The cusps are thickened, distorted and retracted. A few infective vegetations are seen on the free margin of the cusp adjacent to the commissure

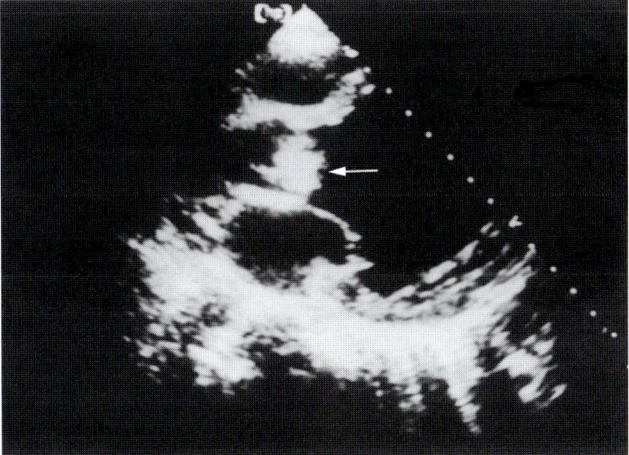

Fig. 5.5b: Echocardiography in parasternal long axis view showing vegetation (arrow) on aortic valve
Note: The patient was a 16 years male who had a bicuspid aortic valve

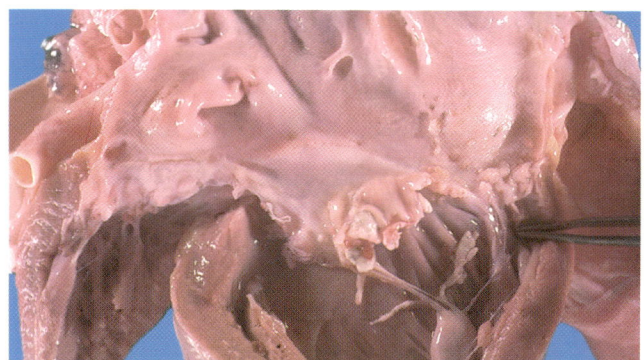

Fig. 5.6a: Infective endocarditis of mitral valve. Suppurative foci in the free margin of the mitral valve extending on to the chordae tendinea are seen. Local destruction of valvular tissue and rupture of few chordae tendinea are present. The mitral valve ring, left ventricle and left atrium are dilated

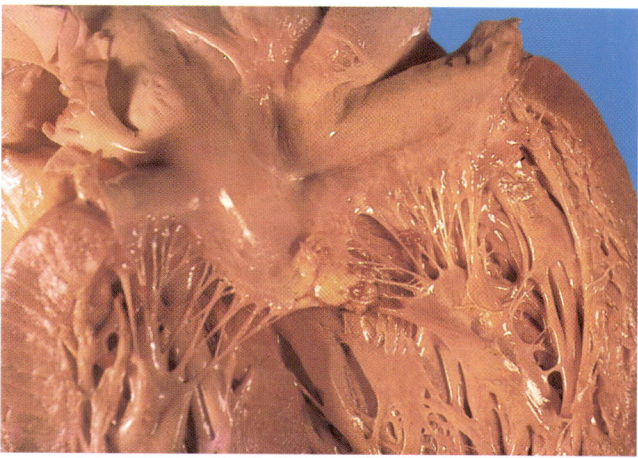

Fig. 5.7: Infective endocarditis of mitral valve to show another morphologic variant. Two yellowish gray, irregular and friable vegetations measuring 1.5 × 1 × 8 cm. are present on the atrial surface of the anterior cusp of the mitral valve at its contact margins. Myocardial abscesses and multiple septic infarcts were present in the spleen and kidney in this case

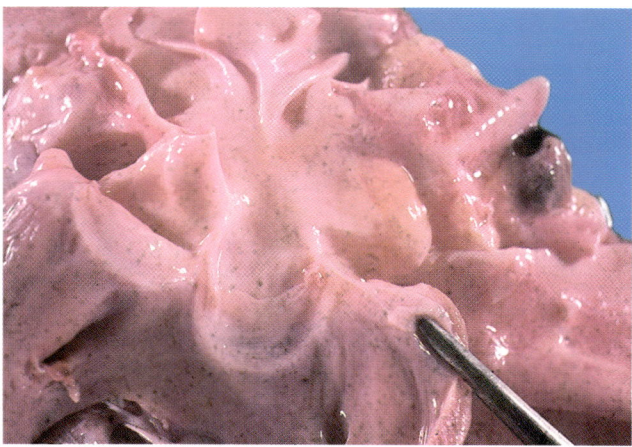

Fig. 5.6b: Infective endocarditis. The pulmonary valve shows small verrucous vegetations along the ventricular surface. Perforation of one of the semilunar cusps is observed (probe)

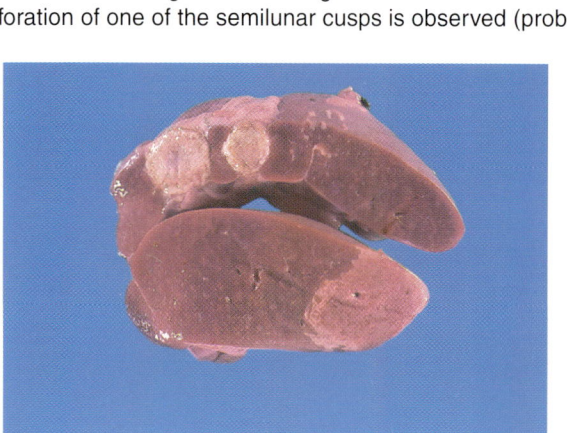

Fig. 5.6c: Infective endocarditis of mitral and pulmonary valves. The spleen shows infarcts (infected) and abscess formation
Note: The patient was a 30 years male who suffered suppurative arthritis. Figs 5.4a to c are from the same case

follow regurgitant jet of blood. Vegetations caused by organisms of low virulence are generally smaller, may be flat or sessile and are less destructive or invasive. **Microscopically,** the vegetations are composed of large clumps of fibrin and platelets in which the causative organism may be recognized (Figs 5.15 to 5.18). The underlying valve shows edema, necrosis and numerous polymorphs in cases of acute IE. Bacteria are seen as dark blue clusters in hematoxylin and eosin sections. Gram's stain is routinely performed on tissue sections to highlight the bacteria (Figs 5.15 to 5.17). Fungi can also be picked up on routine staining but are best appreciated on periodic acid schiff and silver methanamine staining (Fig. 5.19). In cases of infection by low virulence organisms and healing, the underlying valve reveals increased vascularization, chronic inflammation and hyalinization of valve collagen. As stated earlier, RHD is a common risk factor for development of IE. This can be seen on microscopic examination (Fig. 5.20).

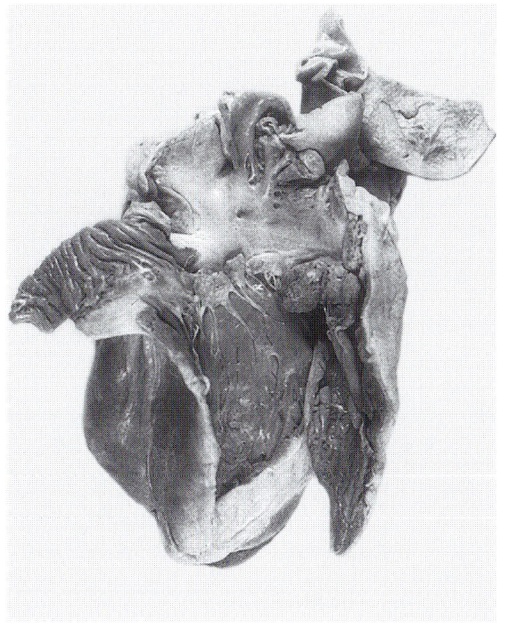

Fig. 5.8a: Infective endocarditis of tricuspid valve. Large bulbous vegetations occupy the valve leaflets. These hang into the right ventricular cavity

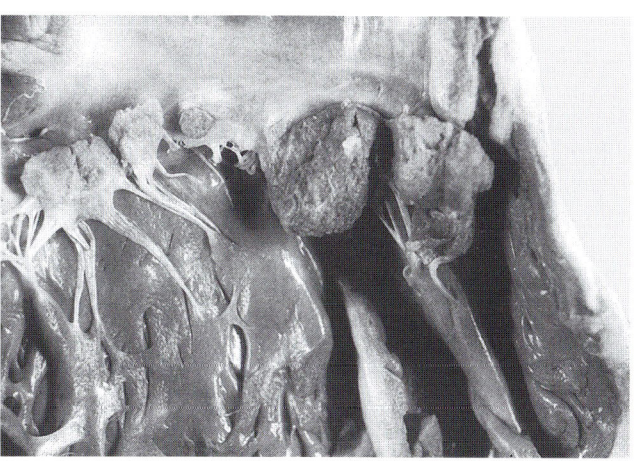

Fig. 5.8b: Infective endocarditis of tricuspid valve. The vegetations are large, dark tan and occupy the entire free margin of the tricuspid valve leaflet

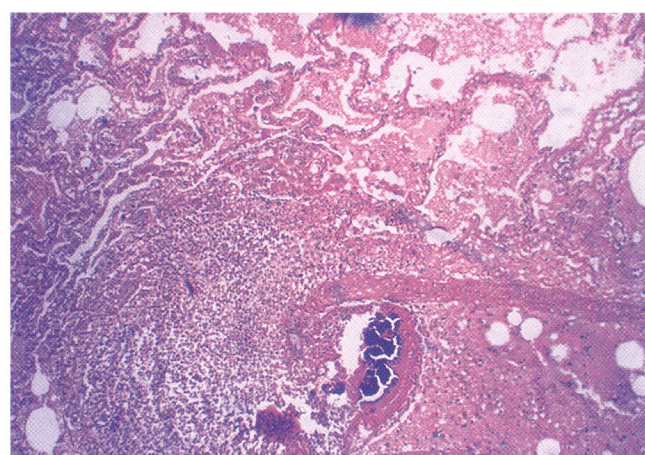

Fig. 5.8c: Infective endocarditis of tricuspid valve. Infected emboli are present in the pulmonary artery
Note: Patient was a thirty years female who presented with fever accompanied with chills and rigors and burning micturition of two weeks duration. She gave history of having had an abortion. She also developed signs and symptoms of acute renal failure. Figures 5.8a to c are from the same case

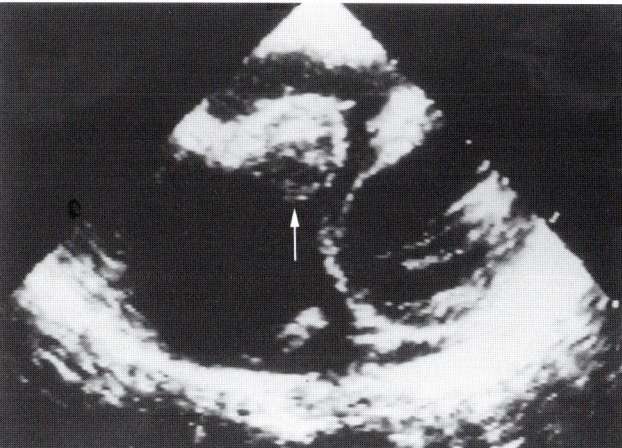

Fig. 5.9: Echocardiography in 4 chamber view showing a large vegetation on tricuspid valve (arrow)
Note: An eight years boy was detected to have a small ventricular septal defect. He was found to have poor orodental hygiene

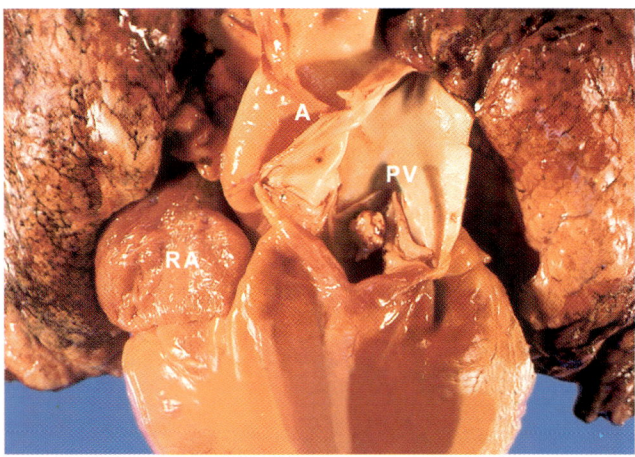

Fig. 5.10: Infective endocarditis. Congenital heart disease. Stenosis of the infundibulum in the right outflow tract was present. Picture shows a ventricular septal defect in the superior margin of which an irregular mass (vegetation) is seen. Lesion is also present on the cusp of the pulmonary valve. The tricuspid valve showed infective endocarditis. RA=right atrium; A=Aorta; PV = Pulmonary valve

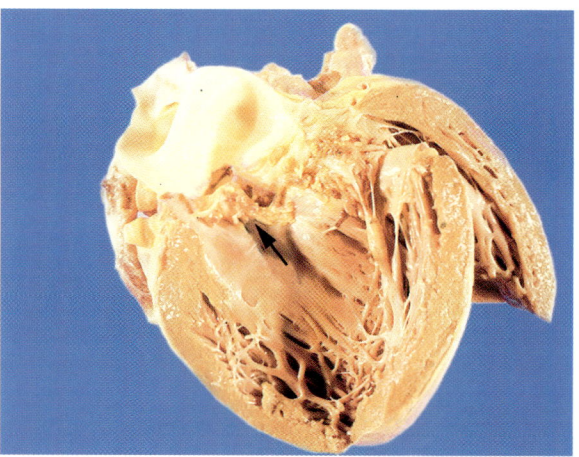

Fig. 5.11a: Infective endocarditis of aortic valve in a case of congenital heart disease. Numerous irregular gray white tags of tissue (vegetations) cover the ventricular surface of the aortic cusps which are seen to encroach upon the aortic surface of the anterior leaflet of the mitral valve. A large ventricular septal defect is seen (arrow in VSD) on the ring of which infective vegetations are present

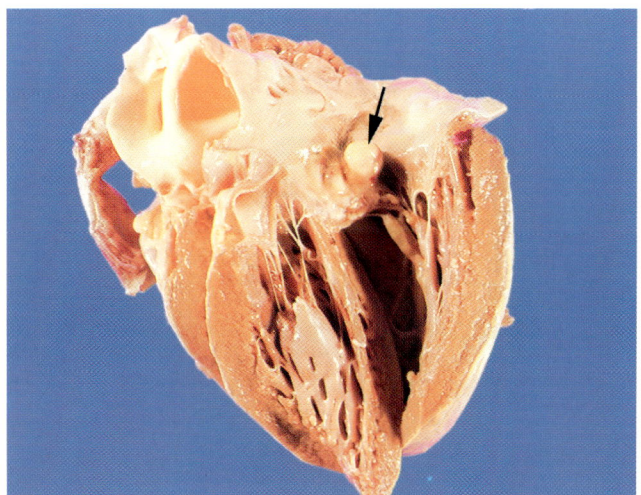

Fig. 5.11b: Healed infective endocarditis of mitral valve is seen as an aneurysmal dilatation of the anterior leaflet of mitral valve near the commissure (arrow)

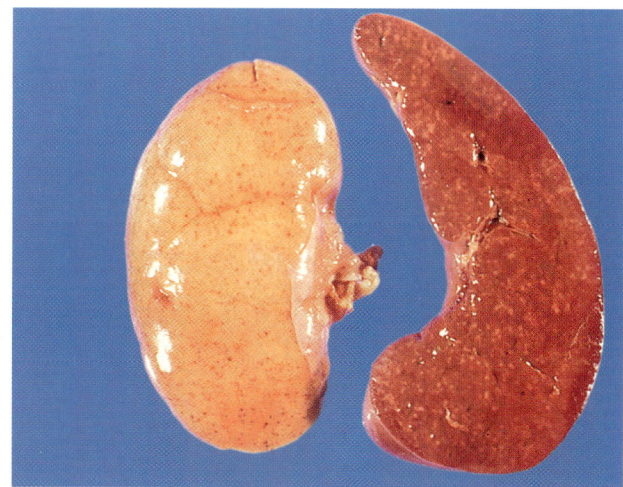

Fig. 5.11c: Healed infective endocarditis, of the mitral valve. The kidneys from this case show multiple punctate hemorrhages (Flea bitten kidney). The spleen was enlarged and soft to feel

Note: Figures 5.11a to c are from the same case

Infective Endocarditis

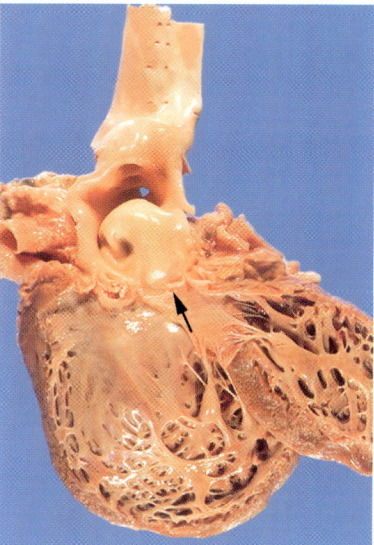

Fig. 5.12: Acute endocarditis of aortic valve. The right coronary cusp shows an irregular vegetation causing erosion of the cusp. The noncoronary cusp shows a perforation (arrow)
Note: A 17 years old female presented with irregular fever for 2 months. A clinical diagnosis of patent ductus arteriosus, aortic regurgitation and infective endocarditis was made. At autopsy, 2 firm vegetations 0.8 cm and 0.5 cm in diameter were present on the noncoronary cusp of the aortic valve. Fenestrations of the aortic valve were also noted

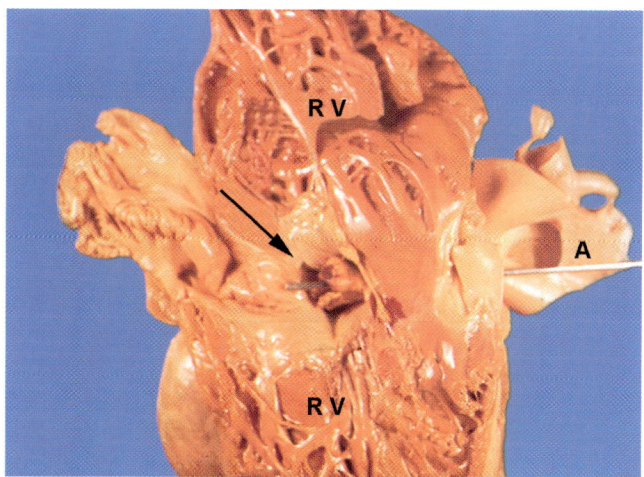 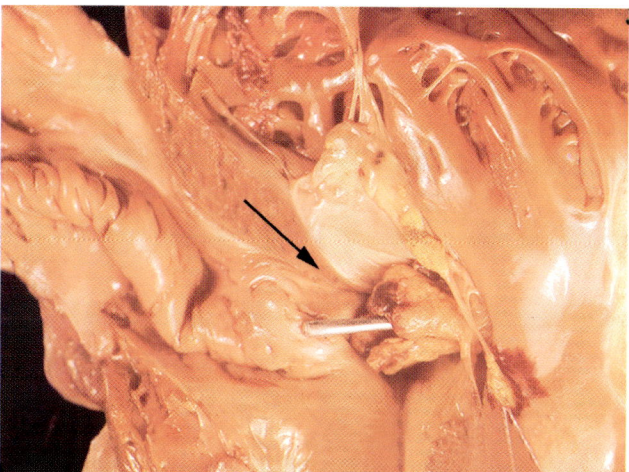

Figs 5.13a and b: Acute endocarditis of the aortic valve resulting in (a) aneurysm and rupture of sinus of Valsalva of right coronary cusp into the right ventricle (RV) at the level of the tricuspid valve (arrow). (b) Latter shows a polypoid projection whose edges are ragged with friable vegetations all around. A—Aorta
Note: Patient was a 26 years old male who presented with fever associated with chills. A clinical diagnosis of aortic regurgitation with ventricular septal defect was made. Patient died of heart failure

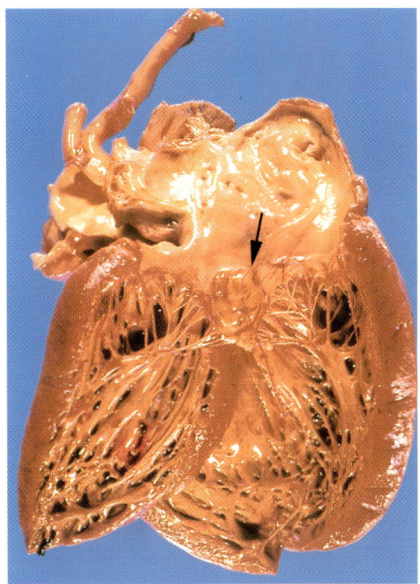

Fig. 5.14: Postinfective endocarditis aneurysm of the anterior leaflet of the mitral valve. Left ventricle shows features of hypertrophy and dilatation (arrow)
Note: Patient was a 22 years male who presented with features of acute gastroenteritis. There was no history suggestive of a cardiovascular disorder. At autopsy, bacterial endocarditis of aortic valve with destruction of all its cusps and aortic surface of the anterior mitral leaflet was detected

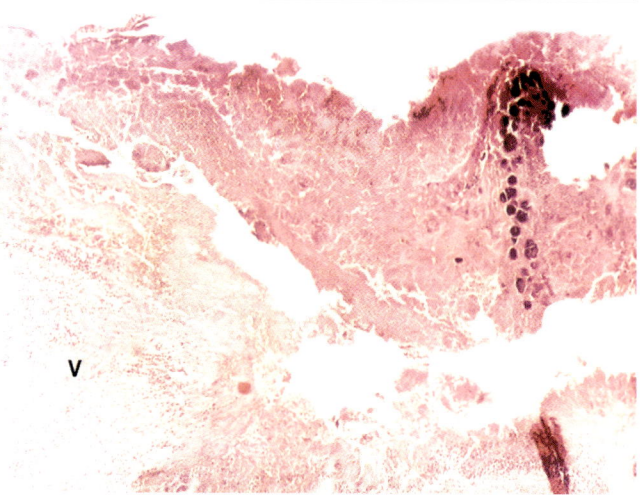

Fig. 5.15: Photomicrograph from the vegetation on the mitral valve. Numerous granular (Gram-positive bacteria) structures mostly in clumps are seen embedded within the clumps of fibrin and platelets. Lower left part of the picture shows part of the valve (v) infiltrated by inflammatory cells. This was a case of rheumatic heart disease who developed infective endocarditis of both aortic and mitral valves

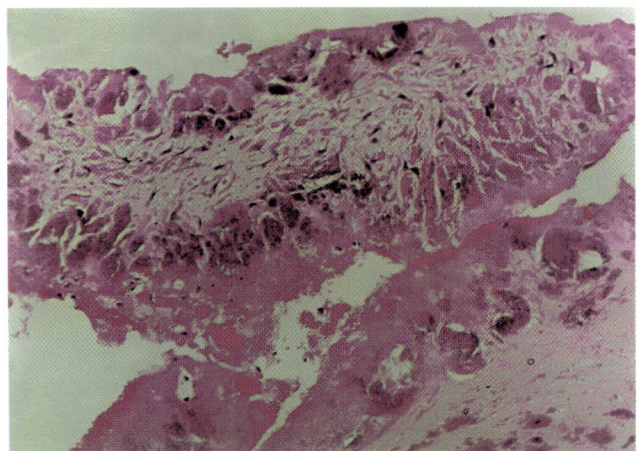
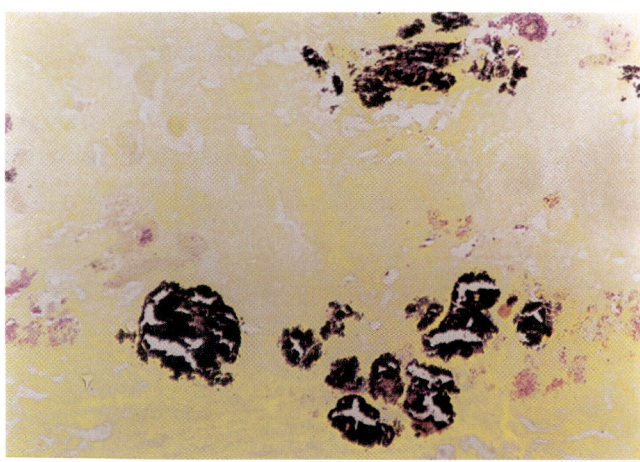

Figs 5.16a and b: Infective endocarditis mitral valve. Photograph shows (a) numerous bacterial colonies and necrosis on the surface of the valve, (b) gram-positive cocci are seen within the vegetation
Note: A 46 years old male a known case of rheumatic heart disease with mitral valve stenosis and regurgitation developed fever following mitral valve replacement

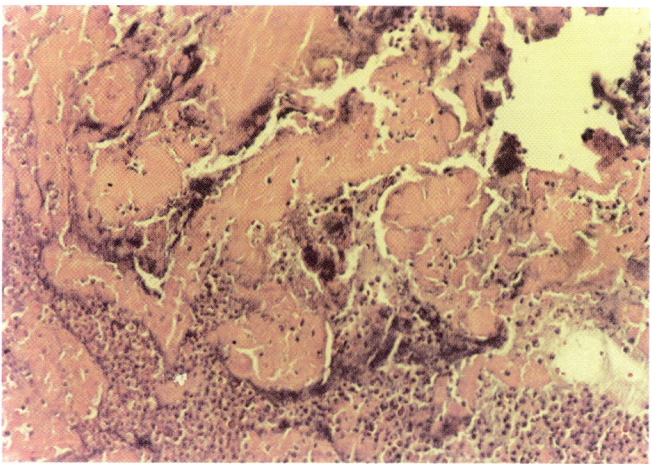

Fig. 5.17a: 3 years old male child a known case of ventricular septal defect. Patient presented with fever. ECHO revealed vegetations on the septal leaflet of the tricuspid valve measuring 2.8 × 1.5 × 1.2 cm. Sections examined show infective vegetations composed of dense clumps of finely granular hematoxylin stained bacteria. Numerous polymorphs were seen within the vegetation and the valve leaflet

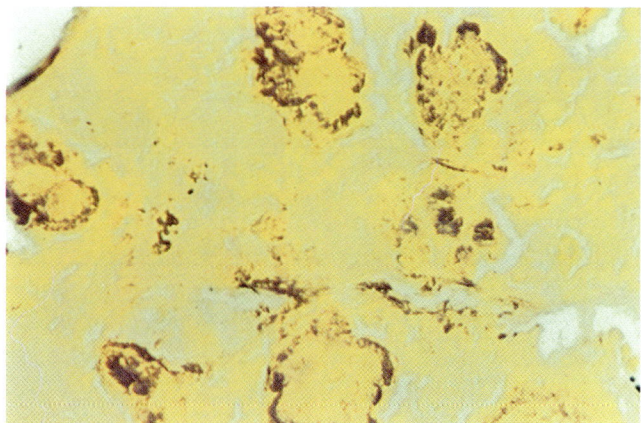

Fig. 5.17b: Infective endocarditis. Gram's stain of the vegetation described in Figure 5.17a. Numerous gram-positive cocci are seen

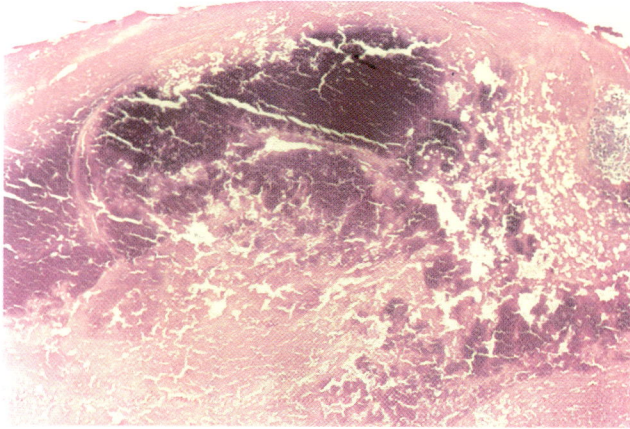

Fig. 5.17c: Infective endocarditis. Sections from other areas of the vegetation revealed focal areas of calcification and necrosis

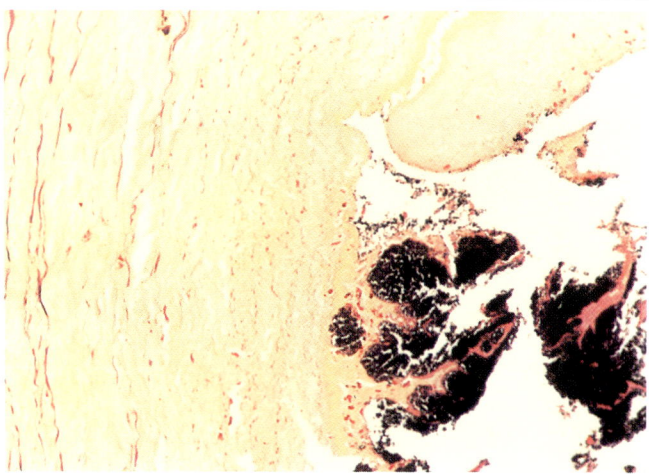

Fig. 5.18: Infective endocarditis of the aortic and mitral valves. The vegetations from the aortic valve extended on to the aortic intima. Photomicrograph to show gram-positive cocci on the aortic intima (intimitis). Patient was a case of rheumatic heart disease with involvement of mitral and aortic valves

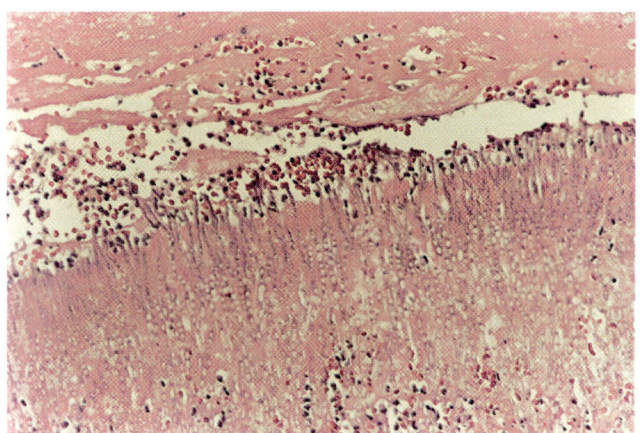

Fig. 5.19a: Infective endocarditis. Microscopic examination of the vegetation show numerous branching septate organisms the histology of which is consistent with Aspergillus species

Note: A 24 years old male was operated for an atrioventricular septal defect. Postoperative ECHO examination revealed a large vegetation (7 × 5 cm) involving whole of atrial septum and extending on to the mitral valve

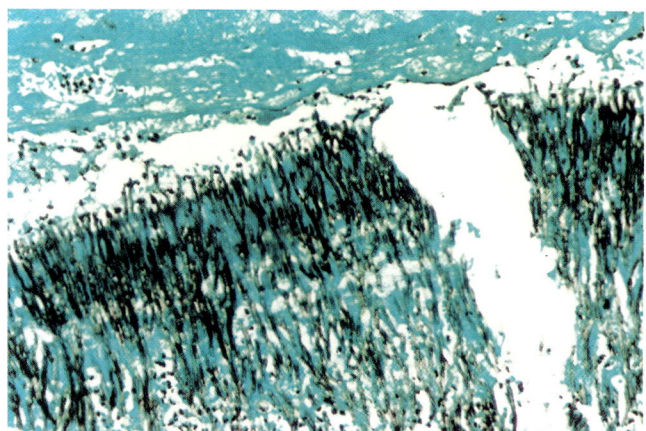

Fig. 5.19b: Infective endocarditis. Silver methanamine stain to highlight the morphological features of the fungus (Aspergillus species)

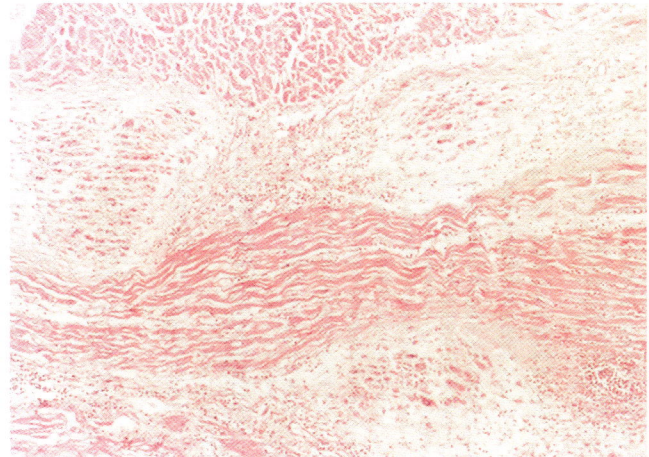

Fig. 5.20a: A case of rheumatic heart disease who developed infective endocarditis. Numerous. Aschoff nodules are seen in the interstices of the myocardium. Myocardial abscess is also seen in the lower right hand corner of the picture

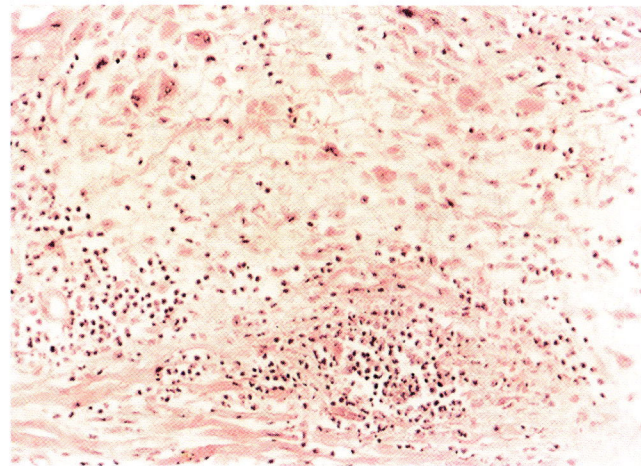

Fig. 5.20b: Higher magnification of Figure 5.20a to show Aschoff nodules and the myocardial abscess

Pathogenesis

Endothelial injury has been demonstrated even in normal valves at sites where they come in contact with each other. The extent and severity of endothelial demage, however, is well-marked in previously damaged valves, e.g. RHD or areas of endocardium exposed to high-velocity jet streams of blood as in small ventricular septal defects, patent ductus arteriosus (PDA) or stenotic valves. Platelet and fibrin aggregates form rapidly at the site of damaged endocardium and provide a trap for infective agents during the course of a bacteremia. The organisms thus colonise and proliferate within the platelet fibrin thrombi to form large masses (vegetations) (Fig. 5.21) which may cause invasion, inflammation and destruction of the underlying valve substance. Normal valvular endothelium in resistant to invasion by most infective organisms. However, overwhelming infection by virulent organisms namely *Staphylococcus aureus* in normal or more commonly in immunocompromised hosts may affect healthy valves as in intravenous drug users, prosthetic valves and other implanted cardiac devices.

Complications of Infective Endocarditis

Most complications occur due to the invasive and destructive nature of the infective organism and the potential for the vegetations to embolize. Healing of infection can cause deformities of the valve.

Cardiac failure can occur due to sudden volume overload consequent to incompetence of the valve resulting from destruction and/or perforation of the valve leaflets, rupture of chordae tendinea, papillary muscle myocardial dysfunction, etc. (Figs 5.2 to 5.4, 5.12 and 5.13). Microembolization into the coronary circulation can lead to **myocardial abscesses** (Figs 5.20 and 5.22). Extension of myocardial abscesses or infective foci into the pericardium may result in **purulent pericarditis.** Additionally, immune complex mediated vasculitis may also contribute to cardiac dysfunction. Erosion and destruction of aortic valve cusps may lead to rupture of sinus of valsalva (Fig. 5.13) resulting in heart failure. Healing consequent to infective endocarditis can result in Valvular deformities, aneurysm of valve leaflets, etc. (Figs 5.11b and 5.14).

68 Illustrated Textbook of Cardiovascular Pathology

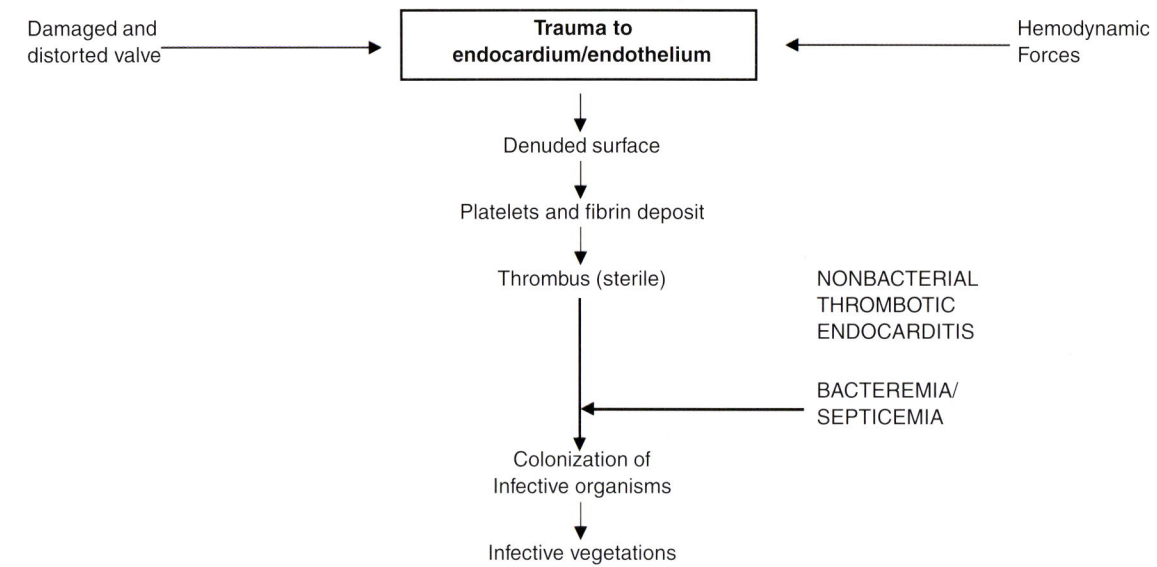

Fig. 5.21: Pathogenesis of vegetations in infective and noninfective endocarditis

Embolic complications This is a major threat in IE. The vegetations are friable and therefore prone to embolize. These cause infarcts and/or abscess formation in the spleen (Fig. 5.6c), kidney, central nervous system, heart and other organs. Mycotic aneurysms may also occur. IE of the valves of the right heart can cause pulmonary embolism leading to infarction or abscess in the lungs (Fig. 5.8c).

Immune complex mediated injury Circulating immune complexes can be demonstrated in cases with prolonged bacteremia usually due to organisms of low virulence (subacute bacterial endocarditis). Immune complex mediated vasculitis in IE is possibly related to the occurrence of arthritis, subungual hemorrhages and focal glomerulonephritis (Fig. 5.23). On naked eye examination, the kidney show tiny petechial hemorrhages (flea bitten kidney) on the external and cut surface (Fig. 5.11c). Petechiae in the skin, conjunctiva and small tender nodules (Osler's nodes) on the finger tips.

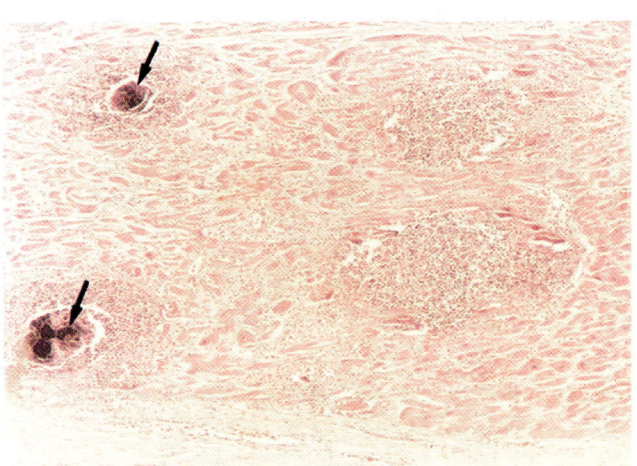

Fig. 5.22: Infective endocarditis of aortic and mitral valves. Multiple myocardial abscesses were observed in this case

Note Numerous bacterial colonies are observed in the midst of the abscess (arrows)

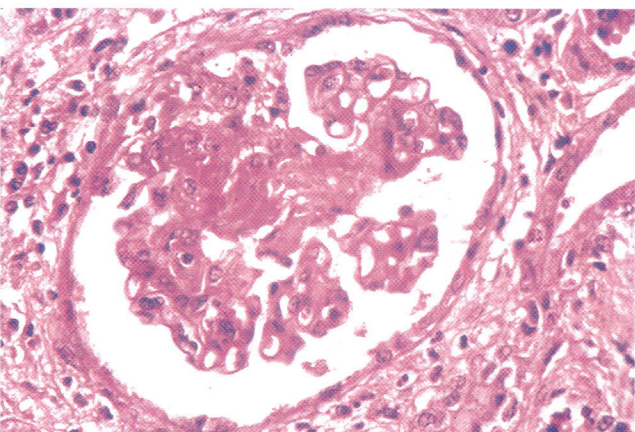

Fig. 5.23: Focal glomerulonephritis in a case of bacterial endocarditis. Part of the glomerular tuft shows a smudgy eosinophilic appearance (fibrinoid necrosis)

Note 28 years female a known case of rheumatic heart disease with involvement of the mitral and aortic valve developed bacterial endocarditis of both the valves and left atrial endocardium

Infective Endocarditis

Prosthetic valve endocarditis (PVE) (Figs 5.24 and 5.25) is a serious complication. Infection occurs generally along the suture line. Endocarditis is a result of contamination introduced at the time of surgery either directly into the wound or via various devices used during surgery. Overall incidence of PVE varies from 1-4%. Early onset endocarditis occurs within 60 days of surgery while late onset develops after 60 days of surgery. About 50% of early onset endocarditis is caused by Staphylococcus (*S. epidermidis* more than *S. aureus*). Streptococcus is the most common causative agent in late onset endocarditis in over 40% cases. Infective endocarditis of the inserted valve can result in abscess formation of the valve ring, valve dehiscence, paravalvular leak, thrombosis, obstruction of the valve, embolic complications, etc. Degenerative changes and deterioration of the prosthesis can also occur. Similar infections can occur in tissue valves (Figs 5.26 to 5.28) and in dacron grafts (Fig. 5.29).

Endocarditis in intravenous drug abusers This group is particularly prone to develop recurrent attacks of infective endocarditis. Right sided valves more commonly the tricuspid valve is affected in over 50% cases. Aortic and mitral valves can be involved in 25% and 20% cases respectively. In 2-3% cases multiple valves may be affected.

Infection of normal native valve is can be caused by highly virulent organisms namely Staphylococcus. *Staphylococcus aureus* is the causative agent in over 50% cases. Streptococci and Enterococci are causative agents in about 20% cases. Fungi mostly Candida and Aspergillus may be isolated in about

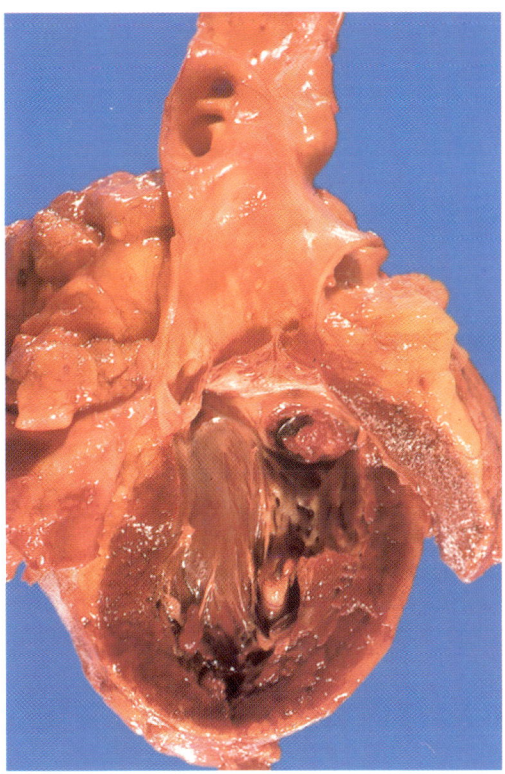

Fig. 5.24: A case of rheumatic heart disease. Prosthetic valve (Björk-Shiley prosthesis) in the mitral position. An irregular mass dark red in color (fresh and organizing thrombus) is seen covering the ventricular aspect of the valve. The stitches were intact

Note A case of rheumatic heart disease. Mitral valve was replaced by Björk-Shiley prosthesis. Patient died 4 months postoperatively. Aortic and tricuspid valves were also involved by the rheumatic process

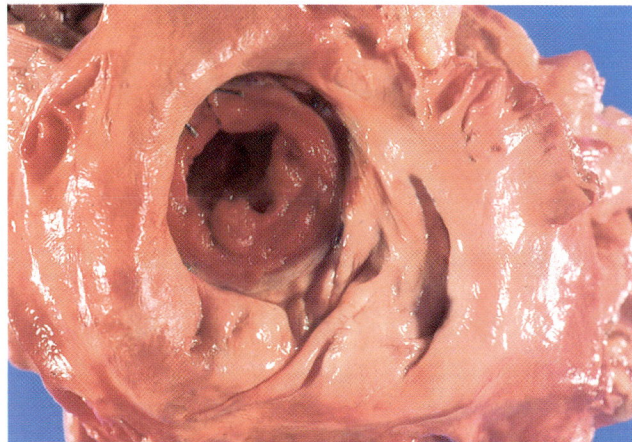

Fig. 5.25: A case of rheumatic heart disease with involvement of mitral and aortic valves. Mitral valve replacement was done by Björk-Shiley prosthesis. A fresh occlusive thrombus is present on the atrial aspect of the prosthesis

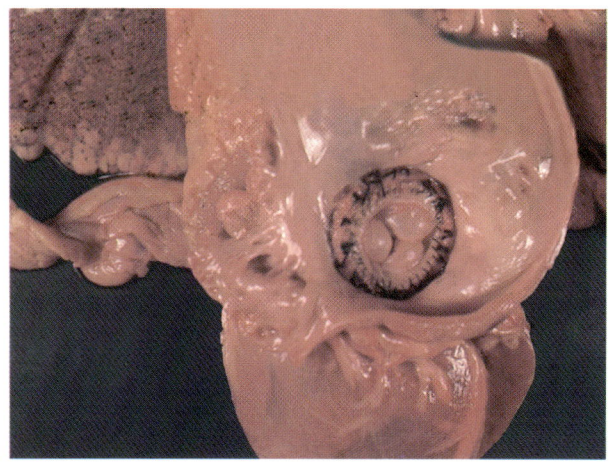
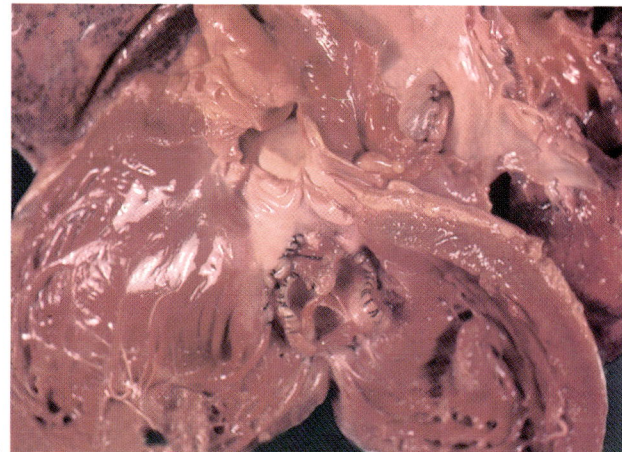

Figs 5.26a and b: Rheumatic heart disease. Patient was a 14 years male who had features of mitral valve stenosis and regurgitation. Mitral valve replacement by autograft (autologous fascialata graft mounted on a titanium support) was done. Patient died of ventricular fibrillation. Erosion of one of the foot processes of the graft was observed (a) atrial view (b) ventricular view

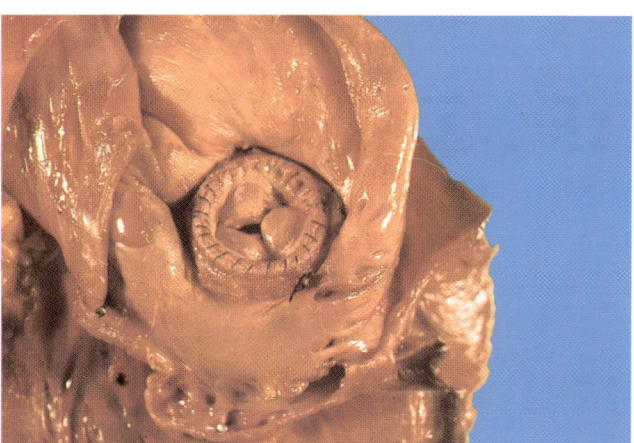
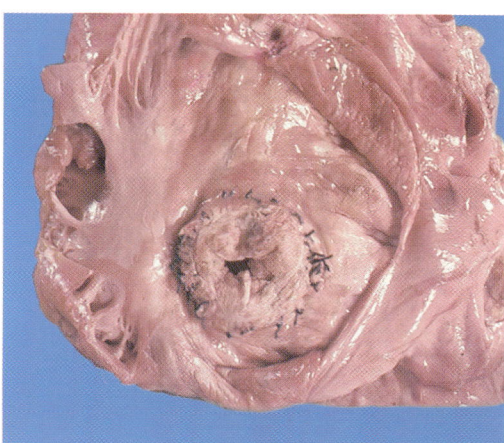

Fig. 5.27: Rheumatic heart disease with involvement of mitral and tricuspid valves. Mitral valve replacement was performed using homograft valve

Fig. 5.28: Fungal endocarditis (Aspergillosis) of the replaced mitral valve (homograft). Atrial view of the homograft which is completely covered by fibrin and light tan tissue. This change was more on the atrial than the ventricular surface

Note: 28 years female a case of rheumatic heart disease presented with features of mitral valve regurgitation. Mitral valve replacement with homograft aortic valve mounted on a stainless steel frame covered with dacron was performed. She developed low grade fever postoperatively and died seven weeks after surgery

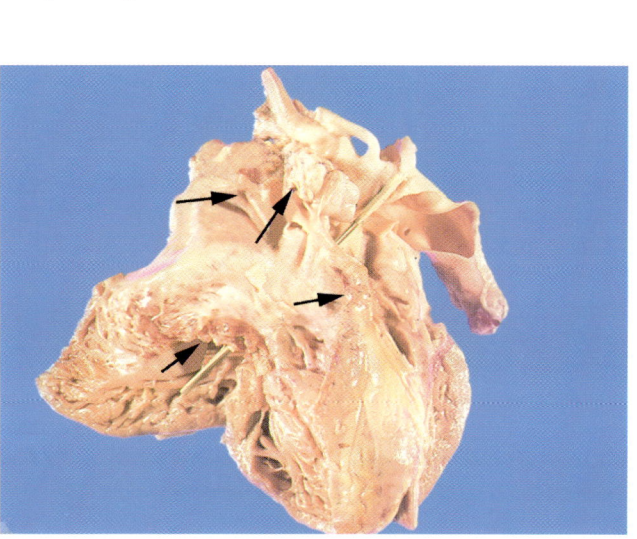

Fig. 5.29: Infective endocarditis. Margin of the dacron patch (arrows) reveals necrotic and friable material which shows focal calcification. Rupture of sinus of Valsalva aneurysm into the right ventricle was also detected.

Note: 10 years male child a case of tetralogy of Fallot underwent surgery for closure of ventricular septal defect by applying a dacron patch on it and a pericardial patch over the stenotic pulmonary infundibulum. Postoperatively he had low grade fever for 3 months

5-8% cases. Gram-negative bacilli usually Pseudomonas are detected in about 5-6% cases. Infection with **multiple organisms** may occur in a number of cases. Most common source of infection is skin, contamination of the needles, syringes and other agents used for injection. Other cause of right sided IE includes thrombophlebitis of the subclavian or femoral venous system. **Complications** of right sided IE are **pulmonary infarction** with or without **abscess** formation (Fig. 5.8c).

Nonbacterial thrombotic endocarditis (NBTE)

This is characterized by vegetations ranging in size from 1 to 4 mm mostly on the mitral valve (Fig. 5.30). They are composed of platelets and fibrin, are not infective in nature (bland) and do not evoke an inflammatory response (Fig. 5.31). These vegetations have the potential to cause embolic complications in brain, kidney, spleen and heart and thus assume clinical importance. Additionally, colonization of these bland thrombi may occur and lead to infective endocarditis. The exact cause of this condition is ill

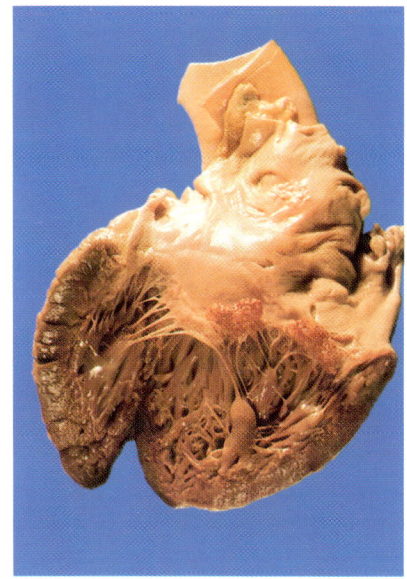

Fig. 5.30: Nonbacterial thrombotic endocarditis. Large reddish vegetations are seen on the atrial aspect of the posterior and part of the anterior leaflet of the mitral valve. The vegetations are present on the contact margin of the leaflets. Spleen and kidney showed multiple healed infarcts

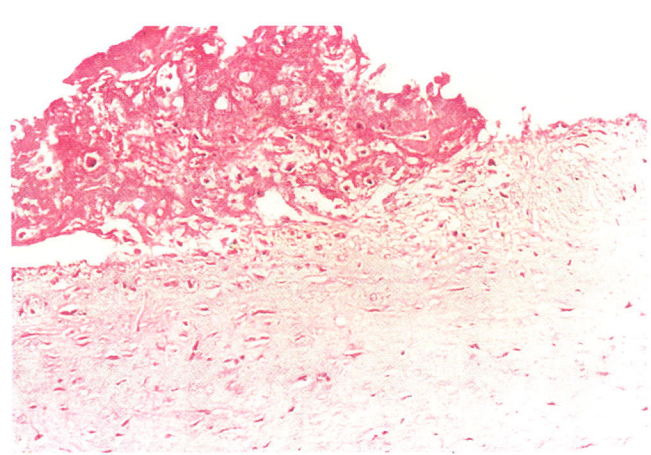

Fig. 5.31a: Nonbacterial thrombotic endocarditis. Microscopically the vegetations are composed of fibrin admixed with platelets and red blood cells. The adjacent valve tissue appears unremarkable

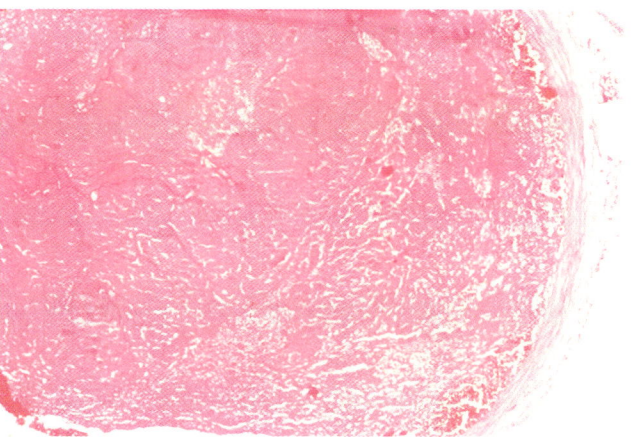

Fig. 5.31b: Nonbacterial thrombotic endocarditis. Photomicrograph of the cerebral artery shows a fresh thrombus. Multiple fresh infarcts were detected in the brain, spleen and kidneys

Note: 12 years old male child presented with fever, recurrent convulsions, weakness of the left upper and lower limbs, headache and vomiting off and on for 3 weeks. A clinical diagnosis of an embolic stroke was entertained. At autopsy the heart was normal except for the aortic valve which showed that free margins of all the three cusps were replaced by multiple grayish white irregular friable vegetations measuring 0.3 cm to 0.6 cm in diameter

understood. Some of the factors implicated include prolonged debilitating diseases, malignancy (carcinoma lung, stomach, pancreas) disseminated intravascular coagulation and other hypercoagulable states. Mechanical wear and tear at the contact point of valve leaflets and cusps leads to trauma of the endothelium which favors deposition of fibrin, platelets, red and white cells to form vegetations (Fig. 5.21).

Libman-Sacks endocarditis This is the endocarditis encountered in about half the cases of systemic lupus erythematosus. It characteristically affects **both** surfaces of valve leaflets where multiple, flat, granular deposits 2 to 4 mm in diameter (vegetations) can be observed. Healing does not produce valvular deformities. Embolic complications generally do not occur. **Microscopically**, the affected valve reveals edema, fibrinoid necrosis, neovascularization and infiltration by lymphocytes and mononuclear cells. Healing is by fibrosis. The vegetations are composed of fibrinoid material and fibrin in which inflammatory cells and blood elements are trapped. Hematoxylin bodies may be seen.

SUGGESTED READING

1. Baddour LM: Infective endocarditis caused by beta-hemolytic streptococci. The Infectious Diseases Society of America's Emerging Infections Network. *Clin Infect Dis* **26(1)**: 66-71, 1998.
2. Bansal RC: Infective endocarditis. *Med Clin North Am* **79(5)**: 1205-40, 1995.
3. Benn M, Hagelskjaer LM, Tveda M: Infective endocarditis, 1984 through 1993: A clinical and microbiological survey. *J Intern Med* **242**: 15-22, 1997.
4. Chopra P, Subramanyam, Bhatia ML: Infective endocarditis—An autopsy analysis of 40 cases. *Ind J Med Res* **72**: 258-68, 1980.
5. Collignon P: Risk factors for infective endocarditis (letter; comment). *Ann Intern Med* **131(2)**: 154-55, 1999.
6. Eiken PW, Edwards WD, Tazelaar HD *et al*: Surgical pathology of nonbacterial thrombotic endocarditis in 30 patients, 1985-2000. *Mayo Clinic Proc* **76(12)**: 1204-12, 2001.
7. Ferincola DJ, Roberts WC: Clinicopathological features of active infective endocarditis isolated to the native mitral valve. *Am J Cardiol* **71**: 1186-97, 1993.
8. Flock JI, Hienz SA, Heimdahl A, Schennings T: Reconsideration of the role of fibronectin binding in endocarditis caused by *Staphylococcus aureus*. *Infect Immun* **64(5)**: 1876-78, 1996.
9. Harris PS, Cobbs CG: Cardiac, cerebral, and vascular complications of infective endocarditis. *Cardiol Clin* **14(3)**: 437-50, 1996.
10. Jiang Y, Magli L, Russo M: Bacterium dependent induction of cytokines in mononuclear cells and their pathologic consequences *in vivo*. *Infect Immun* **67(5)**: 2125-30, 1999.
11. Murphy JG, Steckelberg JM: New developments in infective endocarditis. *Curr Opin Cardiol* **10(2)**: 150-54, 1995.
12. Mylonakis E, Calderwood SB: Infective endocarditis in adults. *N Eng J Med* **345**: 1318-30, 2001.
13. Nettles RE, McCarty DE, Corey GR, Li J, Sexton DJ: An evaluation of the Duke criteria in 25 pathologically condirmed cases of prosthetic valve endocarditis. *Clin Infect Dis* **25(6)**: 1401-03, 1997.
14. Saitoh F, Kawai S, Suzuki H, Okada R, Yamaguchi H, Sawada J, Aoki K, Kato K, Hosoda Y: Surgical pathology of infective endocarditis. *J Cardiol* **27(Suppl 2)**: 91-94, discussion 95, 1996.

6
Ischemic Heart Disease

Heart disease is a significant cause of morbidity and mortality throughout the world. In India while rheumatic heart disease continues to cause major concern, hypertension and ischemic heart disease have attained notable proportions. It is of significance that in the developed world there has been a considerable decline in mortality of coronary heart disease. This is chiefly because of the awareness of the disease, control of risk factors, early diagnosis and management.

Ischemic heart disease is a result of lack of oxygen consequent to inadequate perfusion. There is thus a situation of increased oxygen demand versus the supply. The most common cause of various acute coronary syndromes and ischemic heart disease is atherosclerotic narrowing or occlusion of the coronary arteries. Detailed angiographic, angioscopic and more importantly morphologic analysis of the atheromatous plaque has provided useful information regarding the progression of plaque to cause narrowing/occlusion of the coronary artery.

Atherosclerotic coronary artery disease has a wide spectrum of clinical expressions (Fig. 6.1). While a substantial number of individuals may be asymptomatic, some manifest for the first time with sudden cardiac death. Others present with angina pectoris, a symptom of myocardial ischemia. It is the **acute coronary syndromes**—triad of unstable angina, myocardial infarction and sudden death which lead to significant cardiac morbidity and mortality.

Stable angina is characterized by cardiac pain which is brought on by exertion/exercise. There is no pain at rest. Atherosclerotic narrowing of one or more coronary arteries is present in these cases. The number of stenotic segments and the length of the diseased areas greatly influence coronary blood flow. The stenotic atherosclerotic lesion may be either eccentric or concentric. In eccentric lesions, part of the arterial wall is free of the lesion. It is the latter segment which may undergo spasm and consequently cause significant alteration in the cross sectional area of the lumen. In concentric plaques on the other hand, there is no appreciable alteration the luminal area. In **Prinzmetal variant angina** pain occurs at rest. Coronary artery spasm is well-established in these cases.

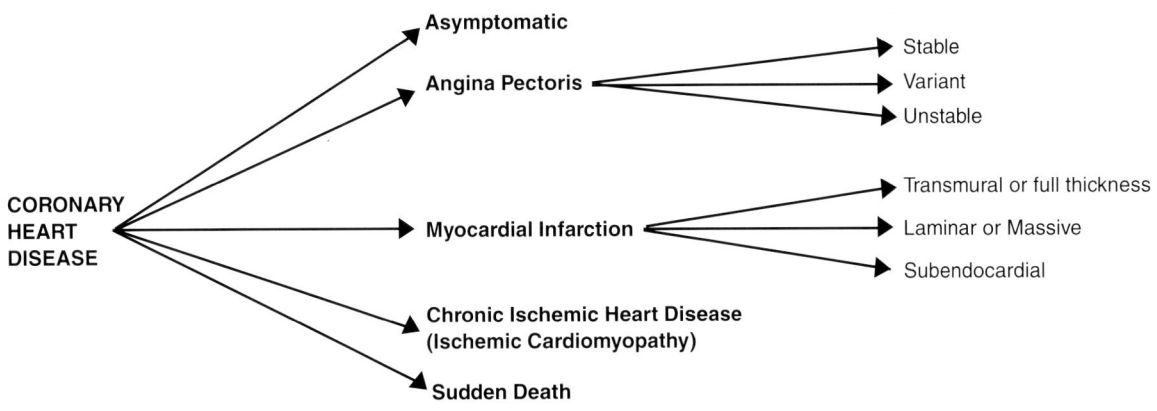

Fig. 6.1: Clinical spectrum of coronary heart disease

74 Illustrated Textbook of Cardiovascular Pathology

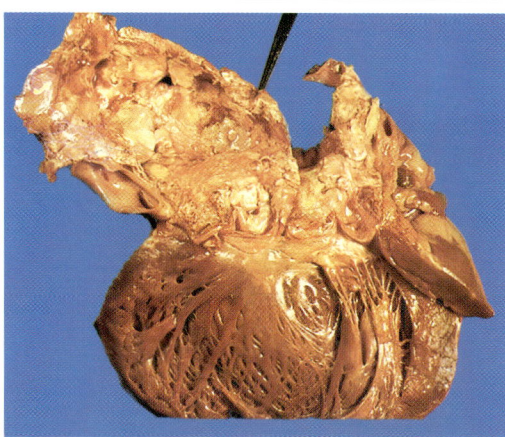

Fig. 6.2: Acute myocardial infarction. The myocardium of the posterior and anterior wall of the left ventricle is diffusely congested. The left ventricle is markedly dilated and the wall is thinned. Ascending aorta shows ulcerated atheromatous plaques which extend to the root of aorta

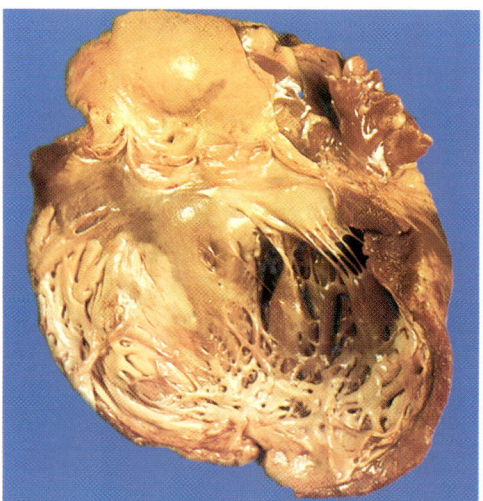

Fig. 6.3: Fresh and old myocardial infarct of left ventricle. A large area of replacement fibrosis of the major part of the posterior wall of the left ventricle and the apex is observed. A dark red congested zone comprising necrotic papillary muscles that have undergone recent infarction are seen. Aorta is unremarkable

Note: The anterior descending branch of the left coronary artery showed atherosclerotic narrowing and an occlusive thrombus in the proximal segment. Microscopic examination of the myocardium revealed congestion and coagulative necrosis of the myofibers

Unstable angina refers to progressively increasing cardiac pain at rest which often is of prolonged duration. This type of angina has a great risk of developing myocardial infarction and therefore is also termed as **"preinfarction angina"**. **Rupture** of an **atheromatous plaque** with **thrombus** formation leads to occlusion of the lumen. Myocardial ischemia results which manifests as pain. The ischemia is generally short lived and therefore does not cause necrosis of the myocardium. Angiographic studies done in unstable angina have shown stenotic lesions in the coronary artery with irregular outlines (ruptured atheromatous plaque) with an intraluminal filling defect (thrombus) demonstrated in a large number of cases. If the occlusion is complete and persistent, myocardial infarction will occur.

Acute myocardial infarction is ischemic necrosis of cardiac myocytes due to lack or loss of blood supply to them.

Pathology

Myocardial infarct cannot be appreciated by the naked eye until about 8-12 hours of onset when the infarcted area may look pale or has a blotchy appearance due to both pallor and congestion (Figs 6.2 to 6.6). Between 18 to 72 hours the infarcted zone appears yellowish and acquires a hyperemic border. The necrotic area is soft and is slightly depressed below the surface of the viable myocardium between 3-10 days. There is progressive collagenization of the necrotic myocardium which is permanently replaced by scar tissue by 7 to 8 weeks (Table 6.1). The healed ischemic myocardium appears pale and is firm to feel (Figs 6.3 and 6.5 to 6.7).

Macroscopic recognition of myocardial infarction in the early stages (4-8 hours of onset of infarction) may be facilitated by staining with tetrazolium dyes-nitroblue tetrazolium (NBT) (Fig. 6.8a) or triphenyl tetrazolium chloride (TTC) (Fig. 6.8b). Due to its dehydrogenase content, the viable myocardium is capable of reducing these dyes to produce a blue (NBT) or red (TTC) color. Ischemic myocardium that has lost its dehydrogenases remains unstained. Staining of myocardium slices identifies distinct zones of ischemic and viable myocardium and thereby helps to delineate the morphology of the infarcts. In experimental studies, either of these

Ischemic Heart Disease

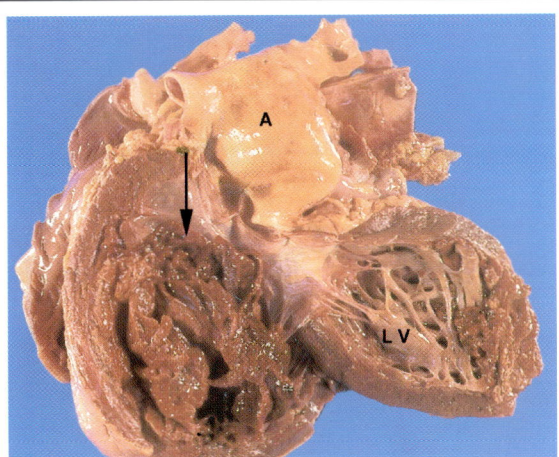

Fig. 6.4: Extensive fresh myocardial infarction involving the entire left ventricle (LV). The infarcted myocardium shows diffuse marked congestion. A large laminated thrombus is occupying the left ventricle cavity (arrow). A—aorta

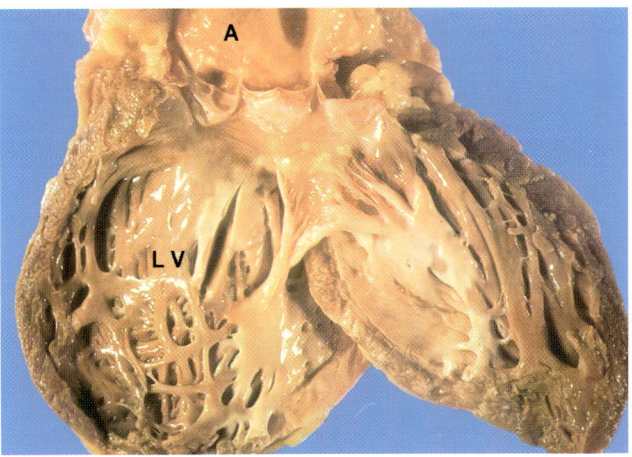

Fig. 6.5: Fresh and healed myocardial infarction of the anteroseptal wall of the left ventricle (LV). The healed infarct is evident by replacement fibrosis of the myocardium and thinning of the ventricle wall. In addition large area of fresh infarction manifest by diffuse congestion of the myocardium is seen. Left ventricle also shows hypertrophy and dilatation. Notice the thinning of the ventricle in the area of recent infarction. A—aorta

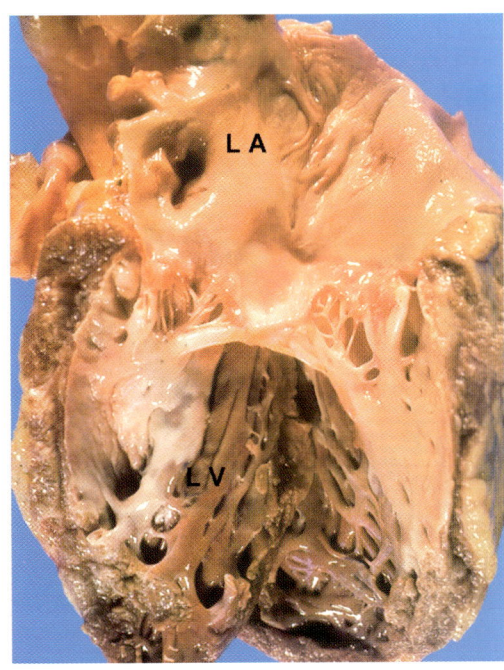

Fig. 6.6: Fresh and healed myocardial infarction of left ventricle. Extensive replacement fibrosis of the myocardium is observed. The chordae tendinea and the anterior and posterior papillary muscles are fibrosed and plastered together. The left ventricle wall is thinned out and streaks of fibrosis are seen within the muscle of the thinned ventricular wall. Additionally, the remaining part of the myocardium is markedly congested (fresh infarct). A fresh thrombus is seen at the apex. LA—Left atrium, LV—Left ventricle

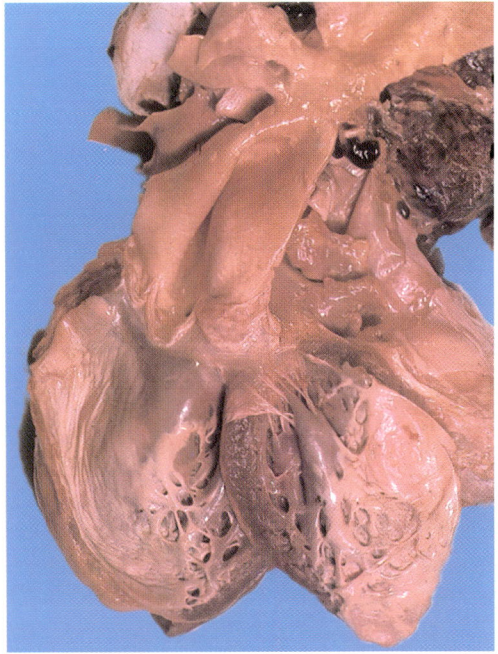

Fig. 6.7: Healed myocardial infarction left ventricle. Marked replacement fibrosis of myocardium evident as a coat of "white paint" is observed. The chordae tendinea, trabeculae carnea and part of the papillary muscle are fibrosed. Endocardium is thickened

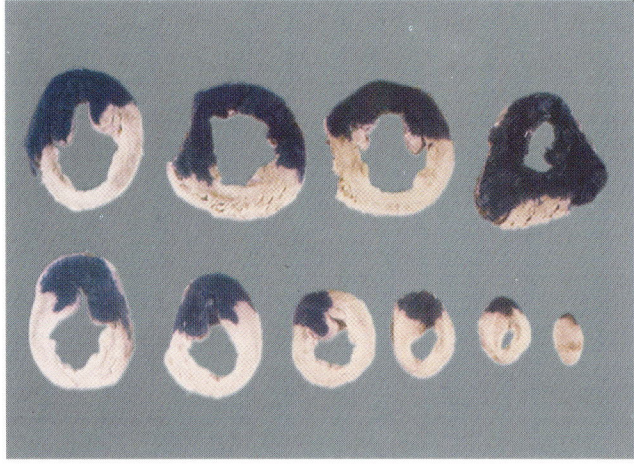
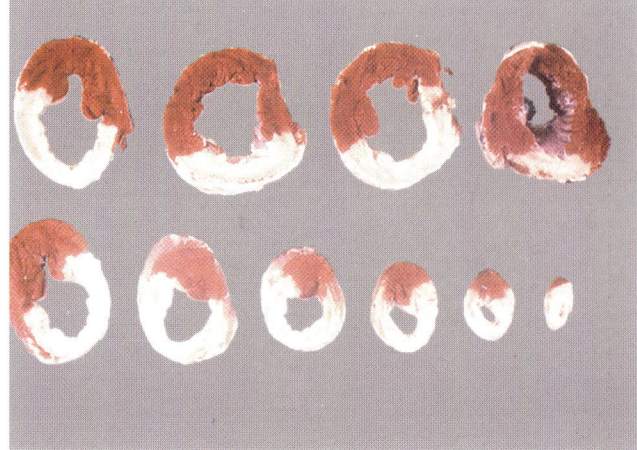

Figs 6.8a and b: Acute myocardial infarction produced in a rat by ligation of the anterior descending branch of the coronary artery. The myocardial slices were treated with (a) nitroblue tetrazolium (NBT) dye or with (b) triphenyl tetrazolium chloride (TTC). The viable myocardium stain blue and red respectively in contrast with pale pink ischemic zone

stains are commonly applied for quantitation of ischemic areas and assess the effect of various intervention modalities to salvage the myocardium at risk (Fig. 6.9).

Myocardial infarcts are commonly referred according to their **extent, location** and **duration**. Coronary artery occlusion leads to ischemic necrosis of the anatomic region of the myocardium supplied by the affected artery (**Regional infarction**). Since the anterior descending branch of the left coronary artery is most commonly diseased (narrowed), its corresponding area of supply namely anterior wall of left ventricle, anterior two thirds of interventricular septum and/or the apex undergoes ischemic necrosis. Regional infarction may be **transmural** or **full thickness** or **nontransmural (massive)** which does not involve the full thickness. Certain definitive features characterise transmural infarction. The entire infarct is generally of the same age and the culprit artery is usually occluded totally with a thrombus. Regional nontransmural myocardial infarction seems to be built up from foci of myocyte necrosis of differing age. This is generally a result of transient occlusive thrombosis of the artery with distal platelet emboli causing small foci of necrosis. **Subendocardial** or nonregional myocardial infarction is ischemic necrosis of the subendocardial region (inner third of the circumference of the left ventricle) and centers of the papillary muscles. The subendocardial region is least perfused and also has scant collaterals and is therefore prone to ischemia. In hypotension and/or shock this region becomes extremely vulnerable to necrosis. Unlike in transmural myocardial infarction, complete coronary artery occlusion is unusual.

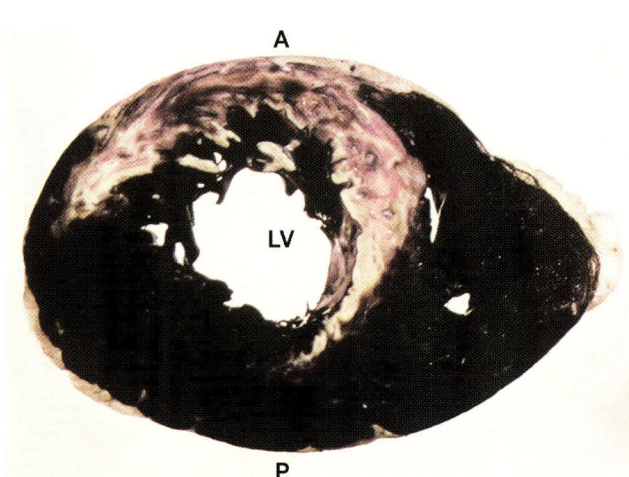

Fig. 6.9: Nitroblue tetrazolium reaction applied to a slice of the heart. The normal myocardium stains blue in color. An anteroseptal infarct of left ventricle is evident by the unstained area. LV—Left ventricle, A—Anterior, P—Posterior

Microscopic changes (Table 6.1) The earliest change described (0-2 hours) is stretching and waviness of the myofibers at the periphery of a myocardial infarct. At 4 to 12 hours **coagulative necrosis** of the myofibers occurs which is seen as homogenous and hypereosinophilic cytoplasm of the myofibers with loss of striations and clumped or pyknotic nuclei. In addition, edema, congestion and/or hemorrhage within the infarcted area is often observed. These changes progress and become well-marked in the following 24 hours. Nuclei undergo further clumping, karyorrhexis and

Table 6.1: Morphologic alterations in myocardial infarction

Time	Macroscopic changes	Light microscopy	Histochemistry	Ultrastructural changes
0-2 hours	Nil	Stretching/waviness of fibers in periphery of infarct.	Decrease in succinic dehydrogenase, phosphorylase, glycogen, oxidases, potassium (K). Increase in Na^+ and Ca^{++} and fat droplets.	Cellular and mitochondrial swelling; distortion of cristae, transverse tubular system and sarcoplasmic reticulum.
4-12 hours	Triphenyl tetrazolium chloride (TTC); Nitroblue tetrazolium (NBT) chloride: Viable muscle stains red or blue respectively. Dead muscle no staining.	Coagulative necrosis+; edema and/or hemorrhage in interstitium+. Neutrophils few.	—	Margination of nuclear chromatin.
18-24 hours	Pallor or blotchiness due to congestion; no softening of ischemic zone.	Coagulative necrosis +– ++ (Homogenous eosinophilic cytoplasm; nuclear changes —pyknosis, karyorrhexis, karyolysis). Edema and hemorrhage +–++; Neutrophils +–++; Lysis of muscle. Contraction band necrosis at periphery of infarct.	—	—
24-72 hours	Pallor+; Hyperemia+; Irregular border of infarct.	Necrosis+++ Loss of nuclei (Karyolysis) Neutrophils+++ Nuclear debris++	—	—
3-7 days	Hyperemic border++. Central yellow brown softening.	Resorption of dead muscle; Macrophages+++ Neutrophils+	—	—
10 days	Center increased softening. Red brown margin.	Reparative tissue (numerous capillaries, fibroblasts), chronic inflammatory cells and hemosiderin pigment (free and within macrophages).	—	—
7 weeks	Scarring. Necrotic area appears pale white and is firm to feel.	Necrotic muscle replaced by hyalinization, scarring.	—	—

karyolysis. The myofibers show degeneration and lysis and there is congestion of capillaries with margination by polymorphonuclear leucocytes, which are also seen in the interstitium of the myocardium (Figs 6.10 to 6.14). The necrotic and inflammatory changes intensify progressively between 1-3 days at which time there is marked myonecrosis, loss of nuclei and an inflammatory cell infiltration predominated by polymorphs and abundant nuclear debris. At the end of first week,

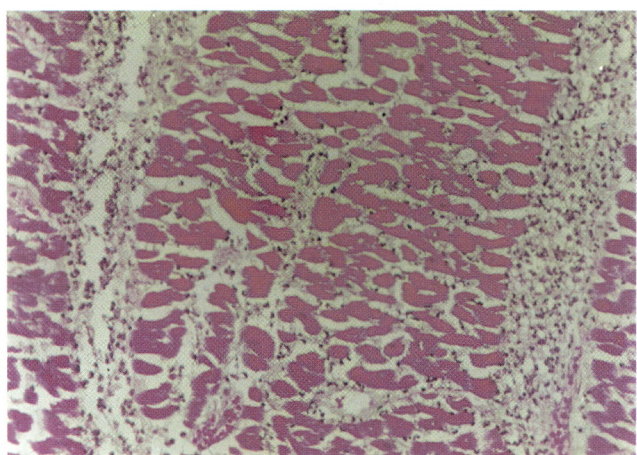

Fig. 6.10: Acute myocardial infarction. Necrotic and degenerated myofibers are present. The interstitium shows necrotic material, nuclear debris and polymorphs

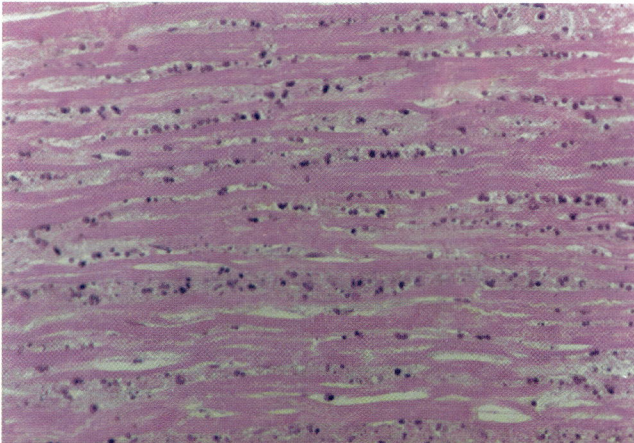

Fig. 6.11: Acute myocardial infarction. The myofibers are necrotic and show coagulative necrosis. Most of them have no nuclei. Interstitium is occupied by necrotic material, nuclear debris and degenerated polymorphs

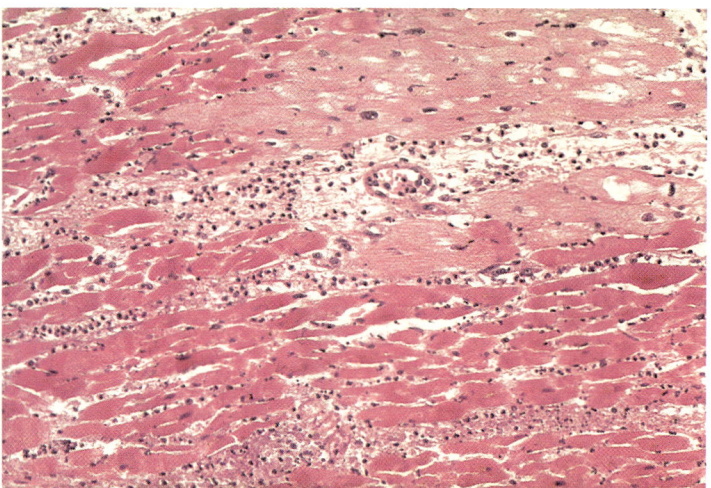

Fig. 6.12: Acute myocardial infarction. The interstitial tissue is widened by an inflammatory infiltrate comprising mostly of polymorphs. Edema and prominent congested capillaries are also present. The myofibers show homogenous light pink sarcoplasm (coagulative necrosis) with loss of striations and nuclei. A group of myofibers (lower part of picture) show hypertrophy and vacuolation of cytoplasm (ischemic change)

Ischemic Heart Disease

the ischemic area shows loss of myofibers and the inflammatory infiltrate is dominated by macrophages. Between 1 and 2 weeks of infarction, myofibers are cleared from the necrotic zone which now shows reparative tissue comprising proliferating capillaries, fibroblasts, hemosiderin pigment and macrophages many of which show hemosiderin within them. From 2 weeks till about 7-8 weeks there is progressive collagenization with scar formation (Figs 6.15 and 6.16).

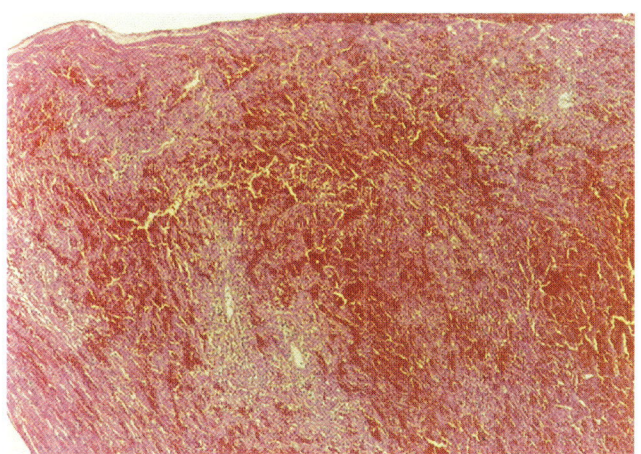

Fig. 6.13: Hemorrhagic myocardial infarction. Marked extravasation of red blood cells is seen in the interstitium of the myocardium

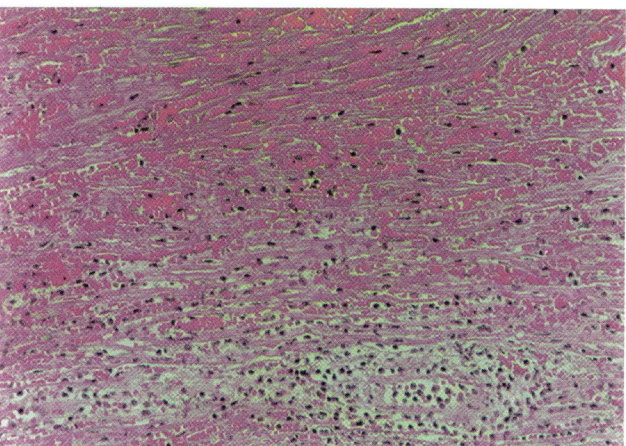

Fig. 6.14: Hemorrhagic myocardial infarction. Extensive fresh hemorrhage and extravasation of red blood cells is seen within the interstitium. Myofibers have homogenous pink cytoplasm with loss of striations and nuclei. Edema and inflammatory cell infiltration chiefly polymorphs are seen in lower third of the photograph

Note: This was a 2 days old full-term baby who had respiratory distress and cyanosis since birth. The baby was a forceps delivery. Possible factors causing hemorrhagic myocardial infarction include prematurity, hypoxia and perinatal sepsis. Hemorrhagic infarction is characteristically seen in reperfusion injury

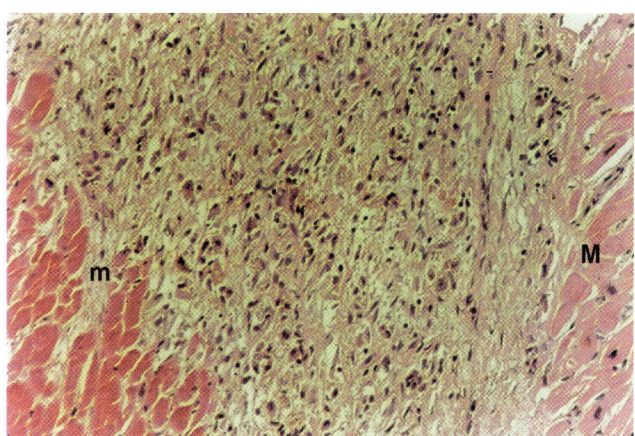

Fig. 6.15: Healing/resolving myocardial infarction. Viable myofibers (M) are seen on right side of picture. Necrotic hyalinized myofibers lacking nuclei (m) are seen on left of photograph. Healing infarct shows replacement of myofibers, few lymphocytes, fibroblasts and numerous histiocytes

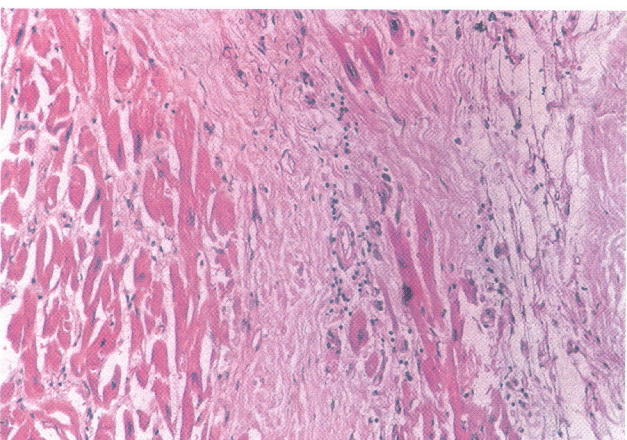

Fig. 6.16: Healed myocardial infarct. Replacement fibrosis of the myocardium with few trapped myofibers and mild chronic inflammation is seen

Besides the typical **coagulative necrosis** which is pathognomonic of acute myocardial infarction, another type of ischemic change known as **colliquative necrosis or myocytolysis** can be seen in ischemic myocardium (Figs 6.17a and b). This change is seen in the myocytes in the subendocardium. These cells though viable suffer chronic ischemia. The cells appear large, vacuolated with intact nuclei. Ultrastructurally loss of myofibers is the predominant change. This change represents hibernation of myocardium which can resume function on appropriate reperfusion. **Contraction band necrosis** occurs in reperfusion injury (described later).

Biochemical changes in myocardial ischemia Biochemical changes can be demonstrated within minutes of onset of ischemia. There is depletion of glycogen stores, progressive decline in high energy phosphate stores and mitochondrial functions, accumulation of lactates and activation of intracellular enzymes such as phospholipases and various lysosomal enzymes.

Etiology and pathogenesis of ischemic heart disease Diseases of the coronary artery which cause either incomplete or complete obstruction of its lumen can cause myocardial ischemia (Table 6.2).

Table 6.2: Causes of coronary heart disease

- Atherosclerosis (over 90% cases)
- Inflammatory diseases of coronary artery
  - Infectious
  - Noninfectious
- Infectious—Bacterial, fungal, tuberculosis, syphilis.
- Noninfectious—Polyarteritis nodosa, thromboangiitis obliterans, Kawasaki disease, rheumatic arteritis, systemic lupus erythematosus
- Embolism
- Thrombotic disorders
- Aneurysms
- Congenital anomalies
- Coronary artery spasm
- Neoplasms
- Trauma
- Conditions that cause increased myocardial oxygen demands (hypertension, valvular heart disease, hyperthyroidism).
- Hemodynamic derangements (shock, massive hemorrhage, anemia).
- Oral contraceptives
- Myocardial infarction with normal coronary vessels.

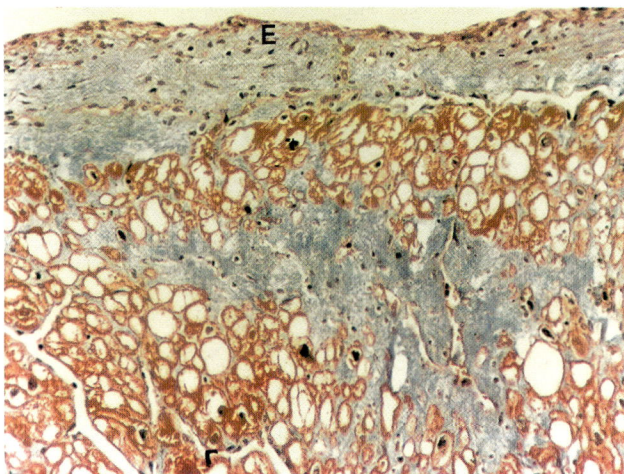

Fig. 6.17a: Ischemic heart disease. Subendocardial (E) myofibers show vacuolar degeneration of myocytes. Focal replacement fibrosis is also seen. Masson Trichrome stain

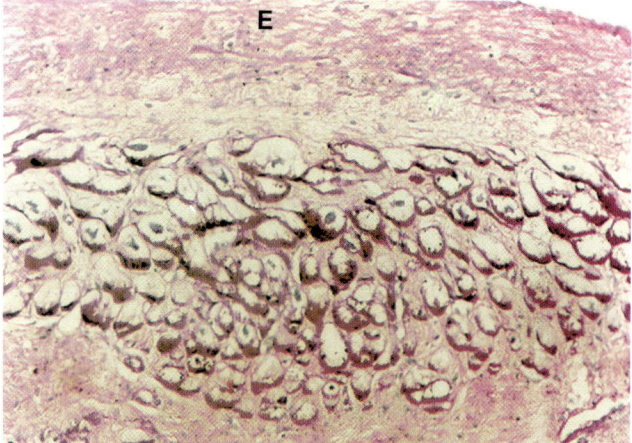

Fig. 6.17b: Ischemic heart disease. Periodic acid Schiff reaction to demonstrate glycogen within the vacuolated myocytes. This was resistant to diastase. E—Endocardium

Note: This change seen in the myocytes in the subendocardium is also termed as colliquative necrosis or myocytolysis and represents chronic ischemia. The myofibers, however, are viable and can resume function

Ischemic Heart Disease

The most common cause in over 90% of the cases is **atherosclerosis** (Figs 6.18 to 6.20). In almost all cases the single most important event leading to myocardial infarction is **rupture** of an **atheromatous plaque** with **coronary thrombosis** (Figs 6.21 and 6.22).

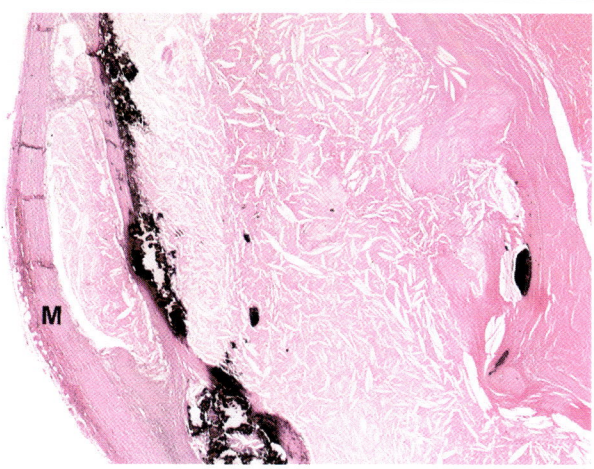

Fig. 6.20: Large calcified atheromatous plaque protruding into and compromising the lumen of the coronary artery. Numerous cholesterol clefts are seen. Media (M) is thinned out

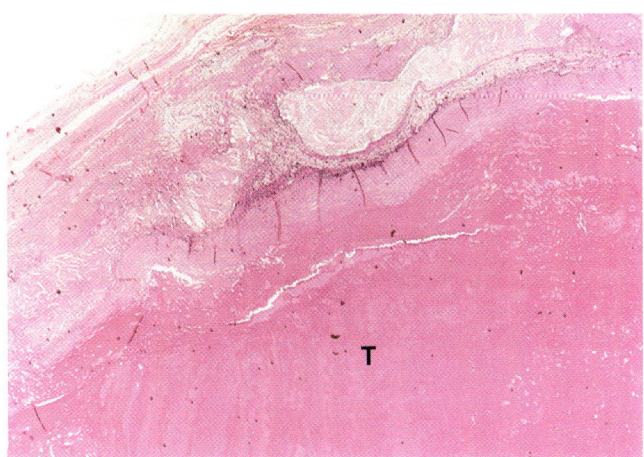

Fig. 6.18: Atheromatous plaque coronary artery. Foam cells and cholesterol clefts are seen. An occluding fresh thrombus (T) is also present

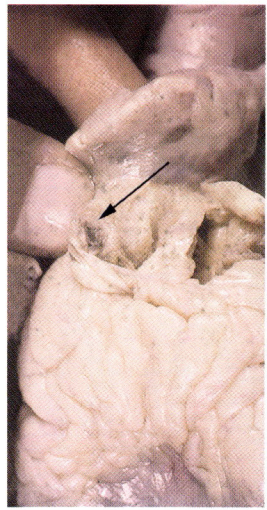

Fig. 6.21: Atherosclerotic narrowing of the coronary artery with an occlusive thrombus (arrow)

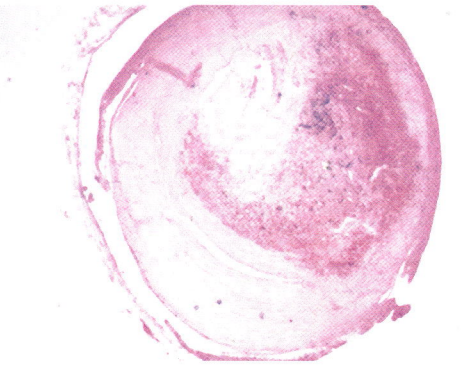

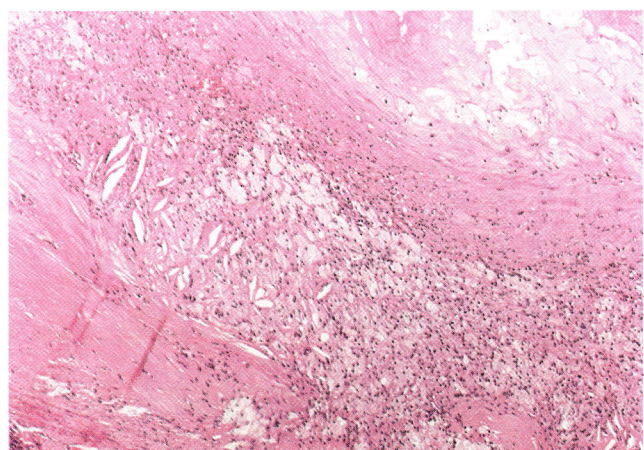

Fig. 6.19: Atheromatous plaque coronary artery. Notice the numerous foam cells and cholesterol clefts within the plaque

Fig. 6.22: Cross section of coronary artery which shows near total occlusion by fibrous plaque (atherosclerosis). Extensive fresh hemorrhage is seen

It has been demonstrated clearly by meticulous reconstruction studies of affected coronary artery lesions in cases of myocardial infarction that various events in an atheromatous plaque lead to coronary artery occlusion. **Fissuring, ulceration** and **rupture** of the **atheromatous plaque** have been clearly demonstrated in a vast majority of cases. Deep intimal injury generally occurs along with fissures and ulcerations of the plaque. The blood from the arterial lumen gushes into the intima where platelets and other elements interact with the exposed collagen leading to thrombus formation within the intima thus causing increase in plaque size. Latter further reduces the blood flow thus favoring intraluminal occlusive thrombus which is rich in fibrin and is susceptible to lysis both natural or pharmacologically induced. The culprit coronary artery is thus totally occluded by a thrombus which is superimposed on a ruptured atheromatous plaque. Coronary angiographic studies done within the first few hours of onset of acute myocardial infarction revealed total occlusion of the artery in about 90% of cases. This figure declined progressively with increasing duration of symptoms thus indicating spontaneous thrombolysis. These observations have revolutionized the management of acute MI and is the basis of aggressive thrombolytic therapy in early acute MI with an aim to salvage the myocardium at risk for better survival of these patients. Minimal injury to the endothelium and/or exposure of the subendothelial collagen leads to platelet adhesion, aggregation and activation. Latter causes release of several vasoactive substances namely histamine, serotonin, and thromboxane which cause vasospasm. Vasospasm is one of the important contributors to ulceration of an atheromatous plaque. Eccentric atheromatous plaque will have a portion of the normal vessel wall which can undergo spasm following vasoconstrictive stimuli.

Much importance has been given to the **plaque type** rather than the **plaque size** in the clinical presentation of coronary atherosclerosis. **Stable plaques** encroach upon the lumen to cause narrowing and may result in stable angina pectoris. The **vulnerable or unstable plaques,** however, are prone to rupture which in turn promotes thrombosis. **Unstability** of the atheromatous plaque seems to be contributed by the core lipid content and the extent of area occupied by it, differing degrees of stiffness between the fibrous cap and the adjacent intima and increased macrophages within the plaque. In addition to various other factors, macrophages also release proteases that can aid in plaque disruption. The size of the thrombus, its location (intramural or luminal) and duration of occlusion result in the various **acute coronary syndromes**. Thus plaque rupture with a labile thrombus which causes transient occlusion may result in unstable angina whereas a large occlusive thrombus may lead to myocardial infarction.

Rarely, myocardial ischemia can be caused by lesions other than atherosclerosis. These conditions are indicated in Table 6.2. In some cases of myocardial infarction coronary arteries are normal and no coronary artery disease can be demonstrated. This group of patients are usually young, often cigaret smokers and may lack the usual factors of atherosclerosis. Vasospasm may play an important role in the causation of myocardial infarction in these patients.

Salvage of ischemic myocardium Occlusive coronary artery thrombosis has been demonstrated in the vast majority of cases of acute myocardial infarction. The aim of management of acute myocardial infarction within the first few hours of its onset is to dissolve the occlusive thrombus in the coronary artery. This is achieved by the use of thrombolytic agents such as streptokinase or tissue plasminogen activator that not only provide reperfusion but also help to salvage the dependent area of myocardium which otherwise would progress to irreversible damage (ischemic necrosis). The rationale of therapy for reperfusion and myocardium salvage have been provided by the elegant experimental observations following ligation of the coronary artery. Injury to myocardium about 15-20 minutes after occlusion is such that if adequate reperfusion is established the changes are completely reversible. The subendocardial region is most susceptible to ischemia. A "wave front" of ischemic necrosis beginning from the subendocardial zone progressively extends to involve the entire width of the myocardium, the subepicardium region being the last to be affected as it is least susceptible to ischemia. The latter region has a rich

Ischemic Heart Disease

network of collaterals which are sparse in the subendocardium. If reperfusion is carried out early enough, the progression of cell necrosis can be checked. Beyond the critical time period, however, reperfusion, or any other intervention does not allow recovery as irreversible changes set in.

Reperfusion injury Reperfusion of ischemic myocardium is done by instilling various thrombolytic agents in the culprit artery. Balloon dilatation of the narrowed coronary arteries also leads to reperfusion (Figs 6.23a, b and 6.24a, b). Ironically, while aggressive measures to induce reperfusion

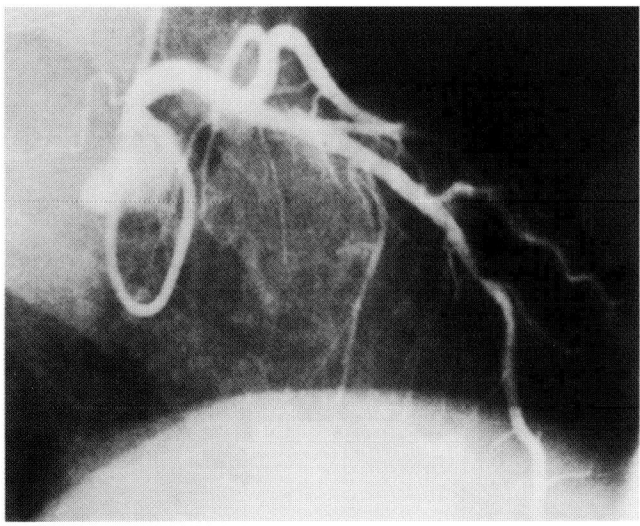
A

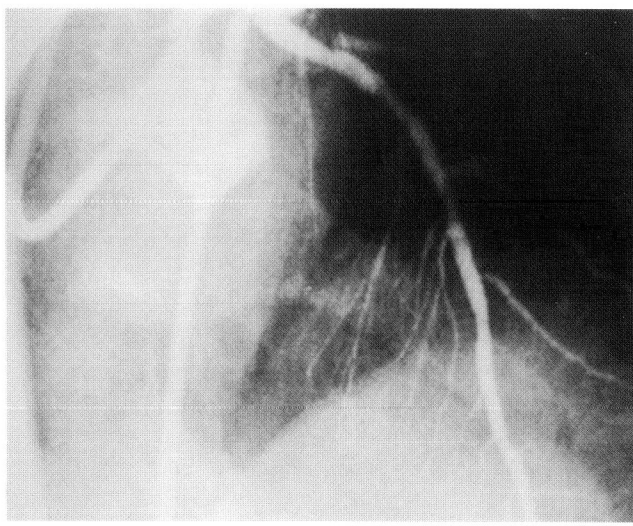
B

Figs 6.23a and b: Cineframe of (a) left anterior descending (LAD) branch of left coronary artery in right anterior oblique with cranial tilt showing tight narrowing (> 80%) in distal LAD and (b) after balloon dilatation the lesion is well-opened

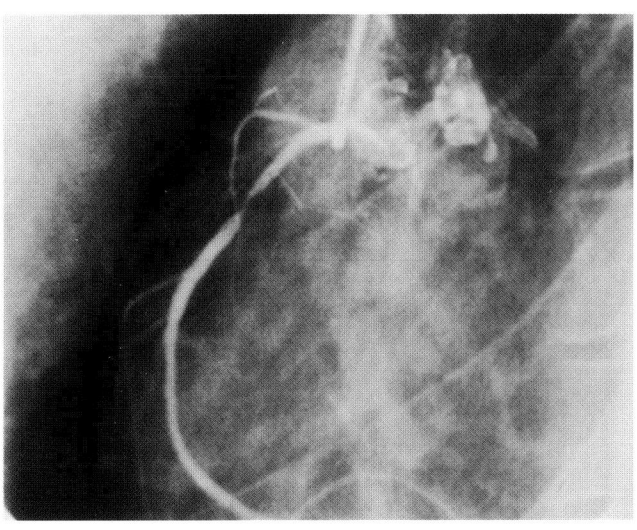
A

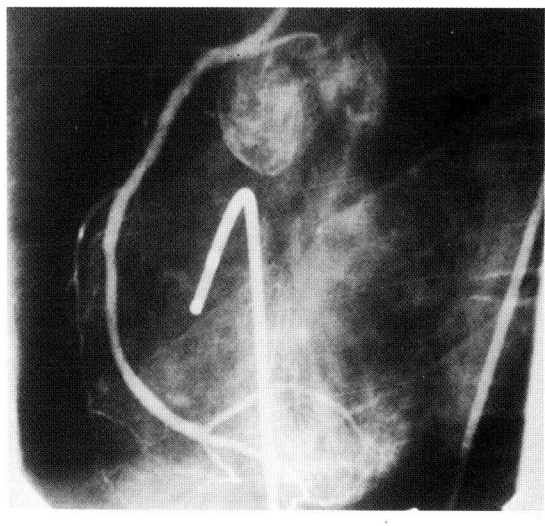
B

Figs 6.24a and b: Selective right coronary artery angiogram in left anterior oblique (LAO), (a) showing tight narrowing of the artery at the origin of sinus nodal branch, and (b) after balloon dilatation right coronary artery in LAO shows good opening of the lesion

have been devised to minimize cell death consequent to coronary artery occlusion, reperfusion can also accelerate necrosis of ischemic myofibers. Following reperfusion the myocytes undergo swelling due to water logging. Calcium ions enter the cell and cause **contraction band necrosis**, disruption of cell membrane and extrusion of mitochondria. Thus, myocardial reperfusion has been likened to a "double edged sword" in that, while on one hand its beneficial effect is undisputed, on the other hand, there is definite evidence of reperfusion induced myonecrosis. Latter is believed to be due to the effect of rapid influx of Ca^{++} and oxygen derived free radicals during reflow of blood. Reperfusion also leads to enhanced production of free radicals which cause cellular damage. Damage to the microvasculature leads to occlusion of the lumen by endothelial swelling and red blood cells. Endothelial damage leads to interstitial hemorrhage and edema.

Morphology of reperfusion injury Since thrombolytic therapy is the mainstay of management of acute myocardial infarction today, it is worthwhile to be aware of the morphologic changes associated with it. Myocardial infarcts consequent to reperfusion injury are invariably **hemorrhagic** possibly due to microvascular ischemic damage which allows extravasation of blood. The irreversibly damaged myocytes reveal **contraction band necrosis** which is due to coagulation of contractile proteins that is seen as transversely oriented, thick eosinophilic bands within myofibers indicating hypercontractile myofibers. This apperance is well-highlighted by phosphotungstic acid hematoxylin (PTAH) stain.

Other therapeutic interventions that can be applied to restore arterial blood flow include (1) Percutaneous transluminal angioplasty; (2) Coronary artery stenting; (3) Coronary artery bypass grafting and (4) Transmyocardial laser and transvascular revascularization.

Diagnosis of myocardial infarction rests on a combination of features such as clinical history, electrocardiographic changes and serial estimation of certain enzymes in the serum (serum cardiac markers). Irreversibly damaged myocardial cells release certain proteins into the circulation which can be estimated. Detection of serum enzymes are extensively used in the diagnosis, clinical monitoring and course of myocardial infarction. The various enzymes that may be estimated are creatinine phosphokinase (CPK), lactic dehydrogenase (LDH) and aspartate aminotransferase (AST). The most frequently estimated enzymes in the laboratory diagnosis of acute myocardial infarction are CPK and LDH. The other serum cardiac markers used to assess myocardial injury include myoglobin and cardiac specific Troponins (Table 6.3).

Table 6.3: Serum markers for diagnosis of acute myocardial Infarction

Markers	Time of			Limitations
	Initial elevation	Maximum activity	Return to normal	
CPKMB	4-8 hours	20-36 hours	3-4 days	Elevated in cardiac surgery, myocarditis, electric cardioversion.
LDH	6-12 hours	3-5 days	10-14 days	False-positive results in patients with liver and renal disease, hemolysis, myocarditis, skeletal muscle disease.
cTnI	4-6 hours	14 hours	7-10 days	—
cTnT	4-6 hours	12 hours-2 days	10-14 days	Elevated in chronic renal disease, skeletal muscle disease or trauma.
Myoglobin	1-3 hours	6-7 hours	24 hours	Elevated in skeletal muscle disease.

Creatinine phosphokinase (CPK) Following acute myocardial infarction, serum CPK rises within 4 to 8 hours, attains a peak at about 24 hours and declines to the normal range within 3 to 4 days of onset of myocardial infarction. Three isoenzymes of CPK have been identified by electrophoresis—MM, BB, and MB. Skeletal muscle contains predominantly MM isoenzyme while the BB isoenzyme is present in brain and kidney. Cardiac muscle contains mostly the MB isoenzyme although some quantities of MM isoenzyme is also present. Small quantities of MB isoenzyme can also be detected in tongue, diaphragm, small intestine, uterus and prostate. It is important to remember that false-positive results may be obtained in muscle diseases namely myopathies, muscular dystrophy, muscle trauma including intramuscular injections, cardiac catheterization, diabetes mellitus, alcohol intoxication, convulsions, etc. These factors need to be discounted when interpreting the values.

Lactic dehydrogenase (LDH) has five distinct isoenzymes, LDH-1 to LDH-5 of which LDH-1 is predominantly located in the myocardium. LDH-1 is elevated in myocardial infarction while LDH-2 is not increased. A LDH-1 to LDH-2 ratio of more than 1 is a good indicator of myocardial infarction. In sharp contrast with CPK, LDH rises later and falls to normal values much later. It rises within 10 to 24 hours attaining peak values at 3 to 5 days and returns to normal anywhere between 8 to 14 days after the onset of infarction. Other conditions in which elevated LDH levels may occur are in hemolysis, liver disease, renal disease, neoplasms, pulmonary embolism, myocarditis, skeletal muscle disease, etc.

Cardiac troponins Cardiac specific troponin T (cTNT) and cardiac specific troponin I (cTNI) are regulatory proteins which are complexed with the contractile apparatus. Increased levels of cardiac troponins in the serum serve as a useful marker for myocardial necrosis. They are more specific as they are not detectable in normal individuals and in skeletal muscle diseases. Additionally small myocardial infarcts which are not detected by CPK-MB estimation may be picked up by troponins. Levels of cTNT and cTNI may remain elevated for about 7-10 days and 10-14 days respectively after onset of myocardial infarction thus highlighting the importance of this test in patients who report 2-3 days after onset of myocardial infarction.

Other laboratory estimations in acute myocardial infarction include polymorphonuclear leucocytosis within the first 3-4 days of infarction, elevated erythrocyte sedimentation rate, hyperglycemia and myoglobinemia. Myoglobin, like the other enzymes, is released from the ischemic myocardial cells. Myoglobin rises early after the onset of infarction but the elevation is for a very brief period and is readily excreted in the urine. Due to these reasons it is of little diagnostic value.

The enzyme of choice to be estimated within the first few hours of infarction is CPK-MB. Serial estimations of CPK-MB in acute myocardial infarction (AMI) are useful not only in diagnosis of early AMI but may also detect reinfarction if the levels do not fall to normal or rise again in the course of hospital stay. In patients presenting 2 to 3 days after onset of symptoms of suspected myocardial infarction, troponins may provide diagnostic help due to the prolonged elevation of these proteins.

Complications of Myocardial Infarction (Fig. 6.25)

Cardiac arrhythmia is one of the most serious complication of acute AMI being present in some form or the other in 70 to 95% of hospitalized patients and accounts for mortality in over 50% of cases. These occur as ventricular tachycardia, ventricular premature beats and ventricular fibrillation indicating electrical instability; sinus tachycardia, atrial fibrillation and paroxysmal ventricular tachycardia due to pump failure and conduction disturbances manifested by sinus bradycardia and partial or complete heart block. **Left ventricular failure and cardiogenic shock** is generally associated with massive MI resulting in substantial loss of contractile myocardium which causes pump failure or cardiogenic shock. **Myocardial rupture** occurs early in the course of acute transmural MI. The most vulnerable period is within the first 2 weeks particularly within 24-72 hours of onset when the necrotic myocardium is soft and friable.

86   Illustrated Textbook of Cardiovascular Pathology

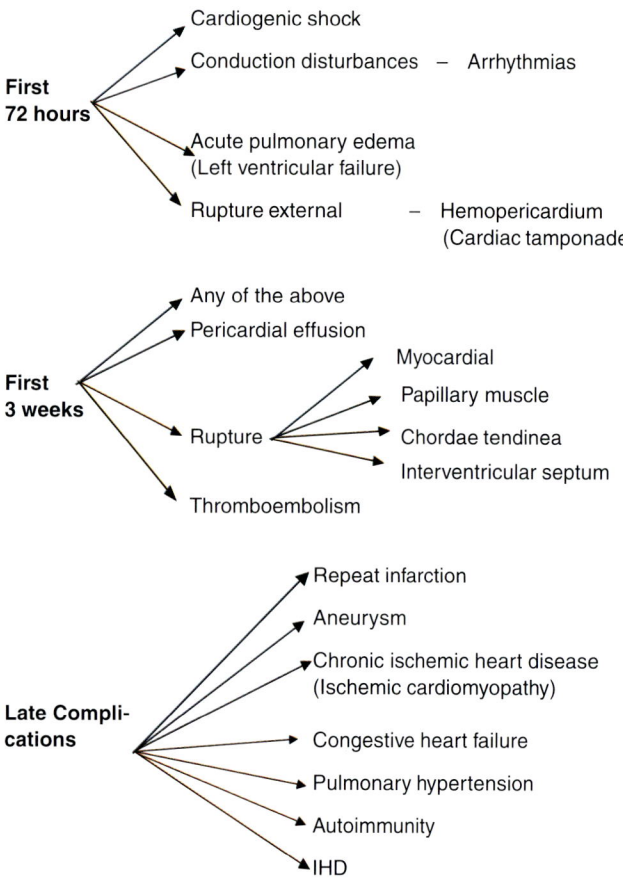

Fig. 6.25: Complications of myocardial infarction

Transmural myocardial infarction associated with hypertension is particularly prone to rupture. This may produce extensive bleeding into the pericardial cavity resulting in **cardiac tamponade** which is often fatal (Fig. 6.26). In a few patients, rupture of interventricular septum may produce features of a **ventricular septal defect** (Fig. 6.27). **Rupture** of the infarcted **papillary muscle** (Figs 6.28 and 6.29) may produce sudden massive **mitral regurgitation** resulting in pulmonary congestion, and **acute pulmonary edema**. **Mural thrombosis and thromboembolism** is a serious complication of MI. Mural thrombi are common in both acute and healed myocardial infarction (Figs 6.4 and 6.30). **Leg vein thrombosis** is a potential complication of bedrest and congestive heart failure which occurs commonly in MI. It also poses a great threat to **pulmonary embolism**. When a myocardial infarct heals the affected area becomes thinned and scarred due to loss of muscle mass. During cardiac systole this area does not contract with the rest of the myocardium but infact bulges out which over the years results **in aneurysm formation** (Figs 6.30 to 6.35). Latter provides for stasis of blood, **thrombosis** and a source of distant **embolism**. Fibrinous **pericarditis** may occur within the first few days of MI. This

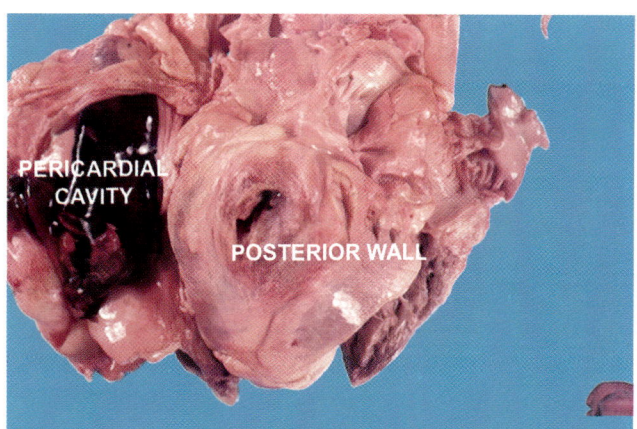

Fig. 6.26: Transmural acute myocardial infarction. A large perforation in the infarcted posterior wall of the left ventricle which has resulted in a blood clot in the pericardial cavity (hemopericardium) is seen. Clinically this caused cardiac tamponade

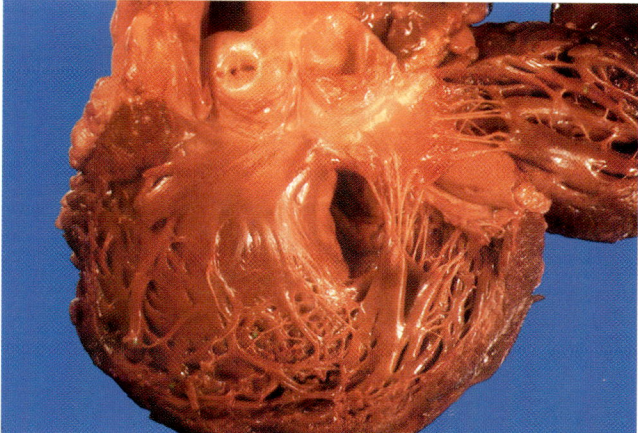

Fig. 6.27: Acute myocardial infarction of interventricular septum causing an internal perforation resulting in features of a ventricular septal defect

Ischemic Heart Disease

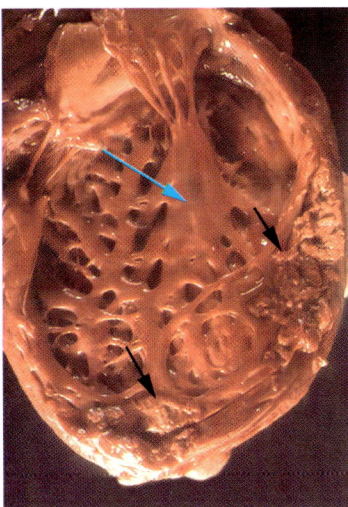

Fig. 6.28: Fresh myocardial infarction of the papillary muscle (blue arrow). Large mural thrombus over the infarct area is seen (black arrows). Hypertrophy and dilatation causing thinning of the wall of the left ventricle is observed

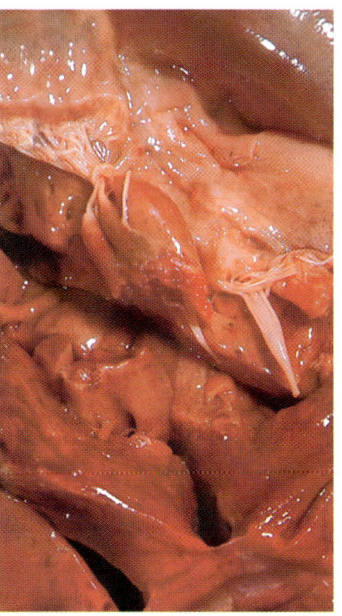

Fig. 6.29: Acute myocardial infarction. The left myocardium is uniformly congested and dark red in color. Rupture of posterior papillary muscle is seen. A few ruptured chordae tendinea are also observed

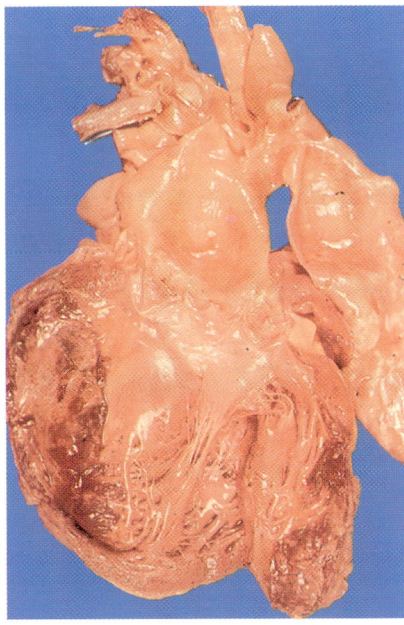

Fig. 6.30: Healed myocardial infarction of apex, septum and anterior wall of left ventricle. There is marked loss of left ventricle muscle with thinning of ventricle wall (aneurysm formation). A large mural thrombus is present

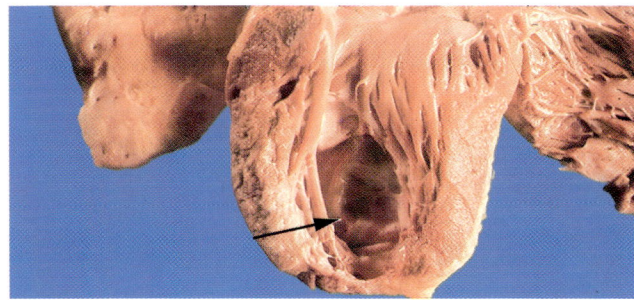

Fig. 6.31: Aneurysm apex of left ventricle consequent to healed myocardial infarction. Fibrosis of the left ventricular wall and the apical region is seen. The wall is thinned out in this area. An aneurysm is present at the apex and posterior wall of the left ventricle (arrow)

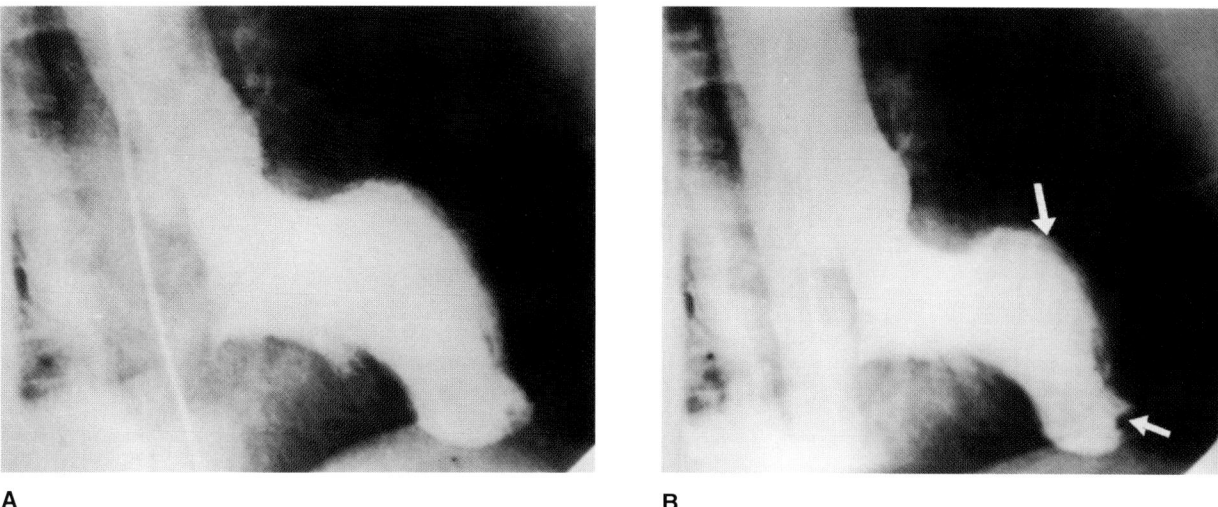

Figs 6.32a and b: Left ventricular angiogram in right anterior oblique. (a) Cineframe in diastole shows bulge on anterolateral border and apex. (b) Systolic frame shows diskinesia of apex (arrow) and anterolateral border (arrow) suggesting aneurysm of left ventricle involving apex and anterolateral border. There is a lucency in the apex suggesting thrombus

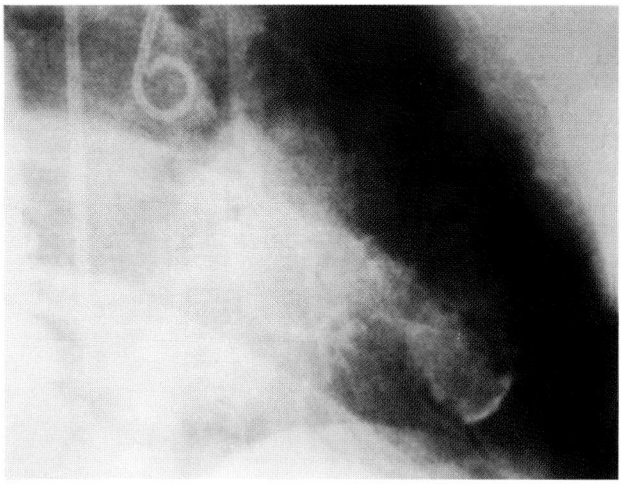

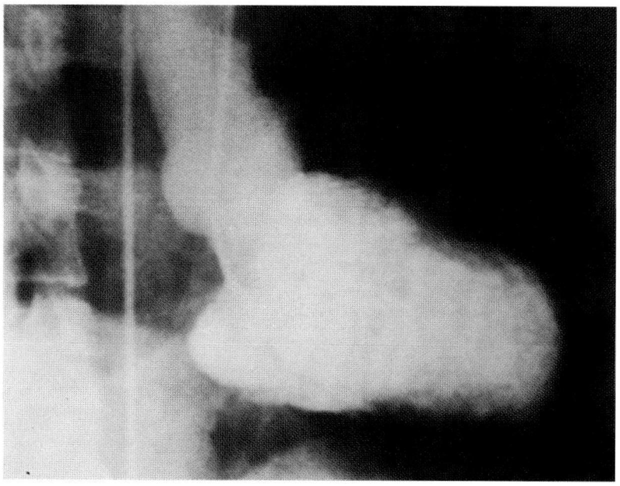

Figs 6.33a to c: (a) Cineframe without contrast shows calcification in the apex. Left ventricular angiogram in right anterior oblique diastole (b) and systole frame (c) showing left ventricular aneurysm involving apex

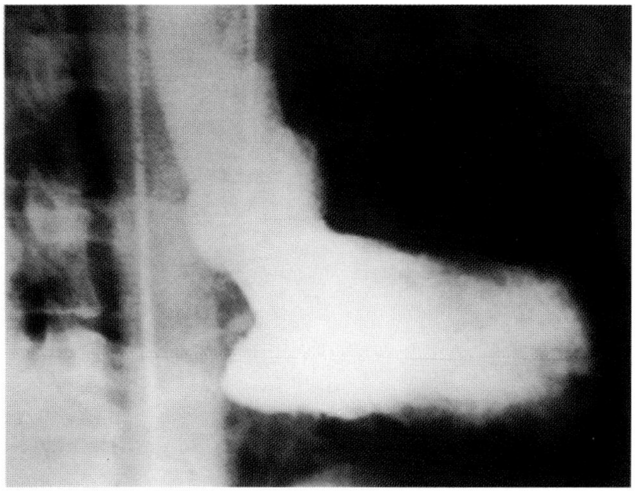

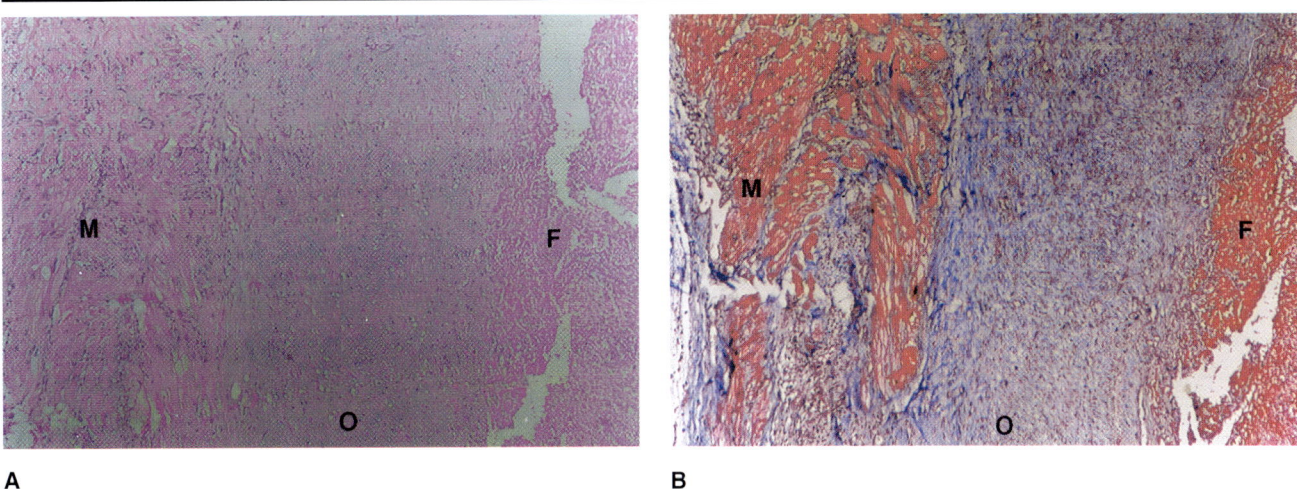

Figs 6.34a and b: Aneurysm of left ventricle (postmyocardial infarction). (a) The left ventricle muscle thickness is significantly reduced (M). Fresh (F) and organized (O) thrombus is present at the aneurysm site (b) Masson trichrome stain

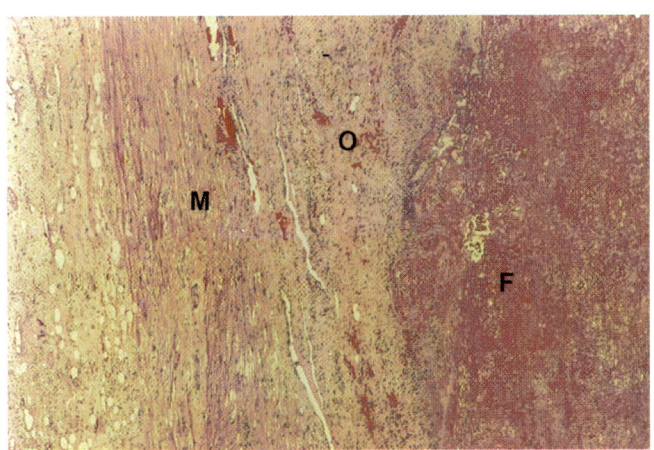

Fig. 6.35: Healed myocardial infarction with aneurysm formation of left ventricle. Muscle (M) of the latter chamber is much reduced. Fresh (F) and organized (O) thrombi occupy the aneurysm

reaction in the pericardium may correspond with an underlying area of myocardial necrosis. Rupture of transmural MI results in hemorrhage within the pericardial cavity. Occasionally pericarditis may develop any time between 2 weeks to 2 years after infarction. This has been termed as **postmyocardial infarction syndrome** (Dressler syndrome) which is characterized by fever, elevated ESR, pericarditis, pericardial effusion, pleurisy and pneumonitis. This condition is believed to be autoimmune in nature.

Chronic ischemic heart disease (ischemic cardiomyopathy) In some individuals with long standing IHD there is a progressive myofiber loss with fibrosis which results in severely impaired ventricular contractility manifesting clinically as dilated cardiomyopathy. The dominant clinical presentation is that of congestive heart failure rather than anginal pain. Generally a previous history of one or more episodes of MI is obtained due to which there is diffuse fibrosis and myocardial dysfunction. Morphologically, the heart may be either normal or increased in size and weight. Evidence of old healed infarcts is usually present. Variable areas of the myocardium reveal fibrosis/scarring. Diffuse, severe coronary atherosclerosis with or without total occlusion is present in almost all cases. Microscopically large area of the myocardium show replacement fibrosis and scarring.

Sudden cardiac death (SCD) One of the major consequences of atherosclerotic coronary heart disease is sudden cardiac death. It may be the first and at times the last manifestation of IHD. It is defined as either instantaneous death without any preceeding symptoms or death occurring within minutes to hours and according to some workers 24 hours after onset of the symptoms. The most common anatomical finding in SCD is coronary atherosclerosis. The mechanism of SCD in most cases is believed to be due to cardiac arrhythmias especially ventricular fibrillation.

SUGGESTED READING

1. Badimon L: The cellular and molecular bases of the acute coronary syndrome. *Rev Clin Esp* 196 (4 Monografico): 3-5, 1996.
2. Chopra P, Sabharwal U: Histochemical and fluorescent techniques for detection of early myocardial ischemia following experimental coronary artery occlusion—A comparative and quantitative study. *Angiology* **39**: 132-40, 1988.
3. Chopra P, Sethi U, Gupta PK, Tandon HD: Coronary arterial occlusion—An autopsy study. *Acta Cardiologica* 38/3 No:3, 183-97, 1983.
4. Chopra P, Sethi U, Talwar JR, Gupta PK, Tandon HD: Pattern of coronary arterial anastomosis and circulation in postmortem angiographic studies of human heart. *Acta Cardiologica* **36**: 249-62, 1981.
5. Christenson RH, Azzazy HM: Biochemical markers of the acute coronary syndromes. *Clin Chem* **44(8 Pt)**: 1855-64, 1998.
6. Hojo Y, Shimada K: Role of cytokines in acute coronary syndrome. *Nipon Rinsho* **56(10)**: 2500-03, 1998.
7. Libby P, Ridker PM, Maseri A: Inflammation and atherosclerosis. *Circulation* **105**: 1135-43, 2002.
8. Libby P: Current concepts of the pathogenesis of acute coronary syndromes. *Circulation* **104(3)**: 365-72, 2001.
9. Logacheva IV, Leshchinskii LA, Zvorygin IA: Immunological characteristics of patients with acute coronary syndrome (unstable angina and myocardial infarction). *Klin Med Mosk* **77(4)**: 23-25, 1999.
10. Michael J Davies: Pathophysiology of acute coronary syndromes. *Indian Heart J* **52**: 473-79, 2000.
11. Muller Wieland D, Faust M, Kotzka J, Krone W: Mechanisms of plaque stabilization. *Herz* **24(1)**: 26-31, 1999.
12. Mulvihill NT, Foley JB: Inflammation and acute coronary syndromes. *Heart* **87(3)**: 201-04, 2002.
13. Peter L Weissberg: Atherogenesis: Current understanding of the causes of atheroma. *Indian Heart J* **52**: 467-72, 2000.
14. Rader DJ: Inflammatory markers of coronary risk *NEJM* 343/16: 1179-83, 2000.
15. Shah PK: Circulatory markers of inflammation for vascular risk prediction. Are they ready for time. *Circulation* **105**: 1758-59, 2000.
16. Shah PK: New insights into the pathogenesis and prevention of acute coronary syndromes. *Am J Cardiol* **26; 79 (12B)**: 17-23, 1997.
17. Takeshita S, Isshiki T, Ochiai M, Ishikawa T, Nishiyama Y, Fusano T, Toyoizumi H, Kondo K, Ono Y, Sato T: Systemic inflammatory responses in acute coronary syndrome: Increased activity observed in polymorphonuclear leukocytes but not T lymphocytes. *Atherosclerosis* **135(2)**: 187-92, 1997.
18. Yutani C, Imakita M, Ishibashi Ueda H, Tsukamoto Y, Nishida N, Ikeda Y: Coronary atherosclerosis and interventions: Pathological sequences and restenosis. *Pathol Int* **49(4)**: 273-90, 1999.

7 Endomyocardial Biopsy

Like the kidney and liver biopsies endomyocardial biopsy (EMB) has evolved as a safe procedure with minimal morbidity and mortality and is performed as a routine procedure. It is safe, easy, convenient and provides useful information in several cardiac disorders. The biopsy is performed via the transvascular approach and is done usually at the time of cardiac catheterization. It may also be done as an individual procedure. Sequential, multiple biopsies can be performed without any side effects. Both ventricles can be subject to the biopsy procedure, however, the right ventricle is preferred as it is easier and safer to biopsy this chamber. Also, right ventricular biopsy is representative of the heart in diseases that are diffuse in nature. Left ventricle biopsies are indicated in cases where the disease affects that chamber, e.g. left sided endomyocardial fibrosis, endocardial fibroelastosis, left sided heart failure greater than right heart failure, left heart radiation, etc.

Under fluoroscopic guidance the catheter is introduced into the right ventricle through the internal jugular vein. This chamber can also be approached through the femoral vein. The configuration of the right ventricular chamber is such that the biopsy forceps is approximated to the right ventricular septum close to the apex. Three to five pieces of the myocardial tissue are obtained as this amount of tissue is necessary to make an adequate interpretation. Tissue thus obtained can be used for evaluation by light and electron microscopy, immunofluorescence, immunohistochemistry, biochemical analyses, molecular studies, etc.

EMB is indicated in a variety of cardiac disorders, however, it is considered as the most useful tool for the diagnosis and monitoring of cardiac allograft rejection. Other important indications of EMB include detection of myocarditis, monitoring anthracycline cardiotoxicity, differentiation between restrictive and constrictive physiology, storage disorders, etc. (Table 7.1).

Table 7.1: Indications of endomyocardial biopsy

Cardiac allograft rejection
Anthracycline cardiotoxicity
Myocarditis (viral, giant cell, granulomatous, rheumatic and drug-induced)
Primary cardiomyopathies (dilated and hypertrophic cardiomyopathy, endomyocardial fibrosis, idiopathic restrictive cardiomyopathy)
Restrictive and constrictive heart disease
Specific heart muscle diseases such as amyloidosis, metabolic disorders (glycogen storage disease, Fabry's disease)
Idiopathic chest pain and arrhythmias
Intracavitary masses
Infections such as cytomegalovirus, toxoplasmosis, Chagas' disease and fungi

For routine light microscopy, three to five pieces of the myocardial tissue are collected in 10 percent neutral buffered formaline. After conventional processing, serial sections of 4-5 μ thickness are cut. It is important to keep in mind to cut the block at at least three levels as at times the lesion may emerge only on deeper sectioning. Spare unstained sections must be prepared and kept to allow for special stains when necessary. When systematically evaluated, a simple hematoxylin and eosin stain provides a wealth of information. However, it is useful to subject other sections to Masson trichrome to assess the degree and extent of fibrosis and myonecrosis. Staining for amyloid should be done in patients presenting with a restrictive/constrictive physiology.

Interpretation of EMB This is a challenging task and adequate precautions need to be taken during collection, processing and cutting of the tissue.

92 Illustrated Textbook of Cardiovascular Pathology

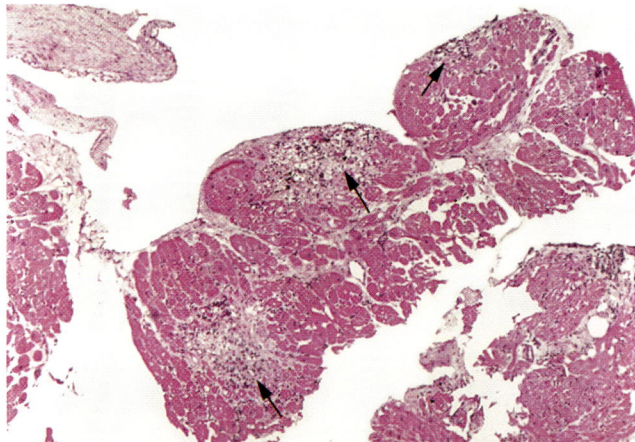

Fig. 7.1: Endomyocardial biopsy of a cardiac allograft. Multiple foci of ischemic injury (arrows) are seen

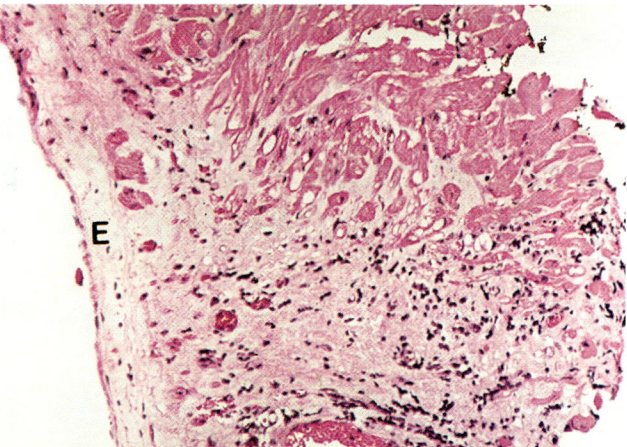

Fig. 7.2: Higher magnification of ischemic change in endomyocardial biopsy of a cardiac allograft. This focus is seen in the subendocardial zone (E). There is loss of myofibers, increased vascularity and infiltration by lymphocytes

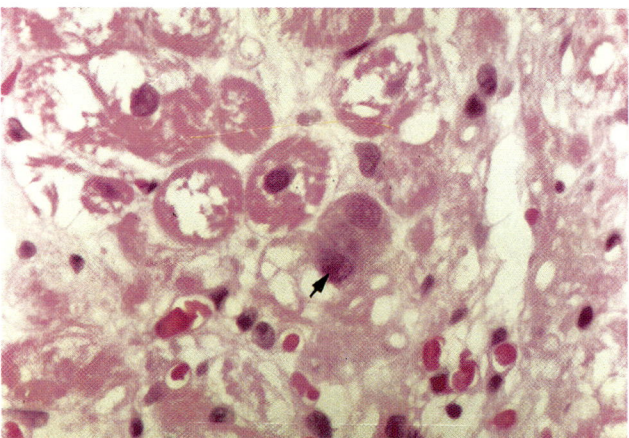

Fig. 7.3: Endomyocardial biopsy of a cardiac allograft. Deep pink eosinophilic intranuclear inclusion suggestive of cytomegalovirus is seen (arrow)

Careful handling of the biopsy tissue goes a long way in evaluation of the biopsy. A number of artefacts often accompany the procedure. The pathologist must be familiar with these as they may create problems during interpretation (Table 7.2). Awareness of artefacts in biopsy along with accumulated experience of reading biopsies can minimize errors of diagnosis. Detailed observations made systematically in relation to the myocardium, endocardium and interstitium provide useful information. Inflammation, its nature, extent and severity must be assessed carefully as reporting myocarditis is treated aggressively by some groups of workers. It needs to be emphasized that stringent criteria (Dallas criteria) must be applied for a diagnosis of myocarditis. Mere presence of some inflammatory cells should not be diagnosed as myocarditis. Inflammatory cell infiltration along with myonecrosis needs to be recognized.

Table 7.2: Problems during interpretation

Sampling error-biopsy may yield negative results due to focal nature of disease (e.g. myocarditis)
Crush artefacts (mechanical trauma)
Contraction bands (mechanical trauma, acute myocardial ischemia, catecholamine-induced injury)
Repeated sampling of same site in sequential biopsies
Myofiber disarray (seen in hypertrophic cardiomyopathy, normally present in right ventricular trabecular carnea and previous biopsy site).
Focal interstitial fibrosis (nonspecific finding; does not imply healed ischemia or myocarditis)
Interstitial mesenchymal cells closely simulate lymphocytes
Endocardial thickening (may be nonspecific; oblique sectioning)
Adipose tissue (normal in right ventricular biopsy)
Mesothelial cells indicate perforation

Important Conditions Diagnosed by Endomyocardial Biopsy

Cardiac transplant rejection Endomyocardial biopsy is considered as a gold standard for the diagnosis of cardiac allograft rejection. Repeated sequential biopsies are done to monitor rejection and other transplant related changes (Figs 7.1 to 7.3). A standard biopsy protocol has been recommended and is followed universally. Monitoring of antirejection therapy is based on the histomorphological findings in the biopsy. The grades of rejection are as per the International Society for Heart and Lung Transplantation.

Dilated cardiomyopathy and lymphocytic myocarditis Endomyocardial biopsy features of dilated cardiomyopathy (DCM) are of a nonspecific nature and the diagnosis is generally clinical. Histologic features include hypertrophy, attenuation (indicating stretching/dilatation), and degenerative changes of myofibers. Varying grades of interstitial fibrosis and inflammatory cell infiltration are observed in some cases (Figs 7.4 to 7.9). The main aim of performing EMB in DCM is to detect myocarditis (Figs 7.10 to 7.13). It is extremely important to make a definitive diagnosis of myocarditis as when present it is treated with immunosuppressive drugs by some centers.

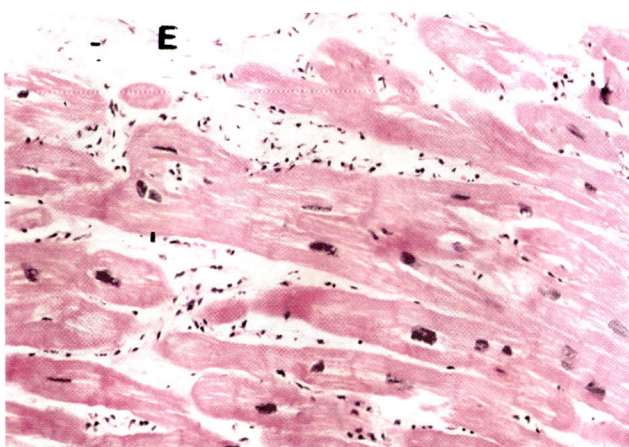

Fig. 7.4: Dilated cardiomyopathy. Prominent anisonucleosis is observed. Mesenchymal cells within the interstitium are striking (These are easily confused with inflammatory cells and a mistaken diagnosis of myocarditis may be given). No myocarditis is present. E—Endocardium

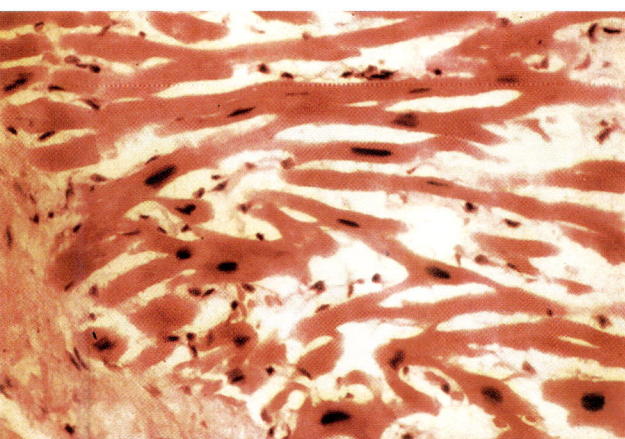

Fig. 7.5: Dilated cardiomyopathy. Marked attenuation of the myofibers is seen. Prominent anisonucleosis signifying myocardial hypertrophy can be appreciated

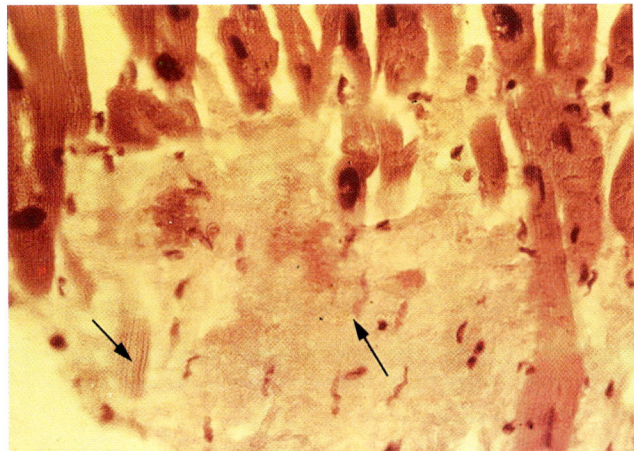

Fig. 7.6: Dilated cardiomyopathy. Large focus of myofiber loss is seen within which remnant degenerated myofibers are recognized (arrows)

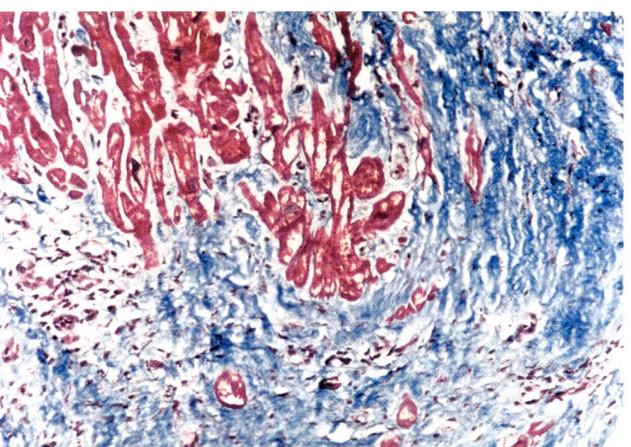

Fig. 7.7: Endomyocardial biopsy from a case of dilated cardiomyopathy. Marked fibrosis is seen. Myofibers show evidence of hypertrophy and degenerative changes. Masson trichrome stain

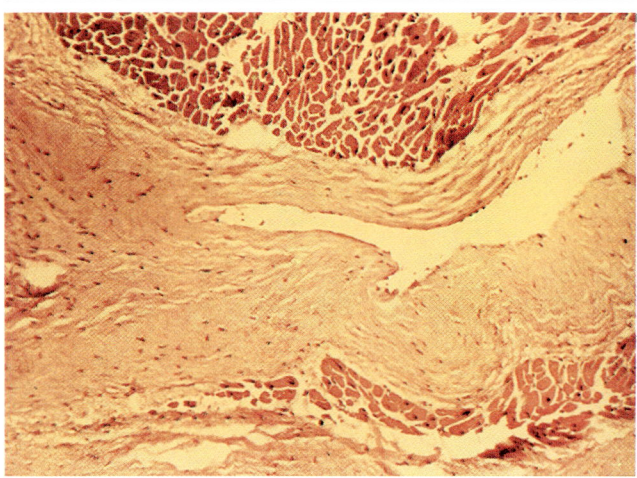

Fig. 7.8: Dilated cardiomyopathy. Photomicrograph shows fibrocollagenous thickening of the endocardium

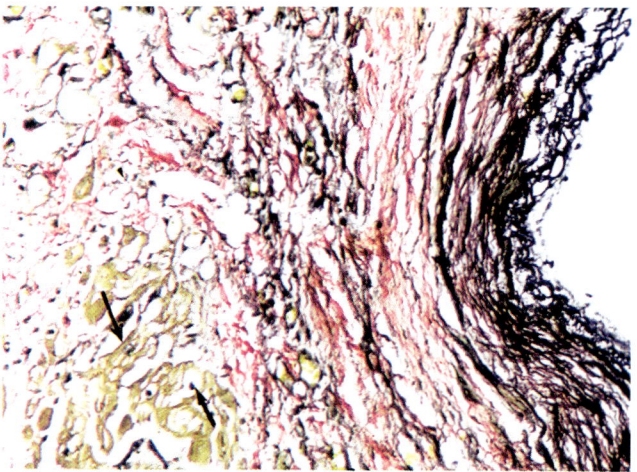

Fig. 7.9: Dilated cardiomyopathy. Endocardium shows thickening by elastic tissue which is arranged in closely packed lamellae. Marked vacuolation of myofibers is also noted (arrows). Elastic van Gieson stain

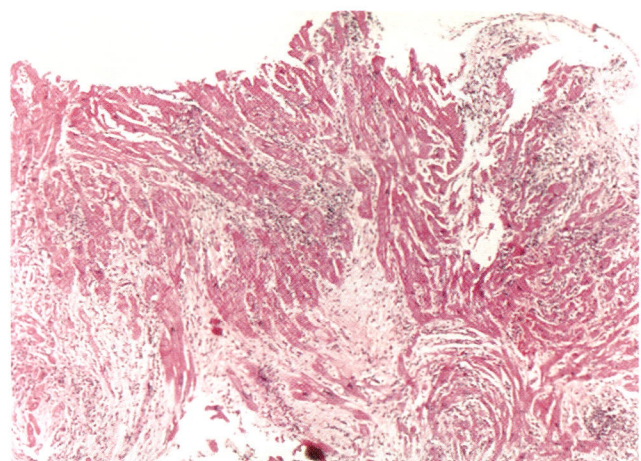

Fig. 7.10: Myocarditis. Endomyocardial biopsy from a case clinically diagnosed as dilated cardiomyopathy. Marked inflammation is seen within the interstitium of myocardium. Myofiber loss is also noted

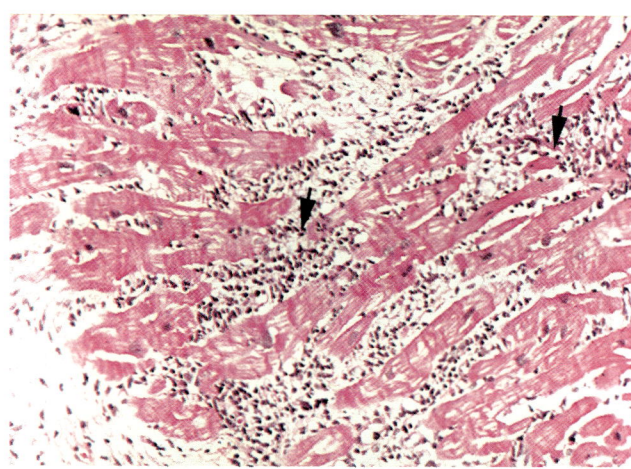

Fig. 7.11: Myocarditis. Higher magnifications of Fig. 7.10 to demonstrate marked lymphocytic myocarditis. Myofiber necrosis (arrows) can be appreciated

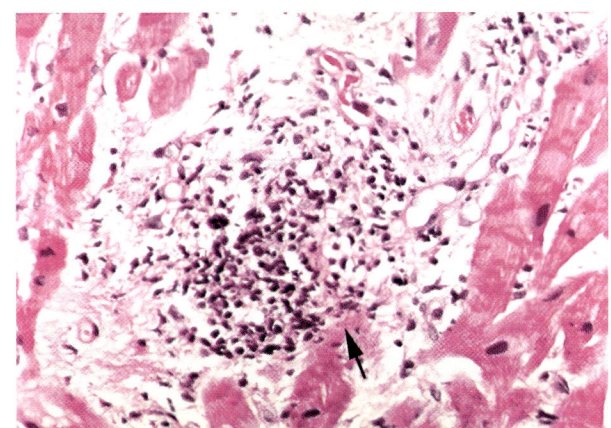

Fig. 7.12: Myocarditis. Another biopsy fragment shows a large focus of inflammatory infiltrate composed predominantly of lymphocytes. Degenerated/necrotic myofibers (arrow) are also present

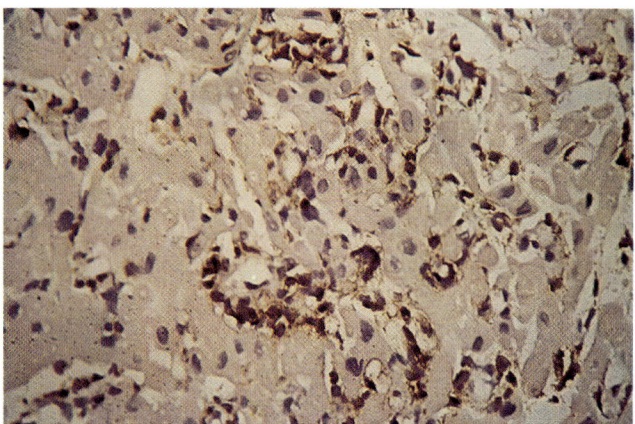

Fig. 7.13: Myocarditis. Antisera to leucocyte common antigen shows positive staining reaction of lymphomononuclear cells which are closely apposed to the myofibers

Note: The patient was a 12 years female child who presented with congestive heart failure. She was a case of diffuse non-specific aortoarteritis

To define myocarditis and its histopathologic criteria a group of eight pathologists met in Dallas Texas. The criteria have thus been designated as the Dallas criteria. The basic aim was to adopt uniformity and reproducibility for the diagnosis of myocarditis. It was recommended that myocarditis be defined as "a process characterized by an inflammatory infiltrate of the myocardium with necrosis and/or degeneration of the adjacent myocytes (Figs 7.10 to 7.13) not typical of ischemic damage (Figs 7.14 and 7.15) associated with coronary artery disease" biopsies. Recommendations for repeated and subsequent is outlined in Chapter 8 (page 108).

There is enough epidemiologic and laboratory data to suggest that myocarditis precedes dilated cardiomyopathy. The principal cause of myocarditis is viral infection importantly coxsackie B virus.

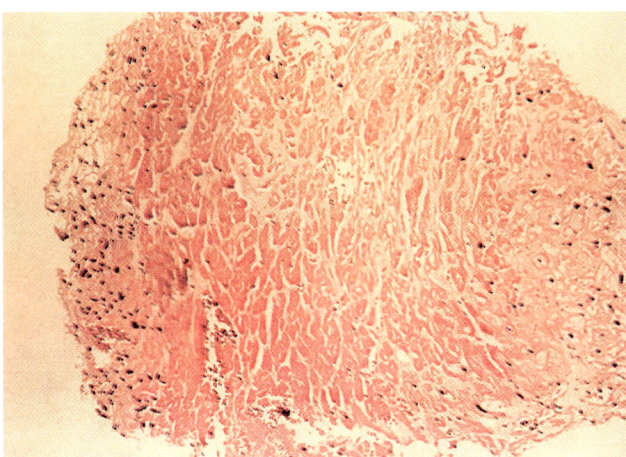

Fig. 7.14: Ischemic necrosis of myocardium. Endomyocardial biopsy from a case diagnosed as dilated cardiomyopathy. Myofibers in the center of the picture are nonviable evident as homogenous pink myofibers with loss of nuclei. The myofibers towards the periphery appear viable

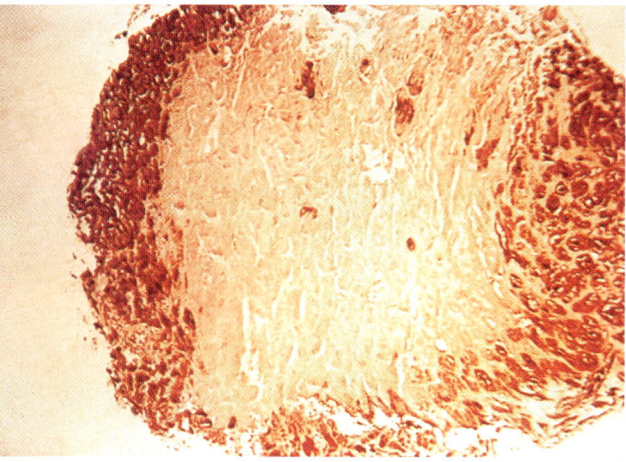

Fig. 7.15: Ischemic necrosis of myofibers to illustrate viable myofibers which stain dark brown with antimyosin antibody. Ischemic myofibers are unstained (Peroxidase-antiperoxidase)

Other enteroviruses like coxsackie A, ECHO and polio can also cause myocarditis. Other RNA viruses which cause myocarditis are influenza, rabies and ARBO viruses, paramyxoviruses, lymphocytic choriomeningitis virus, hepatitic C virus, etc. Certain DNA viruses which have been documented to cause myocarditis are adenovirus, cytomegalovirus, Epstein-Barr virus, vaccinia virus, variola virus, varicella zoster virus. Human immunodeficiency virus has also been shown to cause myocarditis/cardiomyopathy.

Molecular techniques such as *in situ* hybridization and polymerase chain reaction have been used successfully to detect virus specific nucleic acids in heart muscle. It has been demonstrated that myocardial enteroviral infection is detectable in all stages of acute and chronic myocarditis thereby suggesting a possible persistence of enteroviruses in the human heart.

Myocarditis other than lymphocytic myocarditis

a. *Giant cell myocarditis* Endomyocardial biopsy has proven of great value in some cases that present with clinical features of dilated cardiomyopathy. Histologically, myocyte necrosis is associated with a mixed inflammatory infiltrate comprised of lymphocytes, histiocytes, eosinophils and multinucleated giant cells (Figs 7.16a and b). Recognition and reporting of these changes relate to the management of such cases.

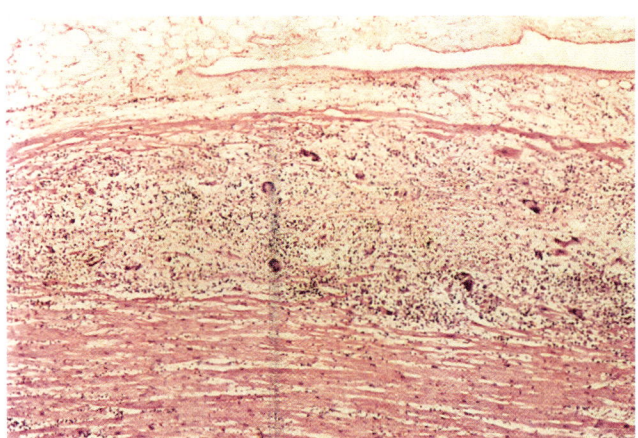

Fig. 7.16a: Giant cell myocarditis. Large area of the myocardium is replaced by an infiltrate of multinucleated giant cells and a mixed inflammatory cell infiltrate

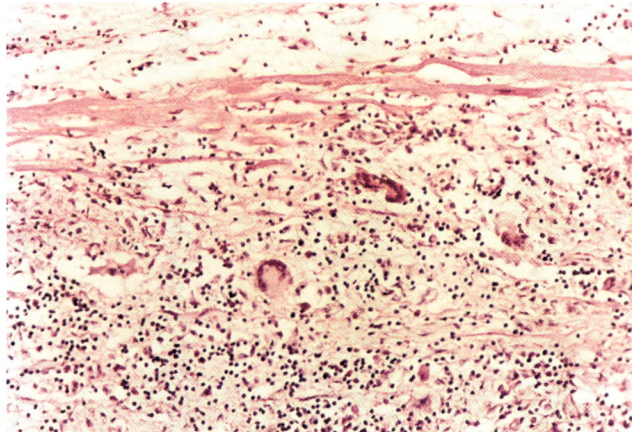

Fig. 7.16b: Giant cell myocarditis. Extensive myocarditis is present. Numerous multinucleated giant cells and a mixed inflammatory cell infiltrate abounding in lymphocytes is observed

b. *Granulomatous myocarditis* This lesion can be easily recognized in endomyocardial biopsy (Figs 7.17 to 7.21). The etiology of granulomatous myocarditis is variable and therefore careful evaluation of histological changes needs to be done for appropriate management.

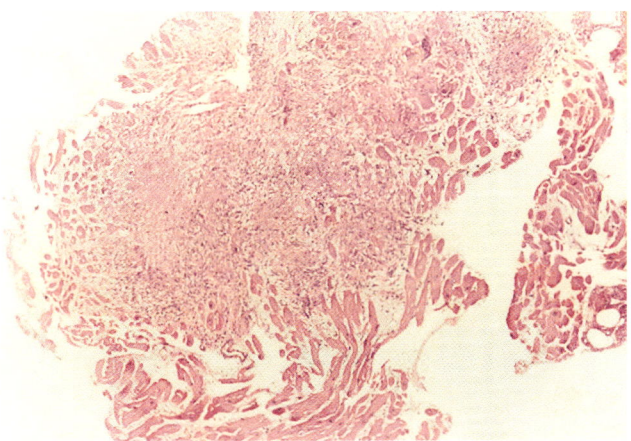

Fig. 7.17: Granulomatous inflammation of the myocardium with necrosis. Endomyocardial biopsy from a case with a clinical diagnosis of dilated cardiomyopathy. Marked destruction of myofibers and areas of necrosis are observed. These findings are suggestive of tuberculosis

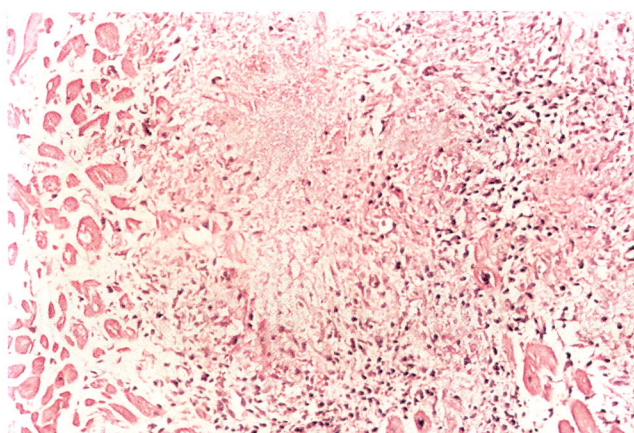

Fig. 7.18: Granulomatous myocarditis. Higher magnification of Figure 7.17 to demonstrate large areas of necrosis bordered by epithelioid cells

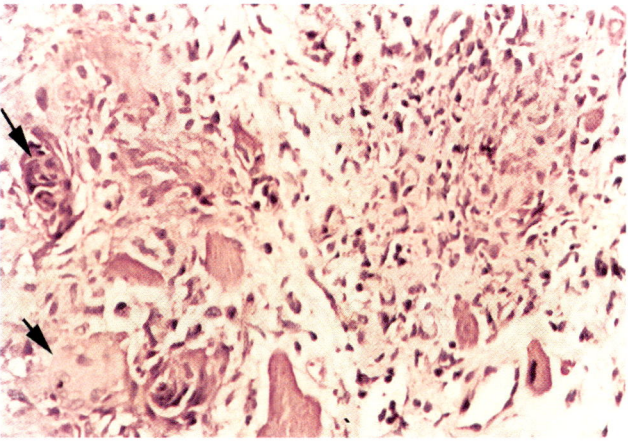

Fig. 7.19: Granulomatous myocarditis. Epithelioid cell granuloma is seen to replace the myocardium. Multinucleated giant cells (arrows) are also observed

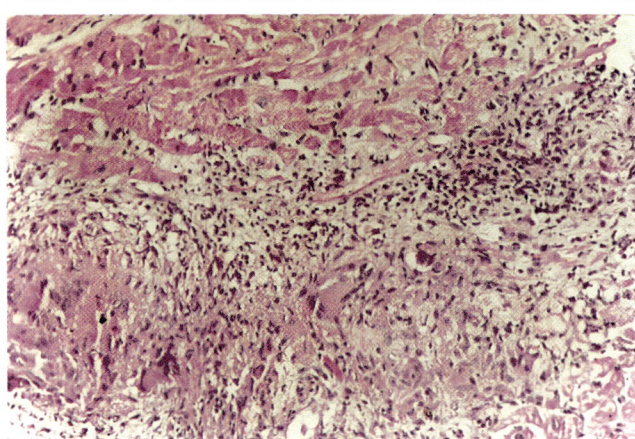

Fig. 7.20: Endomyocardial biopsy from a case with a clinical diagnosis of dilated cardiomyopathy. Granulomatous inflammation is present. Numerous multinucleated giant cells are recognized within the epithelioid cell granulomas. Infiltration by lymphocytes is present. Necrosis of myofibers is also observed

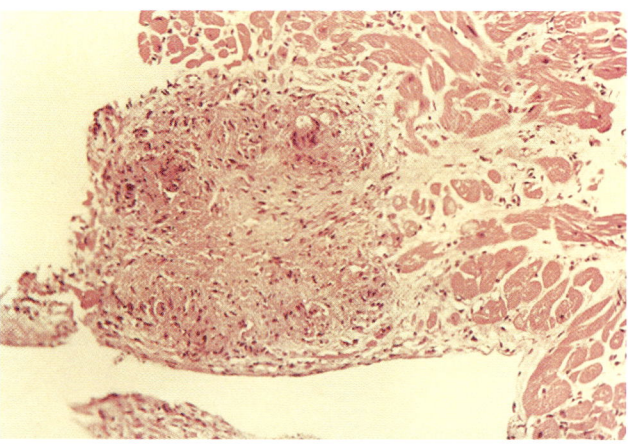

Fig. 7.21: Granulomatous inflammation myocardium. Endomyocardial biopsy showing granulomas in the subendocardium. Tuberculosis and sarcoidosis need to be considered in the differential diagnosis

c. *Rheumatic carditis* (Fig. 7.22) Biopsy done in cases suspected of rheumatic carditis may show certain nonspecific changes and occasionally the specific Aschoff nodule which is diagnostic of the disease. The nonspecific changes include infiltration of the interstitium of the myocardium and/or the endocardium by lymphocytes, eosinophils and macrophages. Myonecrosis may or may not be associated.

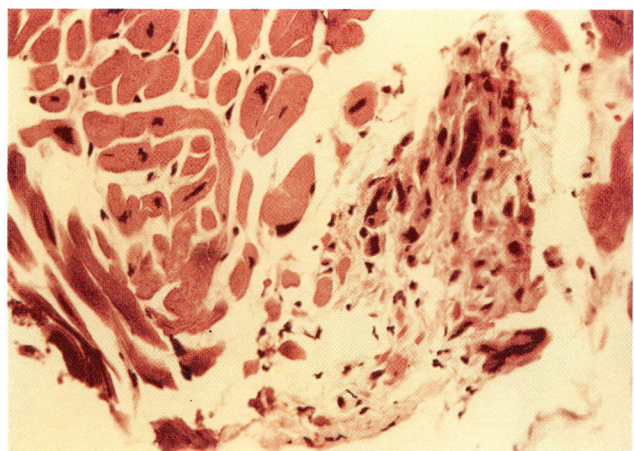

Fig. 7.22: Endomyocardial biopsy from a case of acute rheumatic fever. Well-formed granulomatous phase of the Aschoff nodule is seen in the interstitium of the myocardium

d. *Hypersensitivity myocarditis* This is characterized by infiltration of the interstitium of myocardium by an inflammatory infiltrate dominated by eosinophils (Figs 7.23a and b). A history of exposure/intake of drugs is generally elicited (methyldopa, sulfonamides, penicillin, etc).

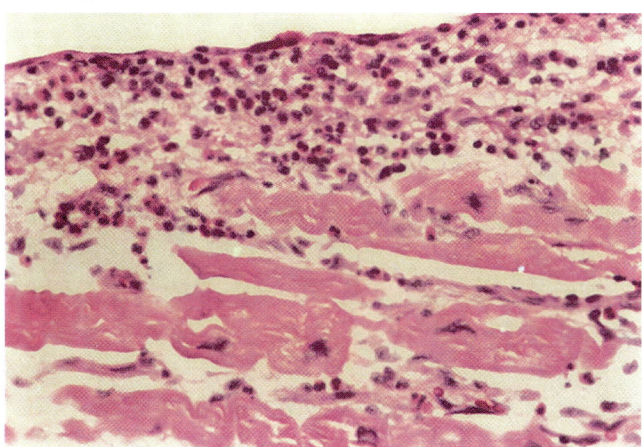

Fig. 7.23a: Eosinophilic myocarditis. Numerous eosinophils are seen in the subendocardium and interstitial tissue of the myocardium. Elsewhere myonecrosis and marked eosinophilic infiltration was observed

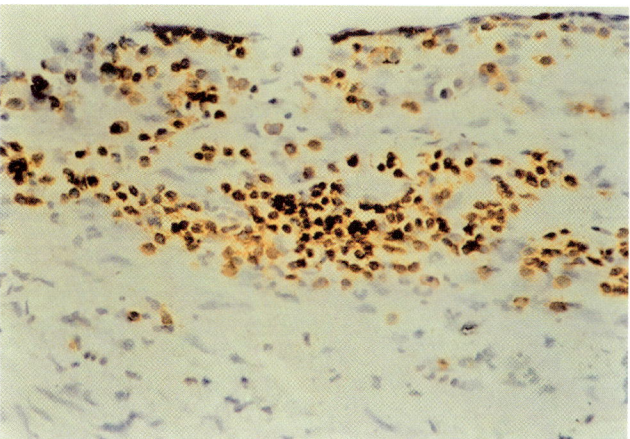

Fig. 7.23b: Eosinophilic myocarditis. The eosinophils show a strong reaction with leucocyte common antigen (Peroxidase-antiperoxidase)

Cardiomyopathies Endomyocardial biopsies are performed commonly in **dilated cardiomyopathy** with the aim to detect lymphocytic or other types of myocarditis as some cases require aggressive therapy (Figs 7.4 to 7.13). A major group in which biopsies are done is the **restrictive cardiomyopathy**. In this group the commoner entities which need to be differentiated are endomyocardial fibrosis, constrictive pericarditis and infiltrative disorders such as amyloidosis. A number of cases who present with features having definitive evidence of restrictive physiology, have no angiographic evidence of endomyocardial fibrosis. The endomyocardial biopsy in such cases do not show features of EMF or an infiltrative disorder. These cases have been designated as **idiopathic restrictive cardiomyopathy** (IRCM).

a. *Endomyocardial fibrosis* Certain biopsy features of angiographically proven cases of EMF suggest this diagnosis. The biopsy generally yields fragments of endocardium and/or thrombus fresh or organized and occasionally fragments of myocardium showing interstitial fibrosis may be included (Figs 7.24 to 7.27). In our experience fragments of thrombus or thickened endocardium are invariably seen in cases of EMF. This is in sharp contrast to the nature of biopsy pieces from cases of dilated cardiomyopathy.

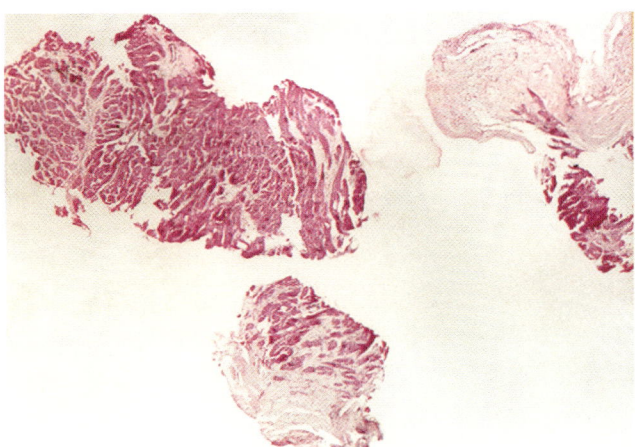

Fig. 7.24: Restrictive heart disease. Endomyocardial biopsy yielded multiple fragments. The lower fragment shows myocardial fibrosis. Tissue in the right upper corner of picture is comprised of marked fibrocollagen thickening of the endocardium. With the clinical background of restrictive physiology the histological features are suggestive of endomyocardial fibrosis

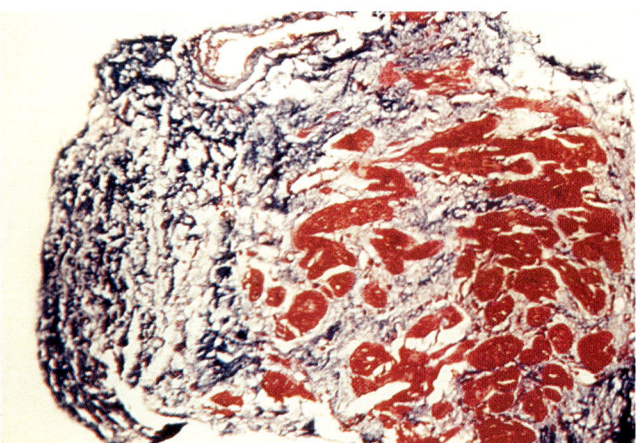

Fig. 7.25: Endomyocardial biopsy from a case of endomyocardial fibrosis (diagnosed on basis of clinical/hemodynamic data). Masson trichrome stain reveals marked fibrosis in the interstitium of the myocardium

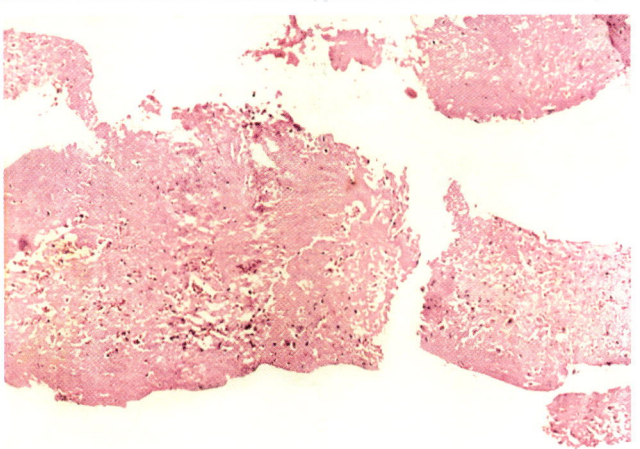

Fig. 7.26: Endomyocardial biopsy done in a case of restrictive heart disease. Fragments of fresh thrombus were obtained. No myocardial fragments were included in the biopsy

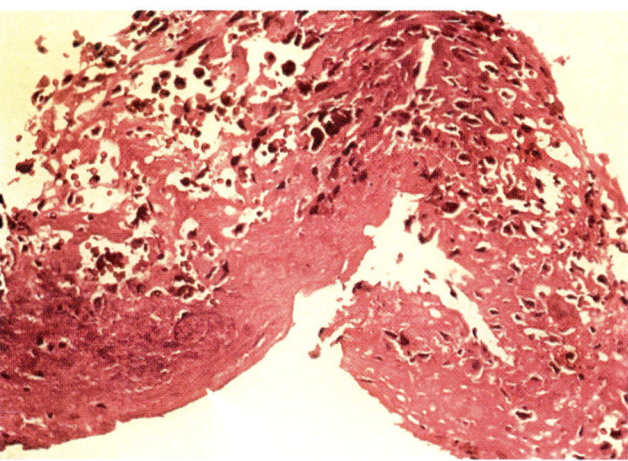

Fig. 7.27: Endomyocardial biopsy from a case of endomyocardial fibrosis showing a thrombus. This was the only material retrieved from the obliterated right ventricular cavity

Note: In endomyocardial fibrosis, the endocardium is markedly thickened with or without an everlying thrombus. The endomyocardial biopsy bioptome therefore is unable to reach the underlying myocardium. Thus in cases of restrictive heart disease, fragments of thrombus and/or endocardial fragments are quite suggestive of the diagnosis of endomyocardial fibrosis

b. *Amyloidosis* As is well-known, endomyocardial biopsy is extremely useful to diagnose this condition. The extent, severity and pattern of amyloidosis is well brought out in the biopsy material. Nodular and/or diffuse deposits of amyloid material have been observed in the subendocardium, interstitial tissue of myocardium, in the perimyocytic region, in the wall of the blood vessels and around adipocytes. Biopsy material can be effectively used for electron microscopy and other special stains such as crystal violet, thioflavin-T fluorescence, congo red for characterising amyloid (Figs 7.28 and 7.29).

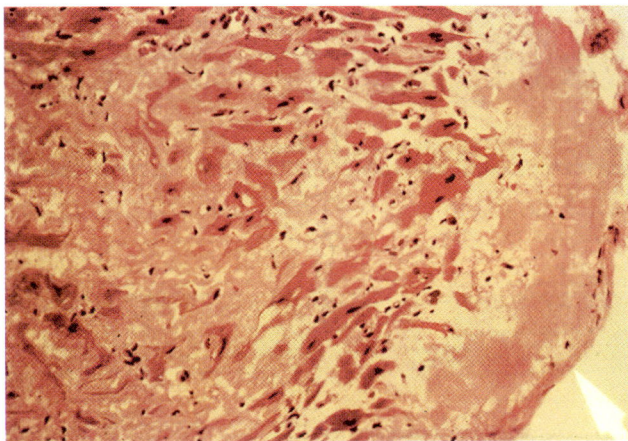

Fig. 7.28a: Cardiac amyloidosis. The amyloid material is present diffusely within the interstitium of the myocardium resulting in loss/atrophy of myofibers. Prominent nodular subendocardial deposits are also present

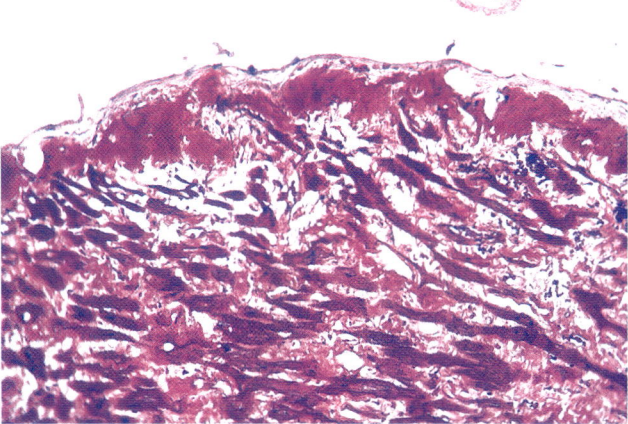

Fig. 7.28b: Cardiac amyloidosis. Crystal violet stain brings out the nodular aggregates of amyloid material in the subendocardium

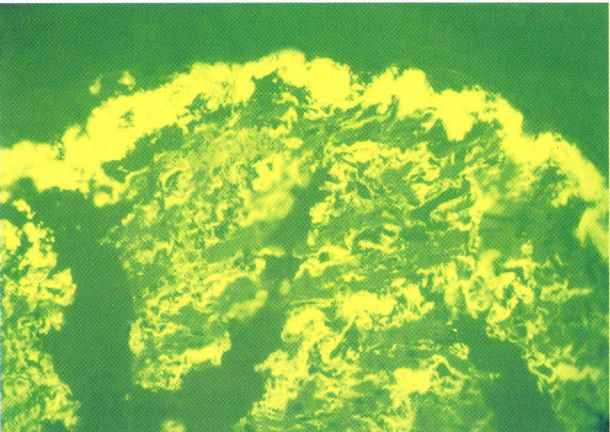

Fig. 7.28c: Cardiac amyloidosis. Thioflavin-T fluorescence of the subendocardial deposits of amyloid

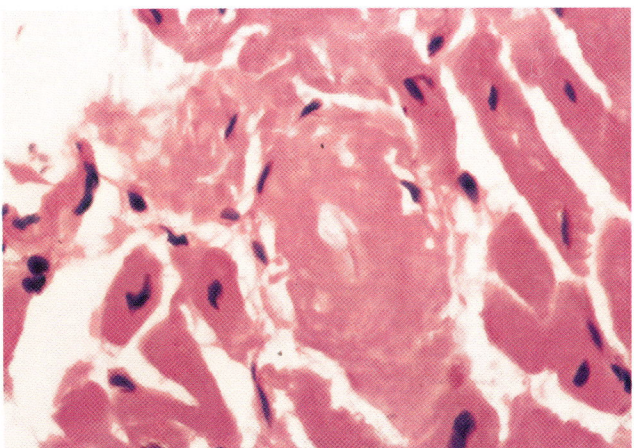

Fig. 7.29a: Cardiac amyloidosis. Pink, homogenous material characterized as amyloid (special stains) is present in the wall of blood vessel

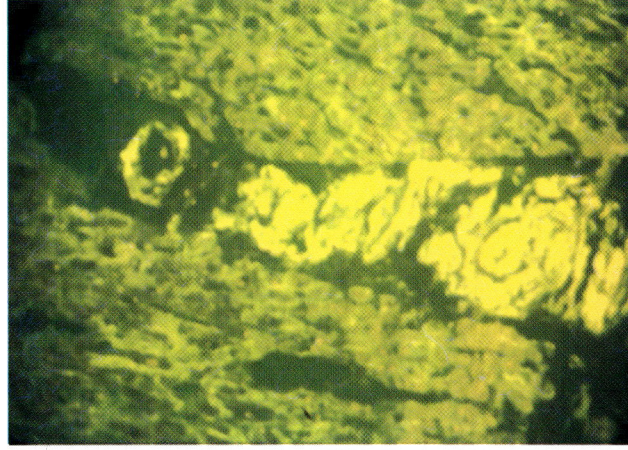

Fig. 7.29b: Cardiac amyloidosis. Thioflavin-T fluorescence to show amyloid deposition in the wall of blood vessels

c. ***Idiopathic restrictive cardiomyopathy (IRCMP)*** This is a specific and definitive entity. Known causes of restrictive cardiomyopathy are not present in the biopsy and instead the biopsy shows certain nonspecific but repetitive features. The endocardium is normal. Myofibers show varying grades of hypertrophy and degenerative changes. Myofibers disarray may be seen in some cases. Interstitial fibrosis is observed usually (Figs 7.30 to 7.33).

d. ***Arrhythmogenic right ventricular dysplasia (ARVD)*** This is a distinct entity and has been recognized as a form of cardiomyopathy. The features on biopsy are described in Chapter 9 (page 136, Figures 9.44 to 9.47).

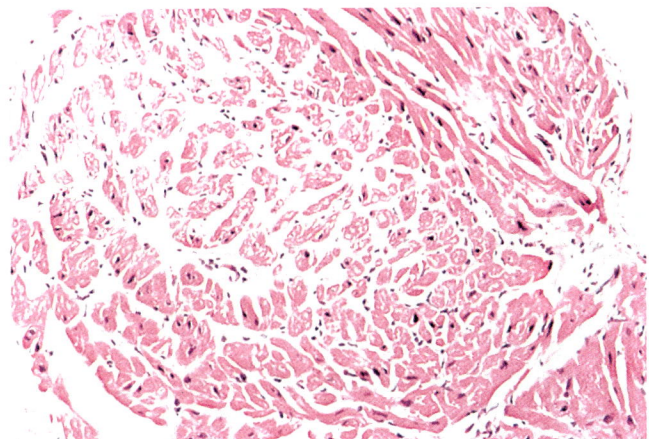

Fig. 7.30a: Idiopathic restrictive cardiomyopathy. Endomyocardial biopsy from a case of restrictive cardiomyopathy (angiographic and echocardiographic data). The endocardium is unremarkable. Myocytes show mild anisonucleosis. Diffuse creeping interstitial fibrosis is present. There were no features of an infiltrative disorder

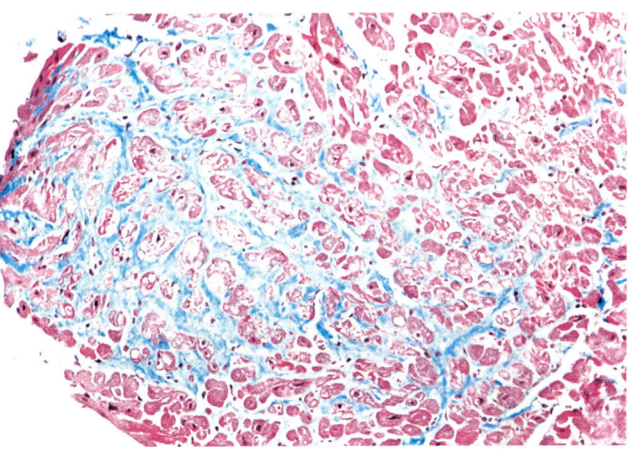

Fig. 7.30b: Idiopathic restrictive cardiomyopathy. Masson trichrome stain highlights the extent and type of interstitial fibrosis of the myocardium

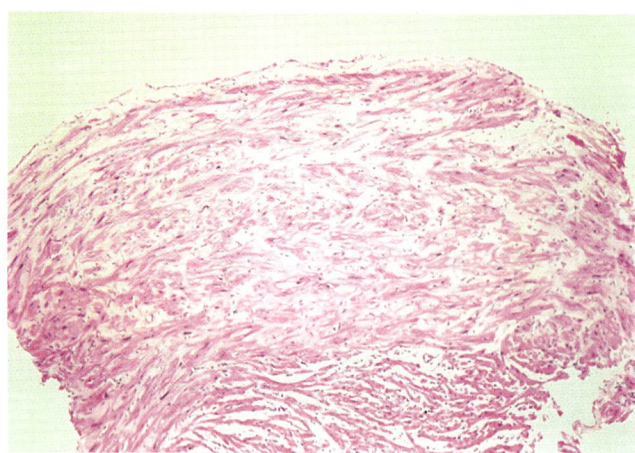

Fig. 7.31a: Idiopathic restrictive cardiomyopathy. The myofibers show marked degenerative changes with prominent cytoplasmic vacuolation. The myofibers appear small and fragmented. Prominent interstitial fibrosis is present

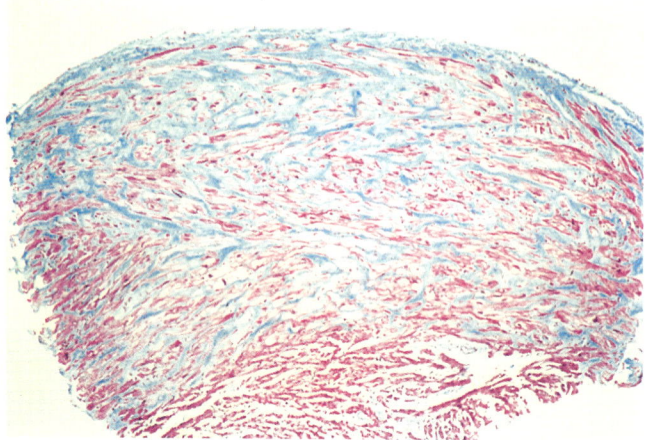

Fig. 7.31b: Idiopathic restrictive cardiomyopathy. Masson trichrome stain brings out the prominent interstitial fibrosis and short fragmented myofibers

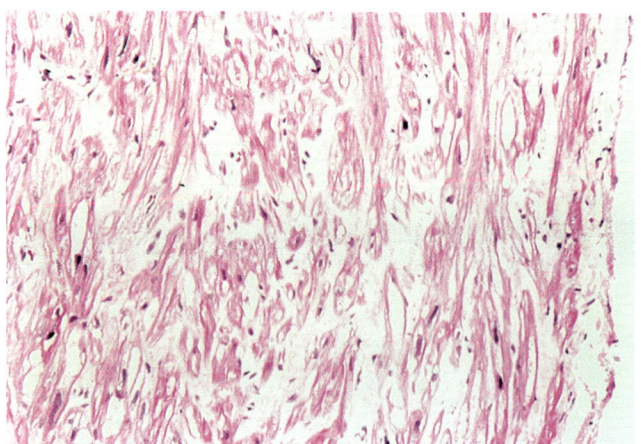

Fig. 7.32a: Idiopathic restrictive cardiomyopathy. The myofibers are short fragmented and show myocytolysis. Interstitial fibrosis is striking. Endocardium is normal

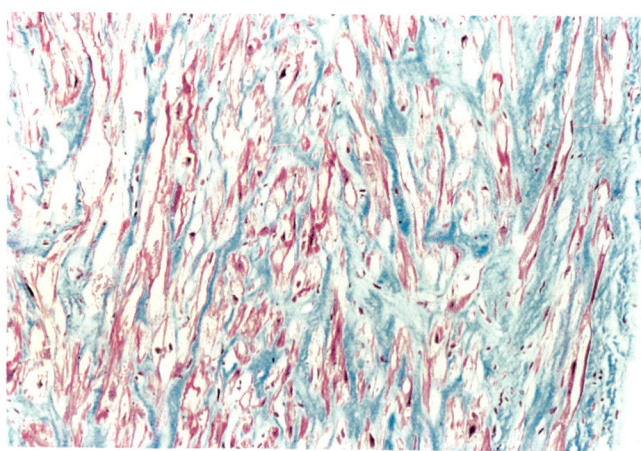

Fig. 7.32b: Idiopathic restrictive cardiomyopathy. Masson trichrome stain highlights short fragmented myofibers separated by fibrous tissue

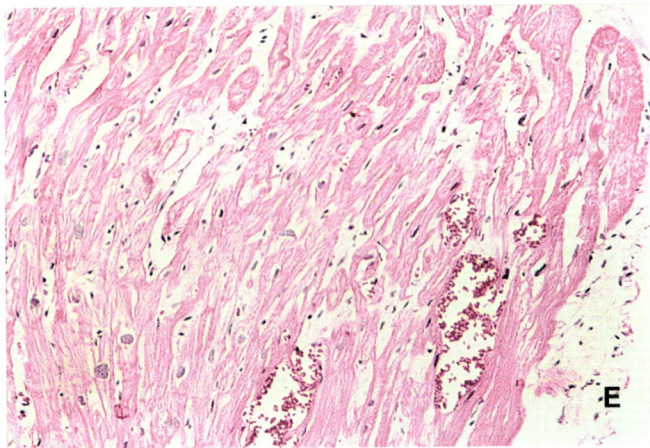

Fig. 7.33a: Endomyocardial biopsy from a case of restrictive cardiomyopathy. Myofibers show anisonucleosis. Focal vacuolation of the cytoplasm is seen. Endocardium (E) is unremarkable. In view of the clinical data, the biopsy was considered to be compatible with idiopathic restrictive cardiomyopathy

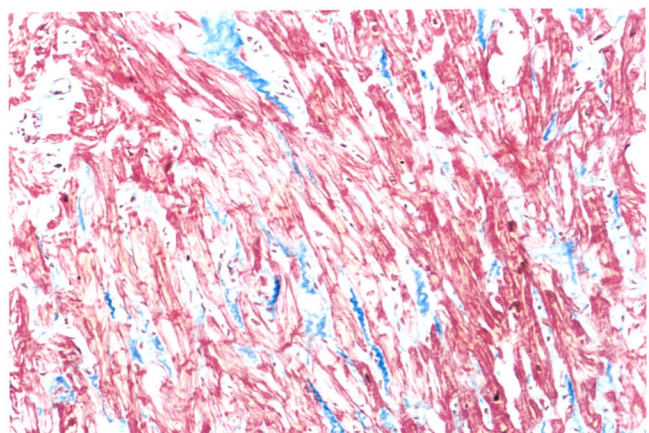

Fig. 7.33b: Idiopathic restrictive cardiomyopathy. Masson trichrome stain brings out the marked degenerative changes of the myofibers and mild interstitial fibrosis

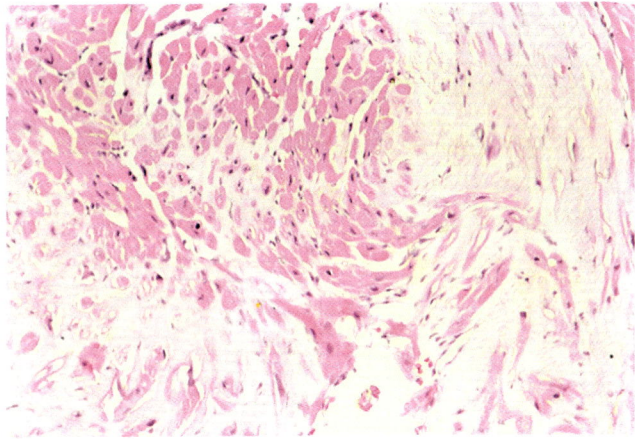

Fig. 7.33c: Idiopathic restrictive cardiomyopathy. Another area from the same biopsy illustrated in Figures 7.33a and b. Large areas of fibrosis of the myocardial interstitium are seen

Tumor and tumor-like lesions Endomyocardial biopsy can be of utility to decide the nature of intracardiac mass lesions (Figs 7.34 and 7.35).

Monitoring anthracycline cardiotoxicity Anthracyclines (Adriamycin or Doxorubicin hydrochloride) are an important group of anticancer drugs used in the treatment of solid tumors and hematologic malignancies. Cardiotoxic effects of this drug are well-recognized and the features are those of dilated cardiomyopathy. Endomyocardial biopsy is an important tool for the diagnosis grading and monitoring of anthracycline cardiotoxicity. It is important to remember that cardiotoxicity of this drug cannot be evaluated on light microscopy. Electron microscopy is mandatory in such cases and therefore the tissue needs to be fixed in an appropriate fixative. The two principal changes of adriamycin toxicity are: (1) myofibrillar loss and (2) swelling and coalescence of the sarcoplasmic reticulum. The extent and severity of the changes in these organelles determine the grade of toxicity.

The dosage of the drug is thus adjusted according to the changes with an aim to prevent irreversible myocardial damage and cardiac failure.

Complications of endomyocardial biopsy Considering the benefits of EMB procedure the complications are few and can be managed conservatively in most cases. EMB is believed to be safer than both liver and kidney biopsy. In experienced hands the morbidity and mortality is insignificant (Table 7.3).

Table 7.3: Complications of endomyocardial biopsy

Hemopericardium
Cardiac tamponade
Pneumothorax
Air embolism
Mediastinitis
Perforation of right ventricular wall
Damage to tricuspid valve and/or chordae tendinea
Premature ventricular contractions
Transient chest pain
Nerve palsies
Hematoma neck

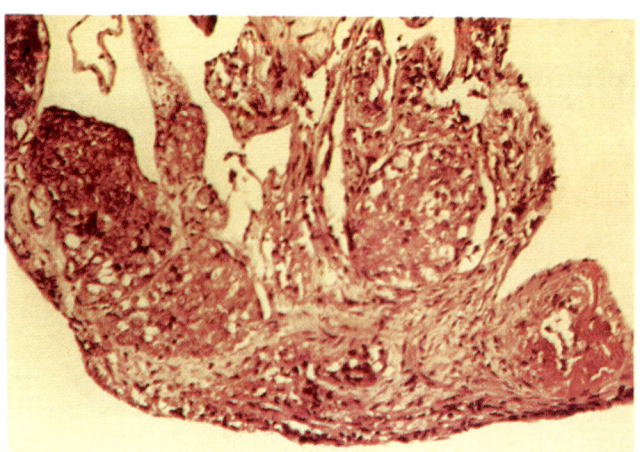

Fig. 7.34: Endomyocardial biopsy from a mass in the left ventricle revealed a malignant epithelial tumor possibly an adenocarcinoma. No obvious primary site could be found

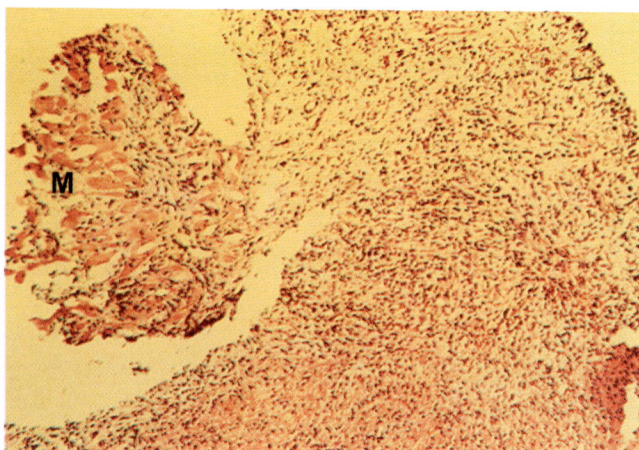

Fig. 7.35: Endomyocardial biopsy from an intraventricular mass. This revealed an organising thrombus which is seen to extend into the myocardium (M). (There was a strong clinical suspicion of a tumor)

SUGGESTED READING

1. Aretz HT, Billingham ME, Edwards WD, Factor SM, Fallon JT, Fenoglio JJ, Olsen EGT, Schoen FJ: Myocarditis: A histopathologic definition and classification. *Am J Cardiovas Pathol* **1**: 3-14, 1987.
2. Barry WH: Cellular and molecular basis of inflammatory myocardial disease. **8(4)**: 499-505, 2001.
3. Chopra P, Talwar KK: Morphological evaluation of endomyocardial biopsy. *Nat Med J India* **9/6**: 279-84, 1996.
4. Chopra P, Ray R: Endomyocardial biopsy—A pathologist's perspective. *Cardiology Today* **4/6**: 341-46, 2000.
5. Cooper LT Jr, Berry GJ, Shabebai R: Idiopathic giant cell myocarditis natural history and treatment. Multicenter giant cell myocarditis study group investigators. *N Engl J Med* **26, 336(26)**: 1860-66, 1997.
6. Feldman AM, McNamara D: Myocarditis. *NEJM* 343 **19**: 1388-98, 2000.
7. Mason JW: Myocarditis: *Adv Intern Med* **44**: 293-310, 1999.
8. Mena I, Perry CM, Harkins S, Rodriguez F, Gebhard J, Whitton JL: The role of B lymphocytes in coxsackievirus B3 infection. *Am J Pathol* **155(4)**: 1205-15, 1999.
9. Micevski V: The use of molecular technologies for the detection of enteroviral ribonucleic acid in myocarditis. *J Cardiovasc Nurs* **13(4)**: 78-90, 1990.
10. Narula JPS, Chopra P, Talwar KK, Reddy S, Vasan RS, Tandon R, Bhatia ML, Southern JF: Does endomyocardial biopsy aid in the diagnosis of acute rheumatic carditis? *Circulation* 88 (Part 1): 2198-2205, 1993.
11. Opavsky MA, Penninger J, Aitken K, Wen WH, Dawood F, Mak T, Liu P: Susceptibility to myocarditis is dependent on the response of alpha-beta T lymphocytes to coxsakieviral infection. *Circ Res* **85(6)**: 551-58, 1999.
12. Seferovic PM, Makoimovic R *et al*: Endomyocardial biopsy: A meta-analysis of diagnostic value. *Postgrad Med J* **70(Suppl 1)**: S21-S28, 1994.
13. Sinagra G, Maras P, D'Ambrosio A, Gregori D, Bussani R, Silvestri F, Morgera T, Pinamonti B, Salvi A, Alberti E, Di Lenarda A, Lardieri G, Klugmann S, Camerini F: Clinical polymorphic presentation and natural history of active myocarditis: Experience in 60 cases. *G Ital Cardiol* **27(8)**: 758-74, 1997.
14. Veinot J: Diagnostic endomyocardial biopsy pathology—General biopsy considerations and its use for myocarditis and cardiomyopathy: A review, *Can J Cardiol* **18(1)**: 55-65, 2002.
15. Veinot J: Diagnostic endomyocardial biopsy pathology: Secondary myocardial diseases and other clinical indications—A review. *Can J Cardiol* **18(3)**: 287-96, 2002.
16. Wu LA, Lapeyre AC 3rd, Cooper LT: Current role of endomyocardial biopsy in the management of dilated cardiomyopathy and myocarditis. *Mayo Clinic Proc* **76(10)**: 1030-38, 2001.

Myocarditis

MYOCARDITIS

Myocarditis is an acute or chronic focal or diffuse inflammatory cell infiltration in the interstitium of the myocardium with myocyte damage/necrosis. The latter component is mandatory for the diagnosis of myocarditis (Dallas criteria). Myocarditis may be caused either by **infectious agents** or in some cases by **noninfectious** agents.

Myocarditis by Infectious Agents

In a vast majority of cases myocarditis is caused by infectious agents the most common of which are viruses (Coxsackie A and B viruses, ECHO viruses, Encephalomyocarditis virus, Human immunodeficiency virus, Cytomegalovirus, Influenza virus, Epstein-Barr virus, etc). Coxsackie A and B virus induced myocarditis is the most frequent one amongst viruses. Pathology of viral myocarditis is discussed in chapter 7. Other infectious agents which cause myocarditis include bacteria, fungi, parasites, Rickettsia, Chlamydia, spirochetes, etc.

Lymphocytic Myocarditis

This is a common type of myocarditis that is invariably of viral etiology. The most frequent viral agents are the coxsackie groups A and B. It is believed that there exists a relationship between viral myocarditis and dilated cardiomyopathy. Well-documented clinical as well as epidemiologic evidences exist to this effect. It has been reported that following coxsackie group B infection of the heart a high incidence of cardiac abnormalities occur. Other studies have reported that about 30% of patients diagnosed as viral myocarditis developed features of dilated cardiomyopathy. Myocarditis has been diagnosed in endomyocardial biopsy specimens from patients of dilated cardiomyopathy.

Microscopically myocarditis is characterized by an interstitial mononuclear infiltrate mostly lymphocytes with damage and/or necrosis of the myofibers (Figs 7.10 to 7.13 and 9.13). The latter feature is mandatory and has been stressed upon in the **Dallas criteria** for the diagnosis of myocarditis. Since repeated biopsies may be done in a case of myocarditis to determine the effect of therapy, etc. the following terminologies were recommended:

First Biopsy

a. **Active myocarditis** with or without fibrosis (inflammatory infiltrate and damage to adjacent myocytes must be present for the diagnosis).
b. **Borderline myocarditis** This is not diagnostic as the inflammatory infiltrate may be sparse and/or no myocyte damage is present. A repeat biopsy needs to be done.
c. No myocarditis.

Subsequent Biopsies

a. **Ongoing (persistent) myocarditis** When the degree of inflammatory cell infiltration is same as or worse than that of the previous biopsy.
b. **Resolving myocarditis** The inflammation is less than the previous biopsy and reparative changes may also be seen.
c. **Resolved myocarditis** No inflammatory infiltrate or necrosis is seen.

As per the Dallas criteria presence of lymphocytic infiltration and myocyte necrosis are mandatory for a diagnosis of myocarditis. Care should be taken to see that merely presence of lymphocytes in the interstitium does not qualify for myocarditis. An additional factor which needs to be remembered is that several mesenchymal cells namely endothelial cells, fibroblasts, macrophages and nuclei of other cells may closely simulate lymphocytes. Appropriate steps must be taken for this at the time of interpretation of the biopsy material.

Molecular techniques like *in situ* hybridization, *in situ* PCR and immunohistochemistry for viral capsid proteins have been used to detect enteroviral genome in the heart muscle both in cases of myocarditis and dilated cardiomyopathy.

Immune-mediated or Noninfective Myocarditis

This type of myocarditis has been documented in various collagen vascular disorders namely rheumatic carditis, systemic lupus erythematosus, polyarteritis nodosa, rheumatoid arthritis, systemic sclerosis and cardiac transplant rejection reaction.

Physical Agents

Myocarditis may also be caused by drugs (e.g. penicillin, sulphonamides, adriamycin, methyldopa, cyclosporine, azathioprine and other immunosuppressive drugs), chemical poisons, irradiation, metabolic disorders (uremia, hypokalemia), etc.

Granulomatous Myocarditis

This condition is characterized by the presence of well-defined granulomas in the myocardium. It is commonly confused with giant cell myocarditis which is a specific condition and entirely different from granulomatous myocarditis. Granulomatous myocarditis can be seen in sarcoidosis, in myocarditis induced by infective agents namely fungal and parasitic disorders and in tuberculosis. Infective agents may be demonstrated in infective myocarditis by employing special staining. In cases suspected of tuberculosis molecular biology techniques may be used if special stains are of no help. Granulomatous response can also occur in response to foreign bodies or devices implanted in the heart.

Sarcoidosis Heart

Sarcoidosis involving the heart appears to be rare in the tropical countries. A spectrum of morphological changes have been described in cardiac sarcoidosis. Patients with clinical symptoms can present with features of dilated and/or restrictive cardiomyopathy. Granulomatous inflammation which may be extensive is commonly encountered in the interventricular septum. This lesion may cause AV block and sudden death. Healing of the involved area can give rise to thinning and aneurysm formation. Microscopically, discrete, non-necrotizing epithelioid cell granulomas replacing the myocardium are present (Figs 8.1 and 8.2). Fibrosis is frequently observed. Lungs and lymph nodes are usually involved.

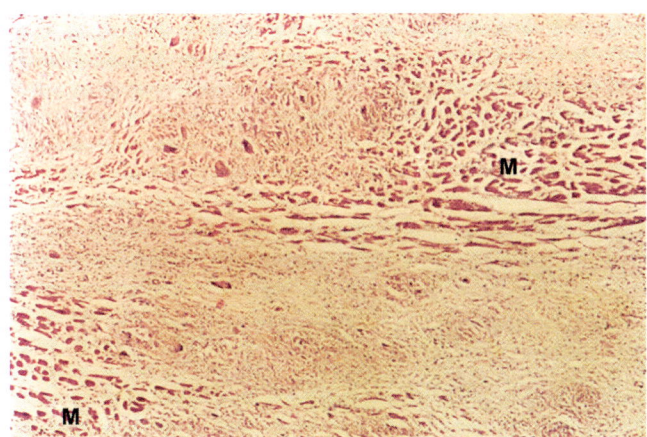

Fig. 8.1a: Sarcoidosis heart. Numerous discrete epithelioid cell granulomas are present in the myocardium which in large areas is replaced by the process. Islands of myocardium (M) are recognized in between the lesion

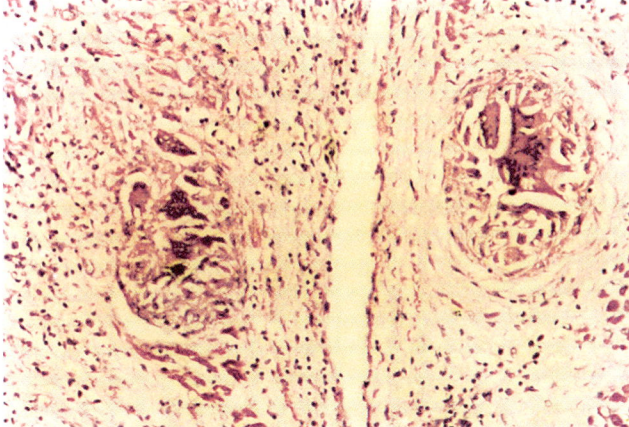

Fig. 8.1b: Sarcoidosis heart. Epithelioid cell granulomas are well-defined and discrete. Multinucleated giant cells and sprinkling of lymphocytes are also seen

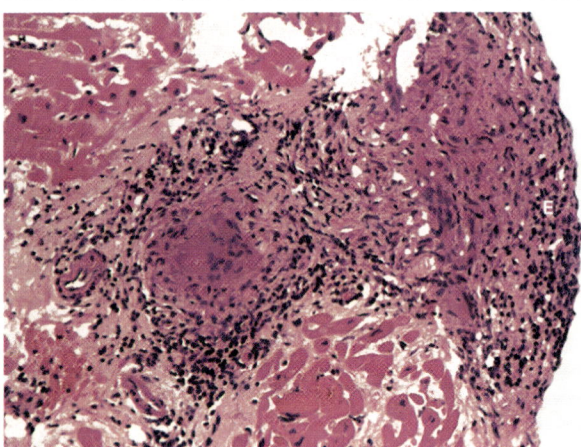
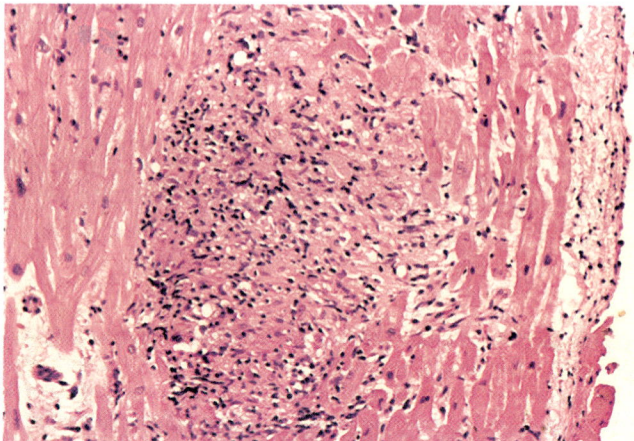

Figs 8.2a and b: Sarcoidosis heart. (a) Photomicrograph of right ventricular endomyocardial biopsy shows, non-necrotizing epithelioid cell granulomas along with multinucleated giant cells within the interstitium of the myocardium and the subendocardial region (E). Multinucleated giant cells and dense lymphocytic infiltration is also observed. Higher magnification (b) shows that the myofibers are destroyed in these areas. Additionally, foci of lymphocytic myocarditis are also observed. Stains for acid-fast bacilli and fungi were negative

Tuberculosis Heart

Tuberculosis is a major problem in developing countries and is fast re-emerging as an infection of great concern. For ill-understood reasons tuberculosis of the myocardium is extremely rare though pericardial involvement is well-recognized. Few case reports have documented myocardial tuberculosis. In a large autopsy series comprising of 32,980 cases only 7 cases of tuberculosis of heart were detected. Tuberculosis in the heart has a tendency to involve the superficially located arteries and the conduction system. Pathological types of myocardial involvement in tuberculosis include nodular variety or tuberculoma, miliary type and diffuse infiltrating form. Microscopically, granulomatous inflammation with or without necrosis is observed (Figs 8.3, 8.4 and 7.17 to 7.21). A careful search for identification of acid-fast bacilli by histochemical stains or culture or both is necessary to confirm the diagnosis. If these are negative, molecular biological techniques could aid in the accurate diagnosis of tuberculosis. In the absence of these diagnostic techniques, sarcoidosis is a close differential diagnosis and needs to be excluded.

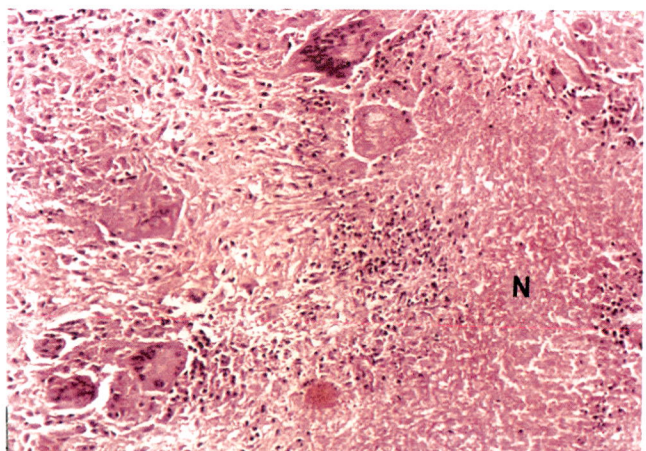

Fig. 8.3: Tuberculoma heart. A large circumscribed nodule measuring 3 cm in diameter was present in the left ventricular myocardium adjacent to the pericardium. Photomicrograph shows extensive necrosis (N) which is bordered by epithelioid cells and giant cells. A few acid-fast bacilli were also demonstrated

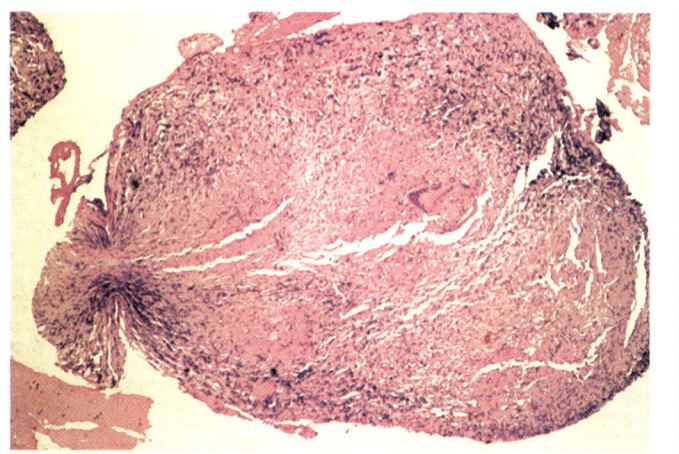
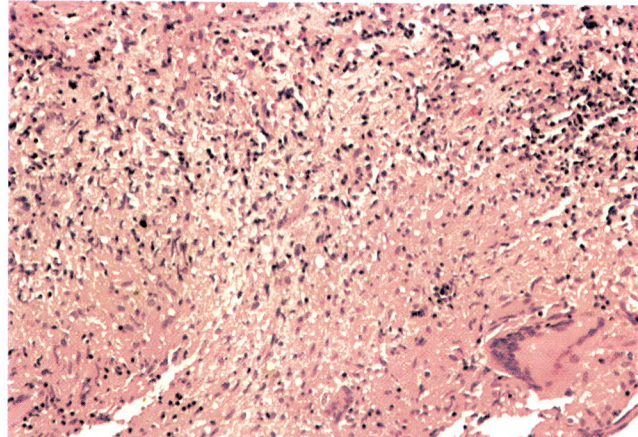

Figs 8.4a and b: Biopsy of the right atrial mass (2 fragments). One of the fragment shows (a) multiple well-formed epithelioid cell granulomas along with multinucleated giant cells, (b) focal areas of necrosis are also present. Histological changes are compatible with tuberculosis

Note: 12-year-old male child presented with features of right sided heart failure. On investigation patient was detected to have a right atrial mass with supraventricular tachycardia and biventricular dysfunction. ECHO revealed a mass occupying 50% of right atrium extending into right ventricle, and superior vena cava. A clinical diagnosis of intracardiac tumor was made

Giant Cell Myocarditis

This is a rare type of myocarditis which has an aggressive clinical course and high mortality. In the acute phase, large areas of myocyte necrosis in a geographic pattern are seen. Numerous multinucleated giant cells are observed in relation to necrotic myofibers. Extensive polymorphic inflammatory cell infiltration comprising of lymphocytes, histiocytes, plasma cells and eosinophils is seen. Epithelioid cell granulomas are lacking. The inflammation may heal by fibrosis (Fig. 7.16). Giant cell myocarditis may occur in association with autoimmune disorders namely thymoma, myasthenia gravis, chronic lymphocytic thyroiditis, giant cell myositis, hypogammaglobulinemia, etc.

Response to immunosuppression has been tried but is poor. Cardiac transplantation is a viable option though the disease may recur after transplantation.

MYOCARDITIS DUE TO FUNGI, PARASITES, PROTOZOA, BACTERIA

Fungal Myocarditis

It can be caused by Aspergillus species, Candida, histoplasma, Cryptococcus and other fungi. It may rarely present as tumorous infiltration of the heart (Fig. 8.5). More commonly fungal colonization occurs as in generalized infection especially in immunocompromised individuals of varying etiology. The tissue response is granulomatous inflammation with foreign body giant cells (Fig. 8.5). Abscess formation may also occur (Fig. 8.6). The causative fungus can be recognized both on conventional staining and on special stains (Methanamine silver, PAS) within the cytoplasm of giant cells.

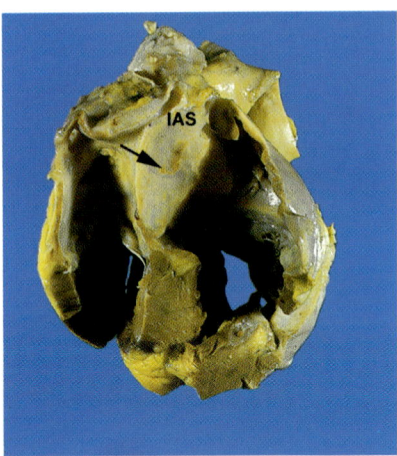

Fig. 8.5a: Fungal myocarditis. The interatrial septum (IAS) is diffusely thickened (arrow) giving an appearance of a tumor mass (Details of the case are provided in the note below)

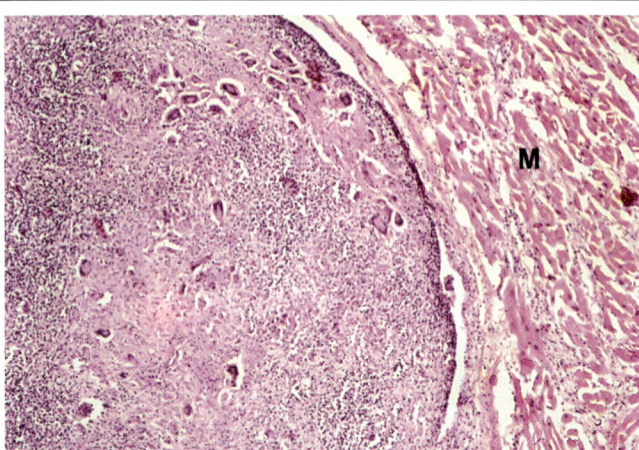

Fig. 8.5b: Fungal myocarditis. Large areas of the myocardium are destroyed and replaced by fibrosis, chronic inflammation and numerous foreign body type of giant cells. The compressed adjacent myocardium is unremarkable (M)

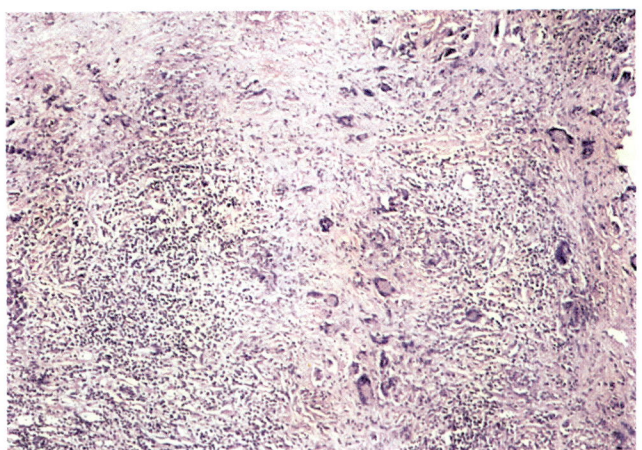

Fig. 8.5c: Fungal myocarditis. The myocardium is replaced by areas of dense fibrosis, inflammatory cells and multinucleated foreign body type of giant cells. Many of the giant cells show fungal hyphae in their cytoplasm

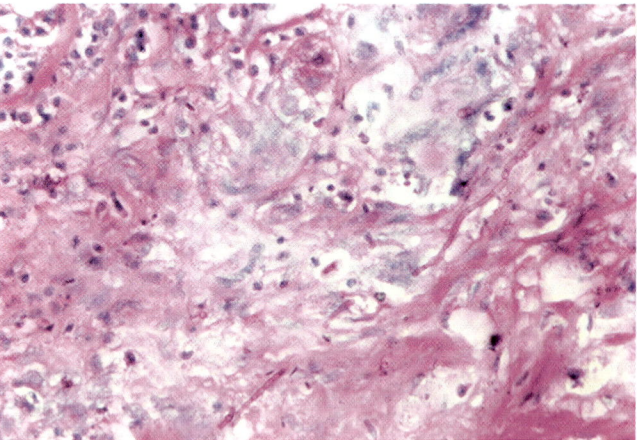

Fig. 8.5d: Fungal myocarditis. Periodic Acid Schiff (PAS) reaction to demonstrate septate and acute angle branching fungal profiles whose morphology is compatible with Aspergillus species

Note: Patient was a forty years male who presented with severe dyspnea for 3 days, palpitations and chest discomfort for 2 days. He had dyspnea on exertion of class II to class III severity for the last 6 months. He was a known case of Wolff-Parkinson-White (WPW) syndrome for the last 2 years. The patient was administered appropriate therapy including DC cardioversion and temporary pacemaker. However, he suffered a downhill course and died 24 hours after admission.

At autopsy, heart was the main diseased organ. It weighed 350 gm. The left and right atrium showed a yellowish white raised plaque like lesion involving the smooth part of the right atrium. The lumen of the superior vena cava was compromised by this lesion which also involved the anatomical site of the SA node and the AV node. The interatrial septum was diffusely and markedly thickened in its entire length. The septum measured 2.5 cm in thickness. It was yellowish white and firm to feel. The anterior leaflet of the mitral valve showed a yellowish white area at the base. Sections from the SA and AV node areas revealed marked fibrosis. No remnants of cardiac conduction system were recognized (Figs 8.5a-d are from the same case)

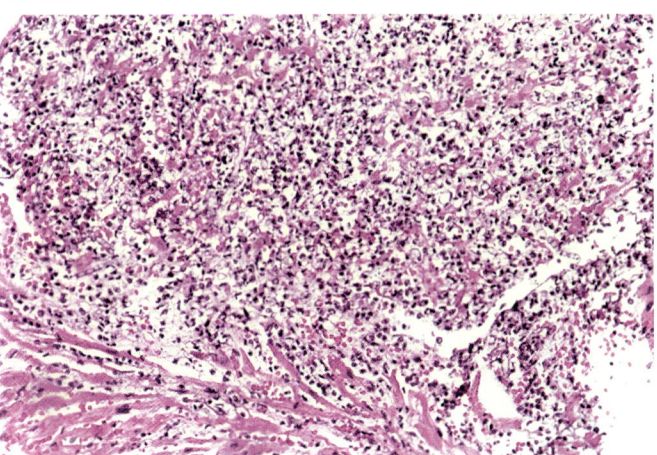

Fig. 8.6a: Myocardial abscess. Large areas of the myocardium are destroyed. Remnants of necrotic myofibers can be seen. A mixed type of inflammatory cell infiltrate consisting of lymphocytes, histiocytes, a few plasma cells and eosinophils is seen. Additionally, a few fungal profiles are recognized amidst the infiltrate. Myocardial fibers are seen in the lower left corner of the picture

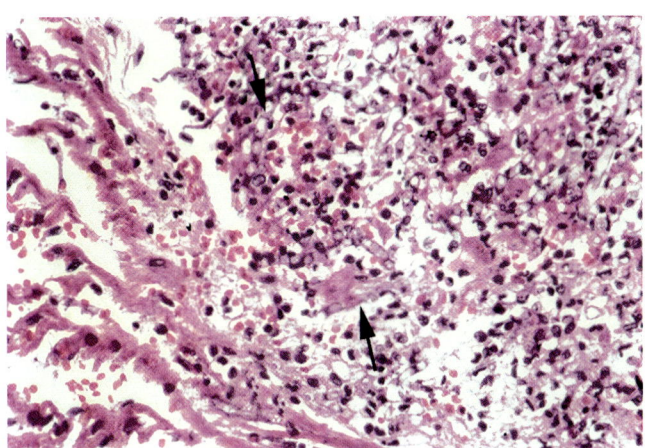

Fig. 8.6b: Myocardial abscess. Higher magnification to show numerous profiles of septate (arrows) fungi (Aspergillus) within the inflammatory infiltrate. A few myofibers are seen on the left of the picture

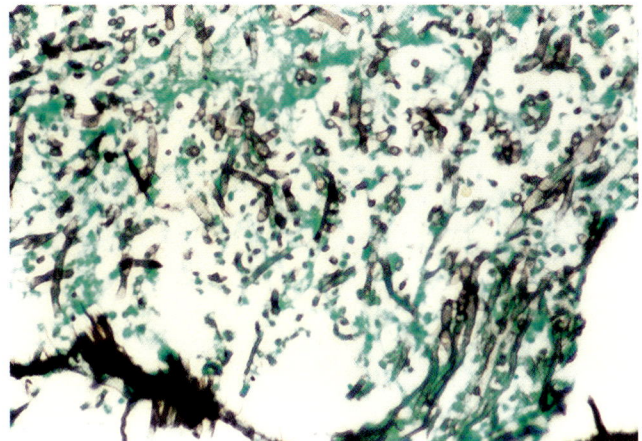

Fig. 8.6c: Myocardial abscess. Silver methanamine stain to demonstrate the morphology of the fungus

Cysticercosis

Cysticercosis (Figs 8.7 and 8.8) is an infection by the larval form of the tapeworm *Taenia solium*. This infection occurs on intake of uncooked pork. It may contaminate vegetables and thus may also occur in pure "vegetarians". Man is the definitive host. The adult worm passes the eggs in stool which are then swallowed by the pig, who is the intermediate host. Eggs hatch in pig's intestine releasing oncospheres which get into the circulation and eventually become encysted as cysticerci in muscle. Ingestion of infected pork meat by man results in development of adult tapeworm. Cysticerci can develop in any organ. Cysticerci are oval pearly white cysts which contain fluid and a single scolex. The scolex has 4 suckers and a double row of hooklets (Fig. 8.8). Cysticerci compress the adjacent structures and when viable do not excite any inflammatory response. When it degenerates, there is inflammatory cell infiltration that is rich in eosinophils. Epithelioid cells characteristically arranged in a palisading fashion are quite characteristic. Giant cells are frequently encountered.

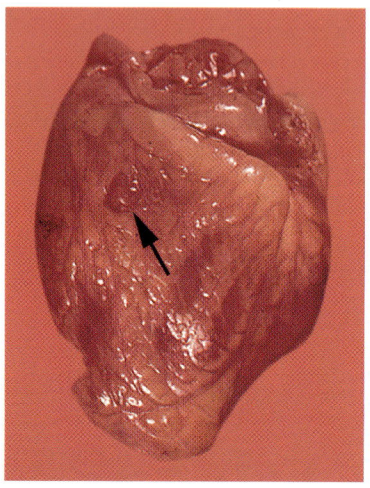

Fig. 8.7a: Cysticercosis heart. The external surface of the heart shows a dark tan well-circumscribed nodule (arrow) on the inferior surface of the heart

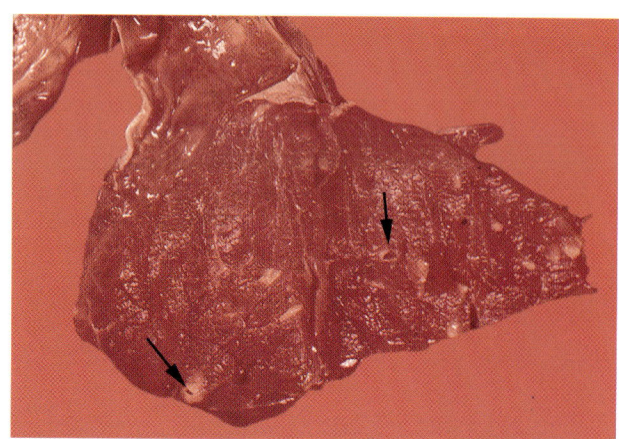

Fig. 8.7b: Cysticercosis skeletal muscle. Multiple gray white nodules with tiny spaces in their center are seen (arrows)

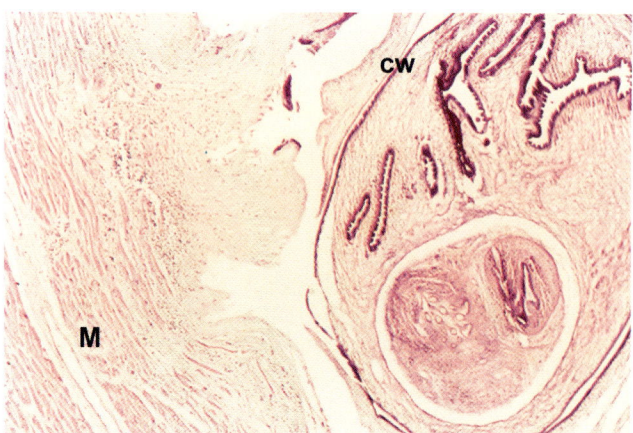

Fig. 8.8a: Cysticercosis heart. Larva of cysticercus is present encysted within the myocardium (M) which is compressed. No inflammatory reaction is seen

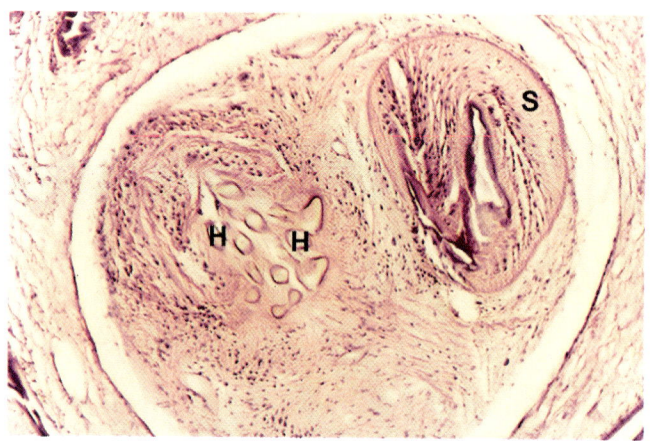

Fig. 8.8b: Scolex of cysticercus showing sucker(s) and hooklets (H)

Note: The patient was a 51 years male who presented with headache, dimness of vision and generalized convulsions. A clinical diagnosis of space occupying lesion in the brain was made. At autopsy, systemic cysticercosis involving brain, skeletal muscle, heart, lung, pancreas, mesentery and intestine was detected

Hydatid Disease

Hydatid disease (Figs 8.9a and b) is a synonym for echinococcosis which is an infection by larval tapeworms of the genus Echinococcus. E. granulosus is most common in man. Dog is the definitive host and the adult worm resides in the small intestine. Eggs are passed in the feces that are swallowed by the intermediate host one of which is man. The oncospheres pass through the intestinal wall, enter the blood stream and develop into hydatid cysts in various organs and tissues. Hydatid cyst of E. granulosus is pearly white, gelatinous and filled with fluid. Microscopically the cyst wall is a laminated membrane lined by a germinal layer which has nuclei. Scolices arise from the inner germinal layer of each brood capsule (Fig. 8.9a and b). Liver is the most common organ to be affected. Cysts can develop in any organ. Heart is affected in 0.5. to 2 percent cases. A dead cyst in any organ shows fibrosis and calcification around it. In the heart the cyst may rupture into the pericardium or into a chamber. Ruptured cyst may produce either a hypersensitivity reaction or metastatic hydatid disease.

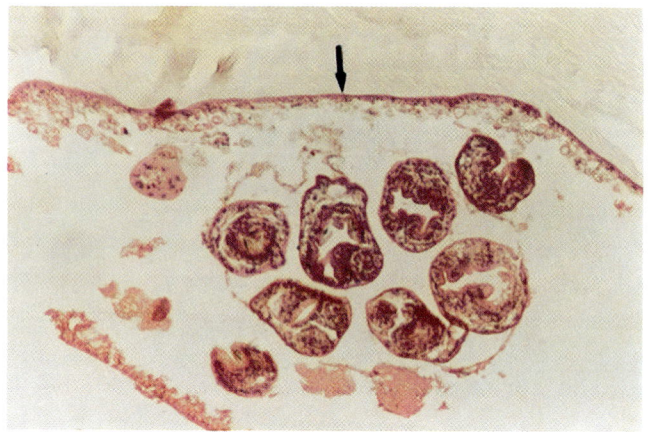

Fig. 8.9a: Hydatid cyst in right ventricular outflow tract. Numerous scolices are seen. Germinal layer (arrow) of the wall of hydatid cyst is recognized in the picture

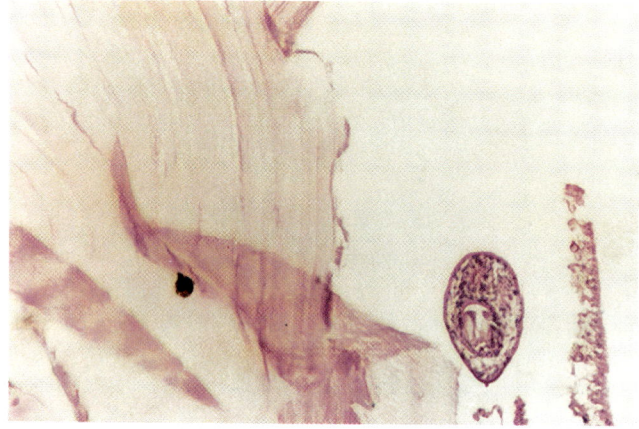

Fig. 8.9b: Hydatid cyst right ventricular outflow tract. Typical laminated membrane of hydatid cyst along with scolex is seen

Note: The patient was a 37 years female who had class II dyspnea. CT and ECHO revealed features of hydatid cyst in right ventricular outflow tract

Malaria

Malaria (Figs 8.10a and b) is caused by a protozoan of the genus Plasmodium. In tropical countries malaria is still widespread and may be associated with high morbidity and mortality. Amongst the four species that affect man namely *P. falciparum, P. vivax, P. ovale* and *P. malariae; P. falciparum* is the most virulent. Sporozoites that lodge in the mosquitoe's salivary gland are inoculated into man when the mosquito next feeds on the human victim. Sporozoites leave the blood and enter hepatocytes where they mature to form Schizonts containing many exoerythrocytic merozoites. In all species except *P. falciparum* relapses occur as merozoites continue to reinfect hepatocytes.

Pathology of malaria is confined to infection caused by *P. falciparum* which is the only species amongst the four which is seen in histologic sections. Patients usually die from cerebral involvement or renal failure. The typical histologic feature is parasitization of red blood cells in all viscera. The parasitized erythrocytes stick to the capillary endothelium thus blocking them (Figs 8.10a and b). These erythrocytes may rupture and there is phagocytosis of malarial pigment and parasites by the reticuloendothelial cells. The cardiac lesion is consequent to capillaries plugged with parasitized red blood cells. Thus focal ischemic changes may be seen in the affected organs.

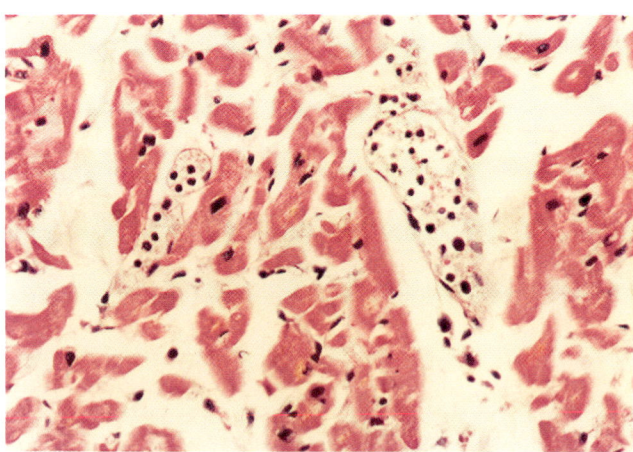

Fig. 8.10a: Malignant tertian malaria *(Plasmodium falciparum)* heart. Capillaries are clogged with numerous parasitized red blood cells

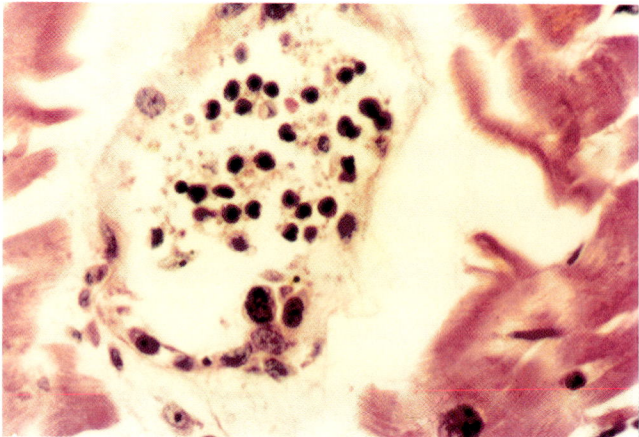

Fig. 8.10b: Malignant tertian malaria affecting the heart. The capillaries show numerous parasitized red blood cells and hemopoietic cells

Note: The patient was a 30 years male who presented with high fever associated with chills and rigors. He deteriorated rapidly and died before any investigations were carried out. At autopsy, severe parasiticemia was observed affecting the brain, liver, heart and lungs

Bacterial Infection

Bacterial infection (Figs 8.11a and b) Myocardial abscesses result most commonly by septic emboli within the coronary circulation. Infective endocarditis is a common source. Bacterial colonies can often be recognized.

Toxoplasmosis

Myocarditis is caused by *toxoplasma gondii* a protozoan and is common in immunocompromised hosts. Parasites are seen within the myofibers. A mixed type of inflammatory cell infiltrate comprising of neutrophils, eosinophils and lymphomononuclear cells is observed.

Chaga's Disease

Chaga's disease is caused by the protozoan *Trypanosoma cruzi*. This disease causes a dilated cardiomyopathy like picture. Microscopically numerous parasites within cells are observed. Infiltration by lymphocytes, plasma cells and macrophages are also seen.

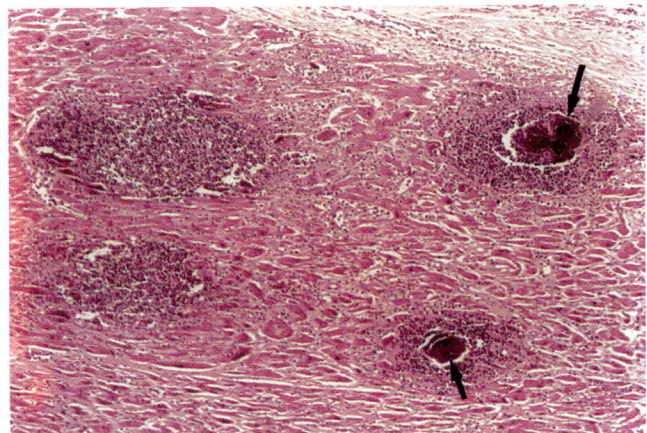

Fig. 8.11a: Multiple myocardial abscesses (bacterial). Bacterial colonies (arrows) can be seen within the abscess. Large areas of the myocardium are necrosed

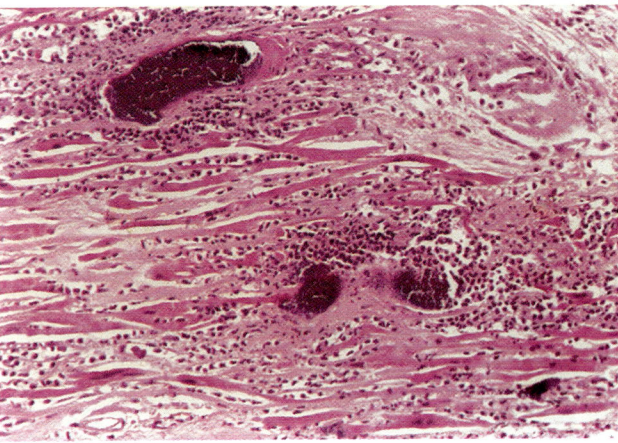

Fig. 8.11b: Myocardial abscess. Septic emboli (bacterial colonies) are seen within the blood vessels. Extensive myocarditis including myonecrosis is present

SUGGESTED READING

1. Archard LC, Bowles NE, Cunningham L et al: Molecular probes for detection of persisting enterovirus infection of human heart and their prognostic value. *Eur Heart J* **12(Suppl D)**: 56-59, 1991.
2. Aretz HT, Billingham ME, Edwards WD, Factor SM, Fallon JT, Fenoglio JJ, Olsen EGT, Schoen FJ: Myocarditis: A histopathologic definition and classification. *Am J Cardiovas Pathol* **1**: 3-14, 1987.
3. Baily GG: Parasitic infections of the heart. *J Infect* **37**: 2, 1998.
4. Datta BN: Parasitic diseases of the heart. In: Silver MD (Ed): *Cardiovascular Pathology* **2**: 1279-96, 1991.
5. Dec GW Jr, Palacios IF, Fallon JT et al: Active myocarditis in the spectrum of acute dilated cardiomyopathies: Clinical features, histologic correlates and clinical outcome. *N Eng J Med* **312**: 885-90, 1985.
6. Feldman AM, Mc Namara D: Myocarditis. *N Eng J Med* **343/19**: 1388-98, 2000.
7. Gore I, Saphir O: Myocarditis: A classification of 1402 cases. *Am Heart J* **34**: 827, 1947.
8. Horn H, Saphir O: The involvement of the myocardium in tuberculosis. *Am Rev Tuberc* **32**: 492, 1935.
9. Kandolf R, Ameis D, Kirschner P: *In situ* detection of enteroviral genomes in myocardial cells by nucleic acid hybridisation: An approach to the diagnosis of viral heart disease. *Proc Natl Acad Sci USA* **84**: 6272, 1987.
10. Kapoor OP, Mascrehans E, Ranaware MM, Gadgil RK: Tuberculoma of the heart. Report of 9 cases. *Am Heart J* **86**:334-40, 1973.
11. Kinare SG: Interesting facets of cardiovascular tuberculosis. *Ind J Surg* **37**: 144-51, 1975.
12. Litovsky SH, Burke AP, Virmani R: Giant cell myocarditis: An entity distinct from sarcoidosis characterised by multiphasic myocyte destruction by cytotoxic. T cells and histiocytic giant cells. *Mod Pathol* **9(12)**: 1126-34, 1996.
13. Pillary SV, Bhigjee AI: Myocardial tuberculosis and polycythemia. *S Afr Med J* **54**: 453, 1978.
14. Ratner SJ, Fenoglio JJ Jr, Ursell PC: Utility of endomyocardial biopsy in the diagnosis of cardiac sarcoidosis. *Chest* **90**: 528, 1986.
15. Silverman KJ, Hutchins GB, Bulkley BM: Cardiac sarcoid: A clinicopathological evaluation of 84 unselected patients with systemic sarcoidosis *Circulation* **58**: 1024, 1978.
16. Valentine H, McKenna W, Mihoyannopoulos P: Sarcoidosis: A pattern of clinical and morphological presentation. *Br Heart J* **57**: 256-63, 1987.

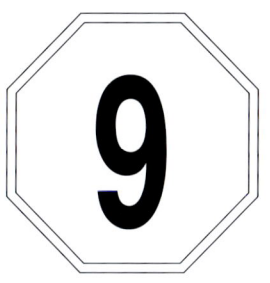

Cardiomyopathy

Cardiomyopathy is a group of heart muscle diseases of unknown cause. The etiology suggested is multifactorial. Four major types have been recognised: (i) Dilated, (ii) Hypertrophic, (iii) Restrictive and (iv) Arrhythmogenic right ventricular dysplasia/cardiomyopathy.

Dilated Cardiomyopathy

Dilated cardiomyopathy (DCM) is characterised by marked dilatation of all chambers of the heart particularly the ventricles. The contractile ability of the heart is much impaired resulting in reduced ejection fraction. Essential to the diagnosis of DCM is a systematic exclusion of coronary artery disease, valvular, hypertensive and congenital heart disease, cor pulmonale and any recognisable infiltrative disorder of the myocardium that results in heart failure.

Gross examination reveals oversized and overweight hearts which are globular in shape (Fig. 9.1). All four chambers are dilated (Figs 9.2 and 9.3). The ventricles show both dilatation and hypertrophy. Often the latter is masked by dilatation and thus hypertrophy may not be appreciated on gross evaluation. Mural thrombi are frequent and may be present in any chamber though left ventricular location is common. Consequently, thromboembolism may occur. Microscopically, a host of nonspecific features are encountered. The myocytes show marked anisonucleosis. Both hypertrophic and attenuated fibers are often admixed (Figs 9.4 to 9.7). Varying degrees of myofiber degenerative changes

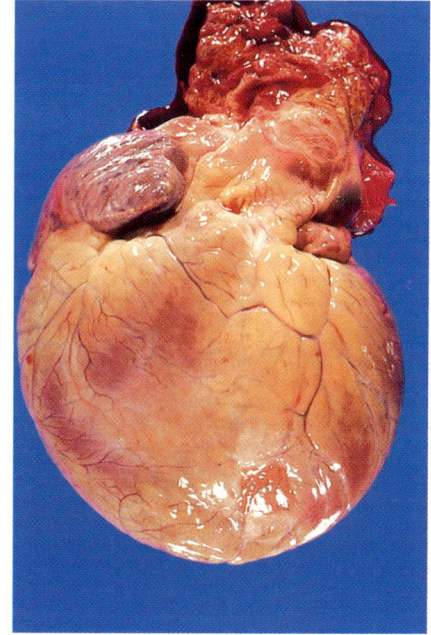

Fig. 9.1: Dilated cardiomyopathy. The heart weighed 550 gm. It is markedly enlarged and shows a globular shape due to dilatation of both the ventricles. The heart was soft and flabby to feel

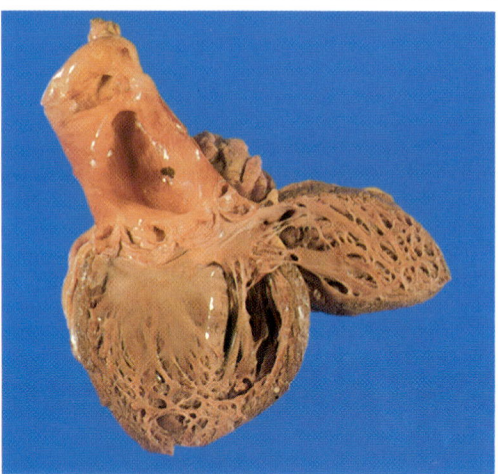

Fig. 9.2: Dilated cardiomyopathy. Left ventricle shows marked dilatation. The left ventricular outflow tract appears widened. The ventricular wall is appreciably thinned. Trabeculae carnea are thickened. The aorta and the aortic valve cusps are unremarkable. The circumference of the aortic valve is increased

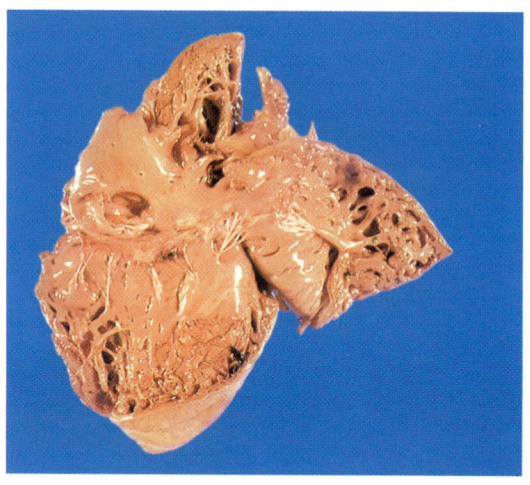

Fig. 9.3: Dilated cardiomyopathy. Opened up right side of the heart to demonstrate dilatation of the right ventricle, right atrium and tricuspid valve ring

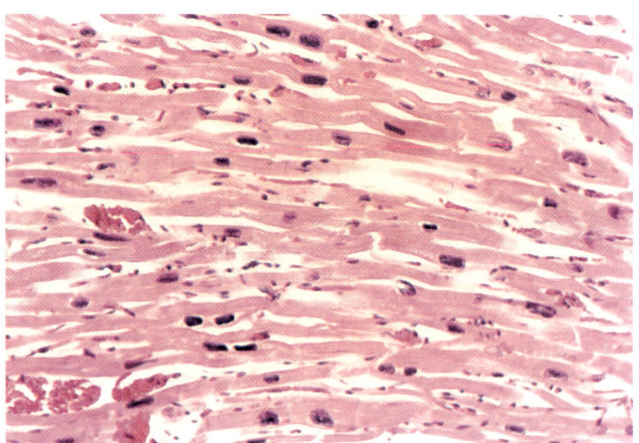

Fig. 9.4: Dilated cardiomyopathy. Myofibers show prominent anisonucleosis indicating hypertrophy

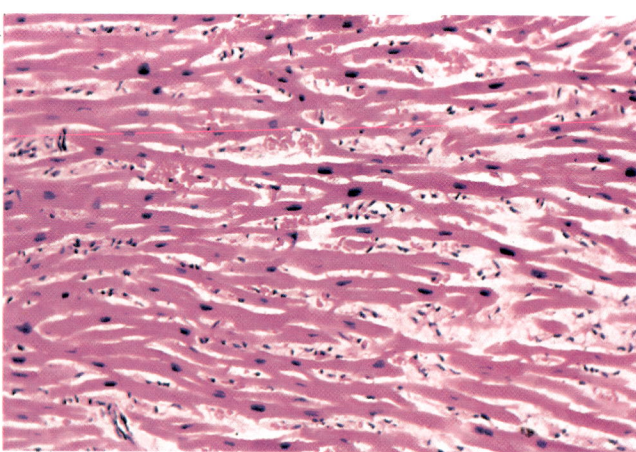

Fig. 9.5: Dilated cardiomyopathy. Hypertrophic and thinned out (attenuated) myofibers are admixed

Cardiomyopathy

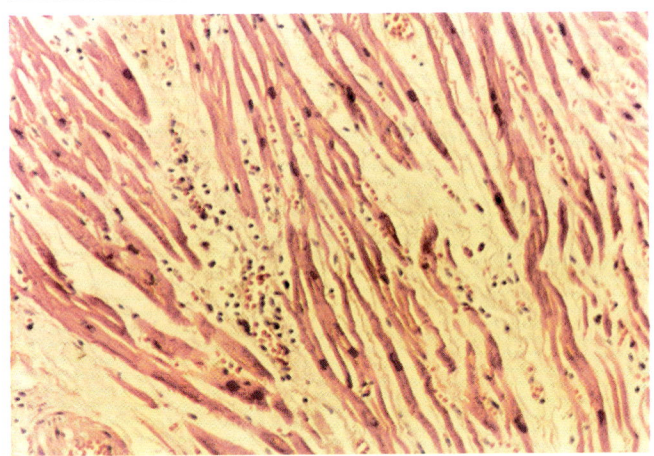

Fig. 9.6: Dilated cardiomyopathy. Attenuated and thickened myofibers are admixed. Anisonucleosis is observed. Mild fibrosis and lymphocytic infiltration is also present in the interstitium

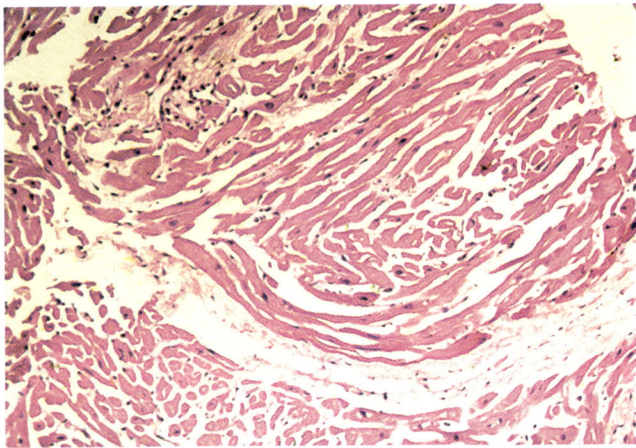

Fig. 9.7: Dilated cardiomyopathy. Hypertrophic and attenuated myofibers are observed. Mild interstitial fibrosis is also seen

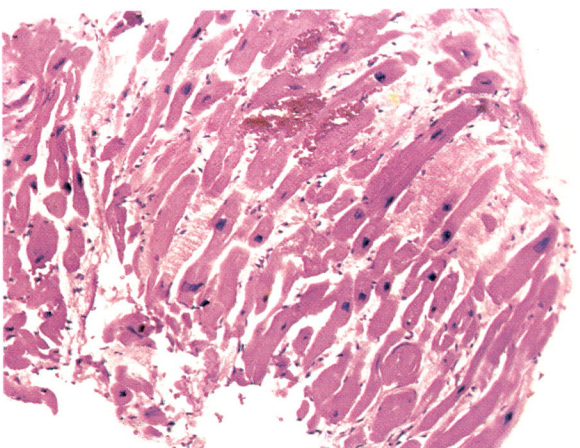

Fig. 9.8: Dilated cardiomyopathy. Myofibers show features of moderate hypertrophy. Prominent focal myocytolysis is also seen

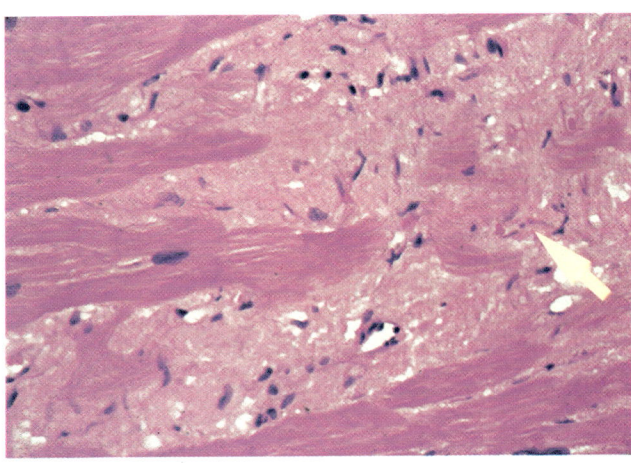

Fig. 9.9: Dilated cardiomyopathy. Myofibers are hypertrophic. Degenerative myofibers evident as tiny broken up fragments are seen (arrow). Fibrosis of the interstitium is observed

and/or myofibrillar loss is present (Figs 9.8 and 9.9 and Figs 7.4 to 7.9). Interstitial fibrosis is evident as perimyocytic or replacement fibrosis. In a few cases, focal myocarditis may be seen (Figs 9.10 to 9.13 and Figs 7.10 to 7.13). Diagnosis of myocarditis has to made using rigid criteria for the same (Ref. pages 95, 108). Prominent mesenchymal and endothelial cells are commonly misdiagnosed as inflammatory cells and therefore caution needs to be exercised. Endocardium is either normal or shows variable degree of thickening by fibrocollagen and some elastic tissue. Smooth muscle in the endocardium is encountered in some cases. **Endomyocardial biopsy** is often performed in DCM. This is with an aim to diagnose myocarditis which is then treated appropriately (Ref. pages 93, 95).

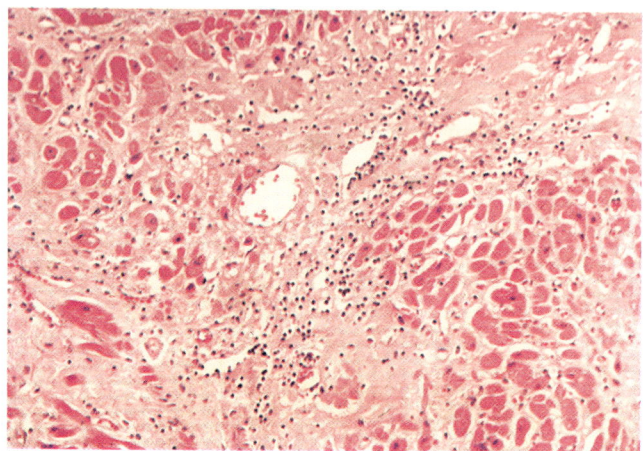

Fig. 9.10: Dilated cardiomyopathy. Large areas of myocardium reveal replacement fibrosis. The latter areas also show infiltration by lymphocytes. The remaining myofibers show features of hypertrophy

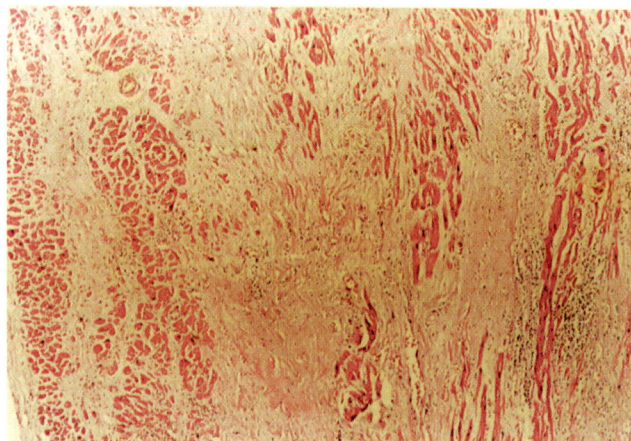

Fig. 9.11: Dilated cardiomyopathy. Extensive replacement fibrosis of the myocardium is noted. Focal infiltration by lymphocytes is observed. Myofibers are thinned and attenuated (right side of picture)

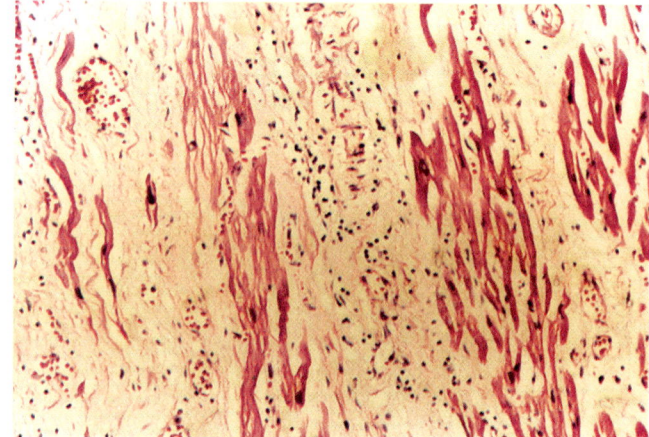

Fig. 9.12: Dilated cardiomyopathy. Prominent replacement fibrosis is observed. Thick and attenuated myofibers are present. These show focal degenerative changes. Infiltration of the interstitium by lymphocytes is also seen

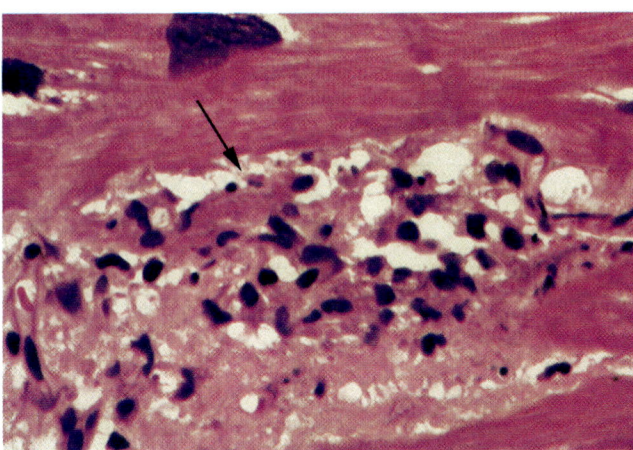

Fig. 9.13: Dilated cardiomyopathy. A focus of myocarditis is seen. Necrotic myofibers (arrow) are recognised amidst the inflammatory infiltrate. The cells consist predominantly of lymphocytes

Note: Changes observed in DCM are entirely non-specific and are observed in any end stage heart disease. The changes must be interpreted in the context of clinical/hemodynamic data

Etiology of DCM is unclear and several factors have been implicated. **Heredity** has a role in DCM and familial clustering of DCM cases is well documented in literature. **Familial** occurrence has been reported in about 20-25% cases. In some familial cases of DCM mutation in the **dystrophin gene** has been described. Familial cases show female preponderance. Mode of inheritance is usually autosomal dominant though X-linked and autosomal recessive patterns have also been described. Various factors/mechanisms are blamed in the etiopathogenesis of DCM. **Viruses** most commonly **coxsackie A and B** are believed to cause myocarditis which culminates in DCM. Viral specific RNA sequences and viral particles in myocardium have been demonstrated in some cases. **Immunologic** mediated injury is another mechanism suggested for the pathogenesis of DCM. Autoantibodies to beta-adrenergic receptors, myosin, M7 molecule and adenine nucleotide translocator carrying ADP/ATP complexes in mitochondria and intercalated discs have been demonstrated in some cases of DCM. Deranged cellular immunity and overexpression of certain cytokines has also been reported. Various genetic causes have been identified in familial cardiomyopathy. These include polymorphisms of MHC class II antigens, mutations in a specific gene involved in control of structural proteins, and genetic abnormalities in mitochondrial genomic material.

Alcoholic cardiomyopathy Alcoholic cardiomyopathy results from consumption of large quantities of alcohol over many years. The clinical picture is that of dilated cardiomyopathy which results from cardiotoxic effects of alcohol that is possibly due to its degradation to acetaldehyde. It has been demonstrated in animal models that acetaldehyde causes decline in mitochondrial function, protein synthesis, abnormalities in myofibrillary ATPase, etc. These biochemical changes result in fat accumulation within myocytes. On naked eye examination, the heart is enlarged with dilatation of all chambers. Microscopically increased fat deposition within myocytes is seen besides other features of dilated cardiomyopathy. Ultrastructurally, mitochondrial swelling, myofibrillar lipid deposition and myelin figures are observed.

Peripartum cardiomyopathy Peripartum cardiomyopathy (PPCM) may manifest at any time during the last trimester of pregnancy or the first 6 months of the post-partum period. This is characterised by signs and symptoms of dilated cardiomyopathy that are related to systolic dysfunction. Incidence of PPCM is greater in multiparous women and with twin pregnancies. In a large number of cases the cardiac size and function return to normal. The cause is not clear but several factors such as nutritional deficiency, myocarditis, small vessel disease, toxemia, response to fetal antigens, etc. has been suggested. Morphological features of PPCM are indistinguishable from dilated cardiomyopathy.

Drug induced cardiomyopathy A variety of drugs and heavy metals such as cobalt and nickel produce features of dilated cardiomyopathy. **Anthracycline derivatives** particularly doxorubicin (**adriamycin**) are antineoplastic agents that are used in the treatment of malignancies particularly in children. High dosages of this agent (550 mg/M2 for adriamycin) is cardiotoxic and causes features of dilated cardiomyopathy and heart failure in about 30% of patients. Cardiotoxic effects can be observed in endomyocardial biopsy which is used to monitor the dosages of this drug. The diagnostic changes, however, are best recognised under the electron microscope. Dilatation of the sarcoplasmic reticulum and myofibrillar loss are the two changes observed in adriamycin cardiotoxicity. The extent and severity of changes are graded for monitoring the dosages of the drug.

Cardiomyopathies associated with neuromuscular disease Cardiac involvement is well documented in various muscular dystrophies namely myotonic dystrophy, Duchenne's and Becker's muscular dystrophy, limb-girdle and fascio-scapulohumeral dystrophy and Friedreich's ataxia. These present commonly as various conduction and rhythm abnormalities. Cardiac involvement occurs in a large proportion of cases of Duchenne's and Becker's dystrophy. Involvement of the heart is also common in Friedreich's ataxia.

Restrictive Cardiomyopathy

Restrictive cardiomyopathy (RCM) is heart muscle disease wherein ventricular filling is impaired with normal or decreased diastolic volume of either or both ventricles. Systolic function is preserved. Increased stiffness of the myocardium results in decreased compliance. RCM includes endomyocardial disease namely endomyocardial fibrosis (EMF) and Loeffler's endocarditis and myocardial disease. Latter are infiltrative disorders ("Secondary cardiomyopathy") like amyloidosis, sarcoidosis, hemochromatosis, storage disorders ,etc. An important group having restrictive heart disease in the absence of the above disorders is termed as "idiopathic" or "primary" restrictive cardiomyopathy.

Hypereosinophilic syndrome (HES) This is also known as Loeffler's endocarditis. This is a systemic disease in which the heart is affected in about 70% to 80% of the cases. Clinical manifestations and hemodynamic data is one of restrictive cardiomyopathy. Endomyocardial involvement occurs. The early stage is characterised by vasculitis, eosinophilic myocarditis and endocarditis and thrombus formation that obliterates the ventricular cavity. In the later stages changes are indistinguishable from endomyocardial fibrosis which is believed to represent end stage of Loeffler's endocarditis.

Cardiomyopathy

Endomyocardial fibrosis (EMF) This disease is endemic in parts of Africa, South India, South and Central America and Asia and is of sporadic occurrence worldwide. Gross examination of the heart reveals biatrial dilatation and normal or decreased ventricular chamber size. Marked thickening of the endocardium is seen to affect either of one or both the ventricles. Inflow tract is affected and the process of fibrosis is diffuse which stops short of the ventricular outflow tract. The valve leaflets and/or chordae tendinea may be plastered by the fibrotic process. Consequently the ventricular cavity is narrowed/obliterated. Thrombus formation compromises the cavity further (Figs 9.14 to 9.22b). The

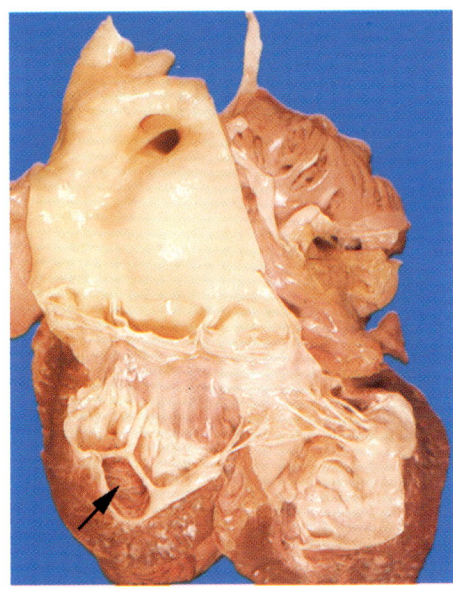

Fig. 9.14: Endomyocardial fibrosis. Opened up left ventricle to demonstrate part of the left ventricular inflow tract, apex, left ventricular outflow tract, the aortic valve and ascending aorta. The endocardium is markedly thickened and appears like a white curtain in the left ventricular inflow tract. A distinct cleavage is seen between the endocardium and the myocardium. Fibrosis stops short as a well demarcated ridge in the left ventricular outflow tract 2 cm below the aortic valve. Mitral valve is enveloped in the fibrotic process. Streaks of fibrous tissue (seen as thin white bands) are observed in the myocardium. Thrombus is seen at the apex (arrow)

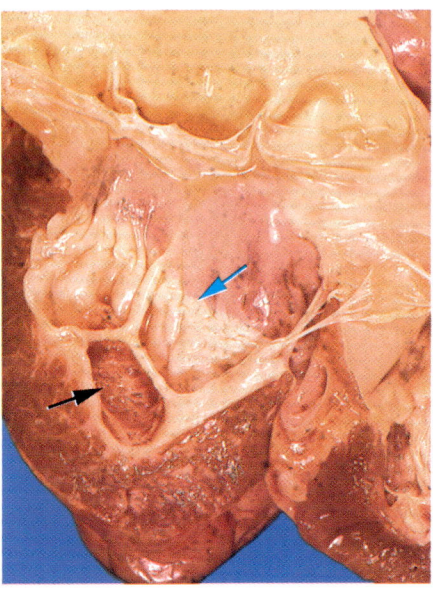

Fig. 9.15: Endomyocardial fibrosis. This picture demonstrates the left ventricular outflow tract. The abrupt ending of the fibrotic process is evident as a ridge (blue arrow). The subvalvular endocardium is normal. Apex shows a thrombus (black arrow head). Whitish specks (fibrosis) are seen in the myocardium. The aortic valve cusps are unremarkable

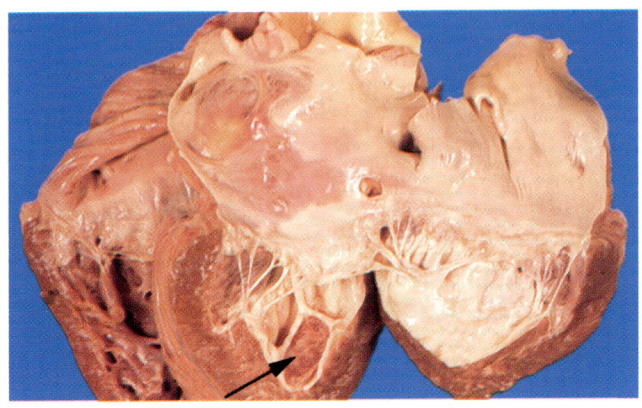

Fig. 9.16: Endomyocardial fibrosis. This photograph focusses on the endocardial thickening of the left inflow tract. The endocardium is markedly thickened and is seen to envelop the mitral valve. Its leaflets and chordae tendinea are plastered with each other and on to the posterior wall of left ventricle. Part of the thickened endocardium in the left ventricular outflow tract and thrombus at the apex (arrow) are also seen in the picture. Notice the fibrotic extensions into the myocardium of the left ventricular wall. The right ventricle is unremarkable

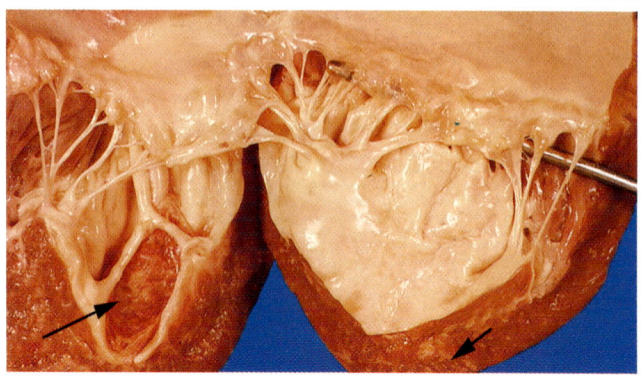

Fig. 9.17: Endomyocardial fibrosis. Higher magnification of figure 9.16 to demonstrate the marked endocardial thickening of the left ventricular inflow tract. The probe has been placed under the posterior leaflet of mitral valve to highlight the fibrosis and plastering of the leaflet and chordae tendinea to the endocardium. Thrombus is seen at the apex (Black arrow). Fibrosis is seen within the myocardium (Blue arrow)

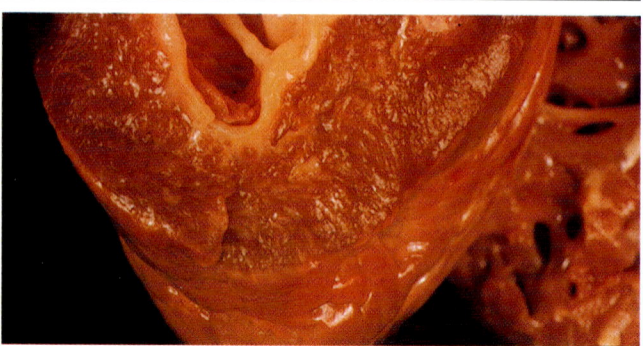

Fig. 9.18: Endomyocardial fibrosis. Photograph shows fibrosis within the left ventricular myocardium which is markedly thickened. Part of the apex with thrombus and thickened endocardium is also seen in the picture

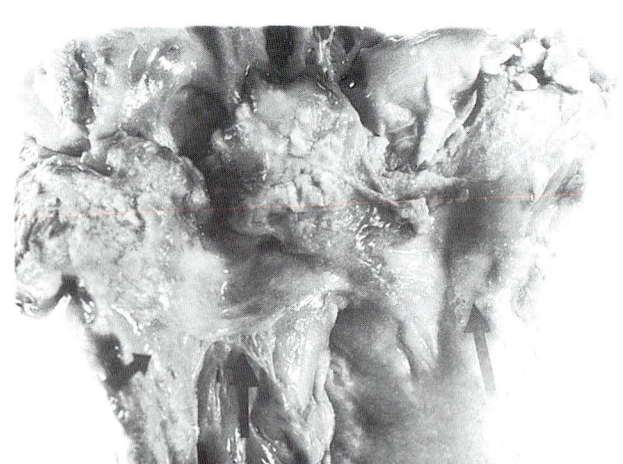

Fig. 9.19: Endomyocardial fibrosis. Opened up right side of the heart. The right atrial cavity including the appendage is filled with large pale yellow irregular masses (thrombus) that are projecting into the cavity and are adherent and incorporated into the wall of the atrium. The normal architecture of the tricuspid valve is lost. It shows fibrous thickening of the leaflets and chordae tendinea with encroachment by the thrombus. The thickened chordae are adherent to the posterior wall of the right ventricle

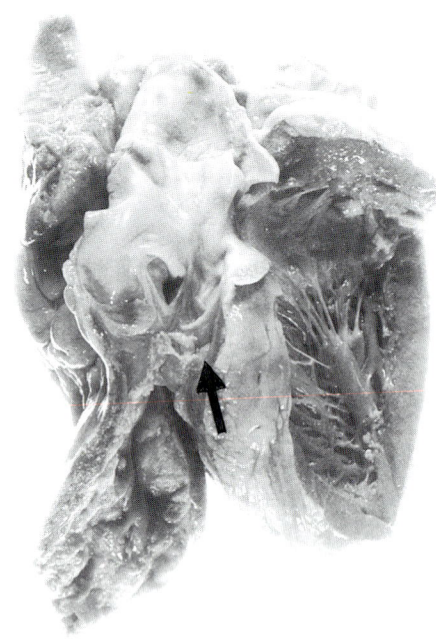

Fig. 9.20: Endomyocardial fibrosis. Opened up right side of the heart showing the right ventricular outflow tract. Latter is occupied by an irregular pale white mass (thrombus) which stops short abruptly below the pulmonary valve. The thrombus is also seen to line the right ventricular wall and is incorporated into it. Left ventricle included in the specimen is unremarkable

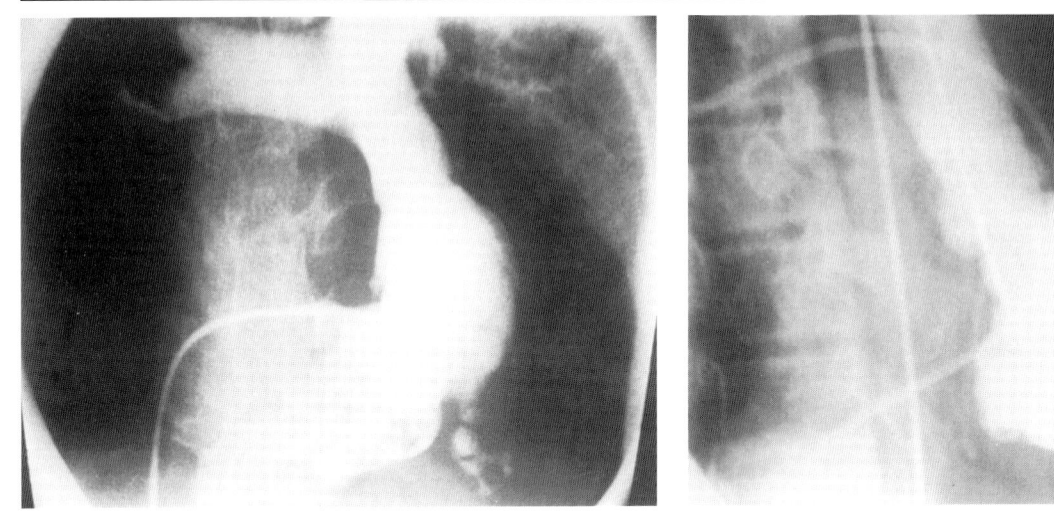

Figs 9.21a and b: (a) Right ventricular angiogram in anteroposterior view demonstrating obliteration of right ventricular apex, dilated outflow tract and small outpouchings (diverticulae within the right ventricular apex). (b) Left ventricular angiogram in anteroposterior view demonstrating apical obliteration with rounding of the left ventricular apex (first appearance)

Note: Patient was a 25 years old female presenting with features of congestive heart failure and dyspnea. The clinical picture and echocardiographic findings were suggestive of restrictive cardiomyopathy. The angiographic features illustrated above are those of biventricular endomyocardial fibrosis

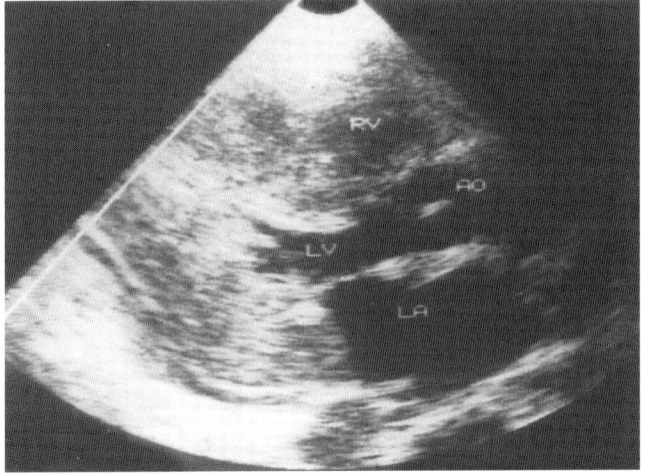 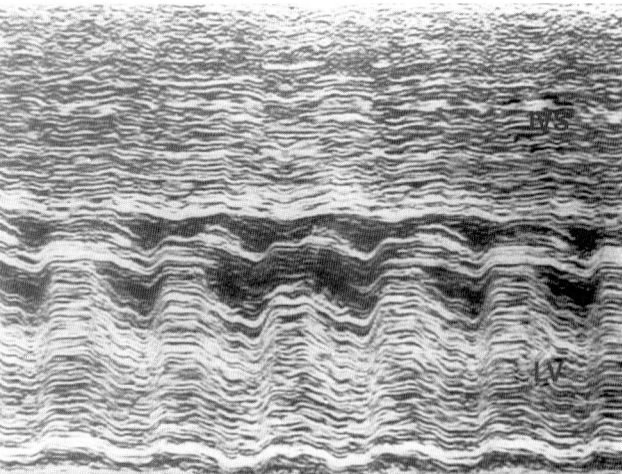

Figs 9.22a and b: (a) Echocardiography in parasternal long axis view showing markedly thickened and echogenic left ventricular wall. (b) M Mode echocardiography in the same patient showing markedly thickened left ventricular posterior wall (LV) and interventricular septum (IVS)

Note: Patient was a 60-year-old female who presented with features of restrictive heart disease

myocardium reveals streaks of fibrous tissue. Microscopic examination shows marked fibrocollagen thickening of the endocardium. Few elastic fibers are also admixed. Deeper endocardium (near the myocardium) shows numerous small and few large sized blood vessels. Inflammation is sparse. No eosinophils are seen. The fibrosis extends into the underlying myocardium and at times extensive interstitial fibrosis is present (Figs 9.23 to 9.33 and Figs 7.24 to 7.27).

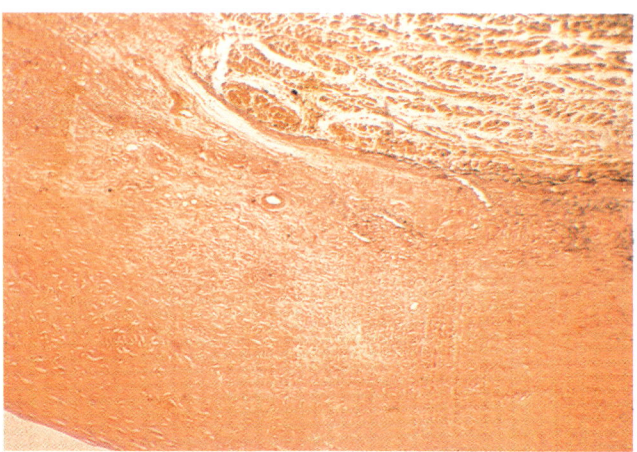

Fig. 9.23: Endomyocardial fibrosis. Photomicrograph shows marked thickening of the endocardium due to fibrocollagen tissue. Some blood vessels are present at the endocardial myocardial interphase

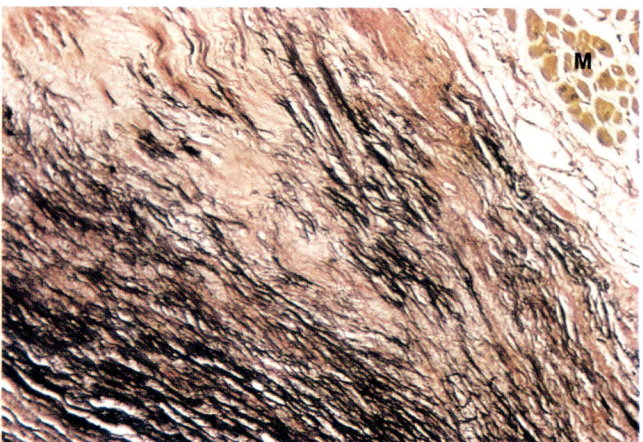

Fig. 9.24: Endomyocardial fibrosis. Endocardium is thickened. Elastic tissue stain shows abundant elastic tissue and interspersed fibrocollagen tissue is also present. Part of the myocardium is also seen in the picture (M)

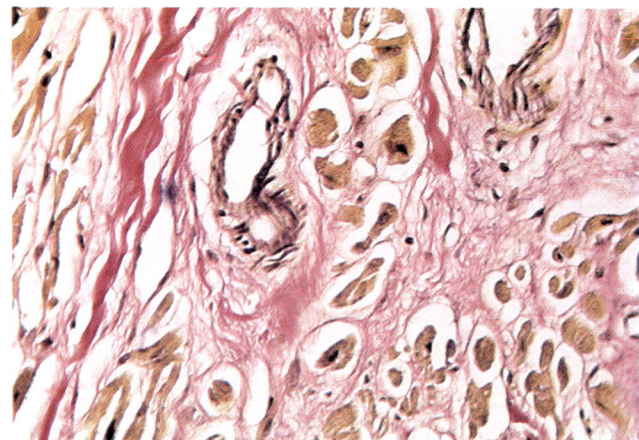

Fig. 9.25: Endomyocardial fibrosis. Fibrocollagen tissue deposition is seen in the interstitial tissue of the myocardium resulting in replacement of some of the myofibers

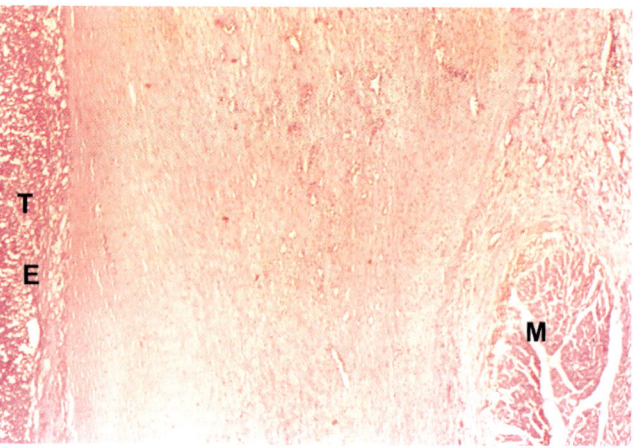

Fig. 9.26: Endomyocardial fibrosis. Endocardium is markedly thickened. Increased vascularity is noted. Inflammation is not present. Myocardium (M) is trapped within vascular fibroconnective tissue. Fresh thrombus (T) is seen on the endocardial aspect (E)

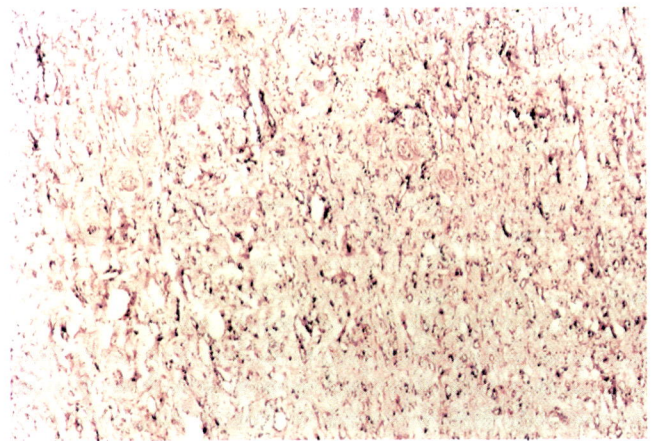

Fig. 9.27: Endomyocardial fibrosis. Part of the thickened endocardium to demonstrate numerous tiny capillaries in the fibroconnective tissue. No inflammatory component is present

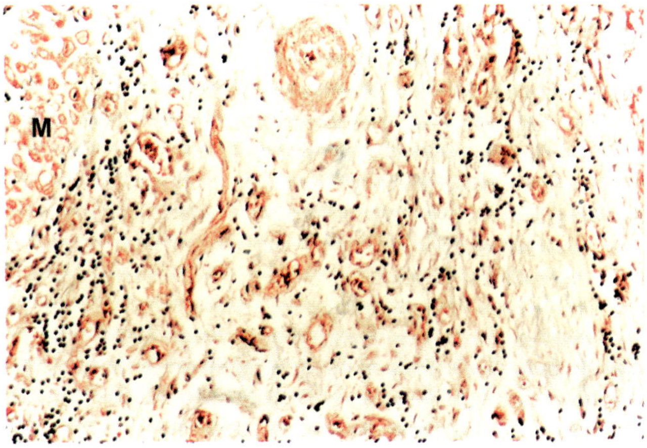

Fig. 9.28: Endomyocardial fibrosis. Masson trichrome stain. Numerous blood vessels and sprinkling of lymphocytes are seen within the thickened endocardium. M–Myocardium

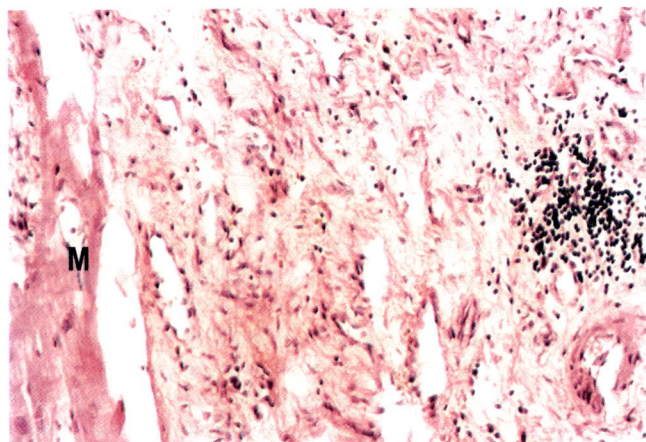

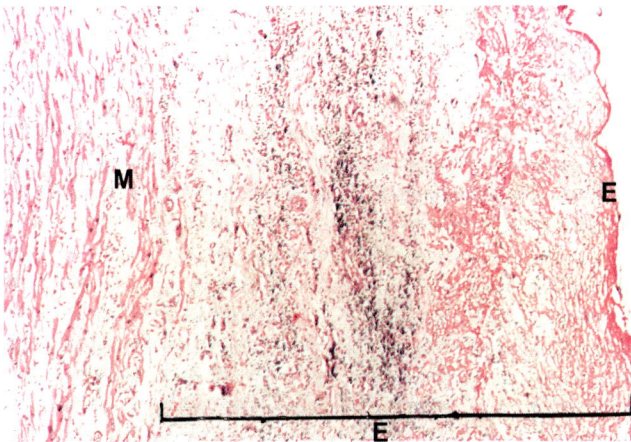

Fig. 9.29: Endomyocardial fibrosis. Numerous blood vessels and a focus of lymphocyte infiltration are seen in the deeper part of the thickened endocardium. M–Myocardium

Fig. 9.30: Endomyocardial fibrosis. Marked thickening of endocardium is observed (E). Note a band of inflammatory infiltrate consisting predominantly of lymphocytes within the thickened endocardium. Fibrosis in the interstitium of the myocardium is present. E–Endocardium; M–Myocardium

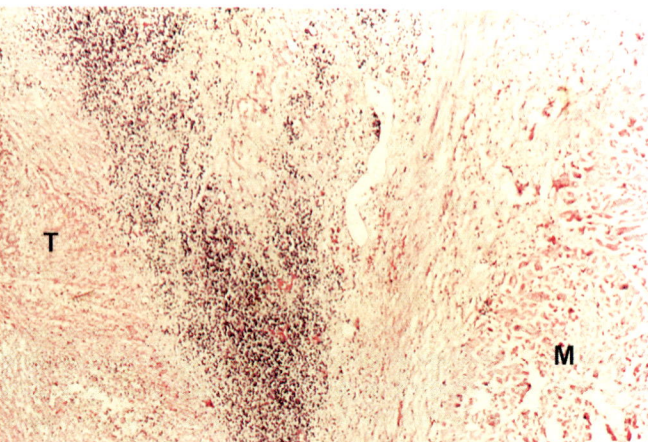

Fig. 9.31: Endomyocardial fibrosis. Dense lymphocytic infiltration is observed within the thickened endocardium. A fresh thrombus (T) is superimposed on the endocardium. M–myocardium

Note: This (Figs 9.27 to 9.31) was a case of right sided endomyocardial fibrosis with unusual morphological features. Patient was a thirty year old female who presented with low grade fever, abdominal pain, progressive development of edema over feet and distension of abdomen for 10 months. On basis of clinical and investigative data a diagnosis of endomyocardial fibrosis was suspected. The patient had a progressive down hill course and despite therapy, died. At autopsy the heart weighed 270 gm. The gross features are illustrated in Figures 9.19 and 9.20.

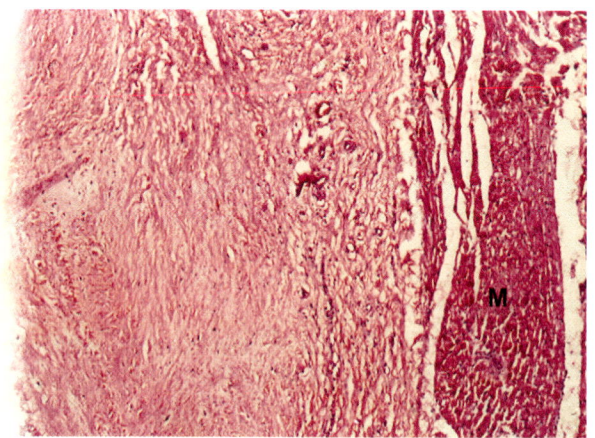

Fig. 9.32: Endomyocardial fibrosis. A young male was detected to have biventricular EMF. Surgical "stripping" of the thickened left ventricular endocardium was done. Photomicrograph shows marked thickening of the endocardium. Increased vascularity is present in the deeper endocardium in close apposition to the myocardium (M)

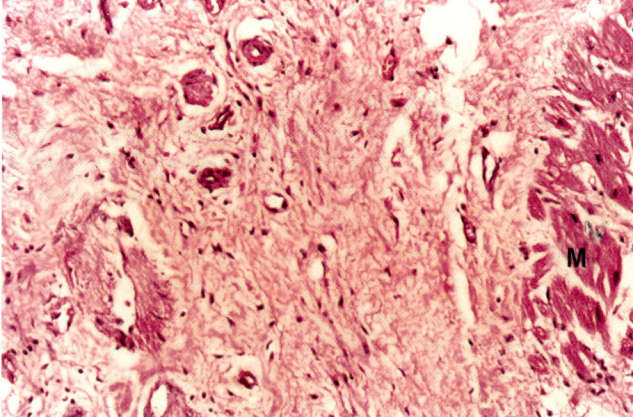

Fig. 9.33: Endomyocardial fibrosis. Prominent blood vessels are present in the deeper endocardium. M–Myocardium

Pathogenesis of endomyocardial fibrosis is far from clear. Hypereosinophilia, serotonins, nutritional deficiencies, excessive concentration or deficiencies of trace elements in tropical soil have been suggested though not proven.

Idiopathic Restrictive Cardiomyopathy

A substantial number of cases presenting with clinical and hemodynamic features of restrictive heart disease do not have any recognised morphological cause. This group has been designated as "primary" or idiopathic restrictive cardiomyopathy. No endomyocardial disease is present.

Gross examination of the heart shows biatrial dilatation while the ventricles are relatively normal sized. The ventricular cavity is normal as are the endocardium and pericardium. Microscopically, a number of non-specific changes are seen namely, myocyte hypertrophy and focal or diffuse perimyocytic fibrosis of variable degree in most cases. Focal myofiber disarray may be observed in a few cases (Figs 7.30 to 7.33).

Etiology of primary restrictive cardiomyopathy is not clear. There appears to be a genetic predisposition. Familial cases have been documented. An autosomal dominant inheritance pattern is seen. Some cases are associated with atrioventricular block and skeletal myopathy. Accumulation of abnormal isoforms of desmin as granulofilamentous material in cardiac and skeletal muscle have been described in some patients. It is believed that collagen network around myofibers limits diastolic relaxation.

Endocardial fibroelastosis (EFE) is encountered in childhood. It is characterised by diffuse thickening of the left ventricular endocardium due to proliferation of fibroelastic tissue. Elastic tissue is arranged in well-oriented parallel profiles. This endocardial change results in decreased compliance and impaired diastolic function of the ventricle. Endocardial fibroelastosis is associated with congenital cardiac abnormalities namely, aortic valve stenosis, mitral valve stenosis and anomalous coronary arteries. Endocardial fibroelastosis may also occur consequent to injury/damage to the left ventricular muscle in childhood. A subset of cases of mumps virus induced myocarditis may culminate in EFE.

Cardiac amyloidosis This is one of the infiltrative disorders of the heart that manifests as restrictive cardiomyopathy. Cardiac amyloidosis affects more commonly men than women and occurs usually in later life. Amyloid deposition in heart occurs in the following forms:

Primary amyloidosis amyloid is immunoglobulin type comprising of immunoglobulin light chain (amyloid AL) and is associated with immunocyte dyscrasia.

Secondary amyloidosis amyloid deposition is consequent to long standing infection in the body and the amyloid material comprises acute phase serum amyloid A (amyloid AA).

Genetic/familial form in which the deposits are parts of the prealbumin transthyretin protein which normally binds thyroxin (amyloid AF).

Senile amyloidosis Involvement is either confined to the atria (IAA) or affects both atria and ventricles. Isolated atrial amyloidosis originates probably from atrial natriuretic factor of atrial myocytes. Amyloid deposition is variable and may be silent or extensive enough to result in cardiac failure.

Primary (AL) and heredofamilial (AF) amyloidosis are commoner than secondary amyloidosis (AA).

Regardless of the type of cardiac amyloidosis the morphological appearances are identical. Atria are mildly dilated. The ventricular walls are thickened, firm and rubbery. In some cases asymmetric thickening of the septum may be present thus simulating hypertrophic cardiomyopathy. Microscopically amyloid deposits are seen in the interstices of the myofibers causing myocyte atrophy and/or loss. Endocardium, wall of blood vessels, valves and the epicardial fat is also involved in a large number of cases (Figs 9.34 to 9.38 and 7.28 to 7.29). Amyloid deposition may also occur in the SA node, AV node and the bundle branches. Latter is associated with conduction disturbances which are more frequently observed in the familial form.

Clinical manifestations of cardiac amyloidosis include features of restrictive cardiomyopathy, congestive heart failure due to rigid and non-compliant ventricles and cardiac conduction disturbances. Orthostatic hypotension occurs in some cases either due to the amyloid infiltration of the autonomic nervous system or blood vessels.

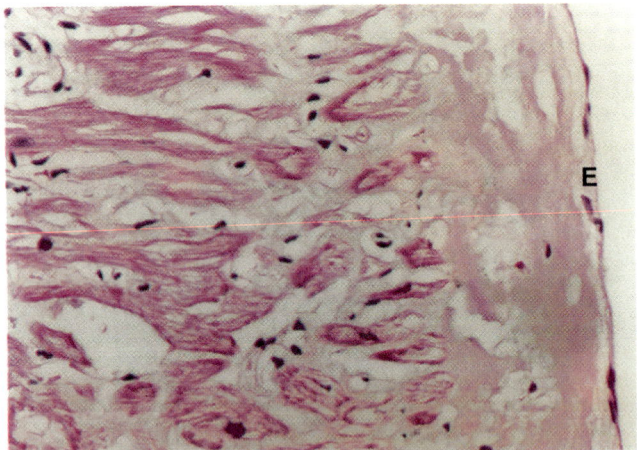

Fig. 9.34: Cardiac amyloidosis. Pale pink homogeneous material characterised as amyloid is present in the subendocardial (E) and interstitial tissue of the myocardium. This material is in close apposition to the myofibers

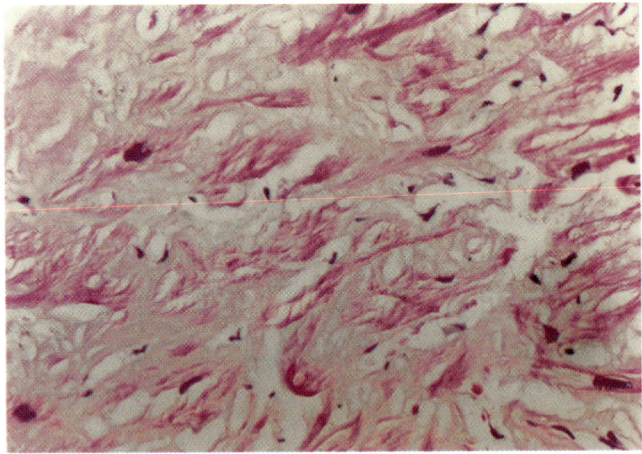

Fig. 9.35: Cardiac amyloidosis. Pale pink material is deposited in the interstitium in the perimyocytic region. The myofibers show varying grades of compression by the material. Latter showed positive birefringence on congo red staining and fluorescence with thioflavin T

Cardiomyopathy

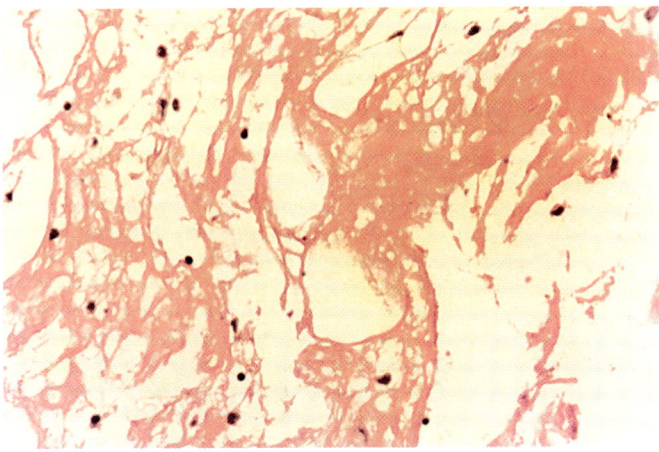

Fig. 9.36: Cardiac amyloidosis. Amyloid material deposits are present in the wall of adipocytes

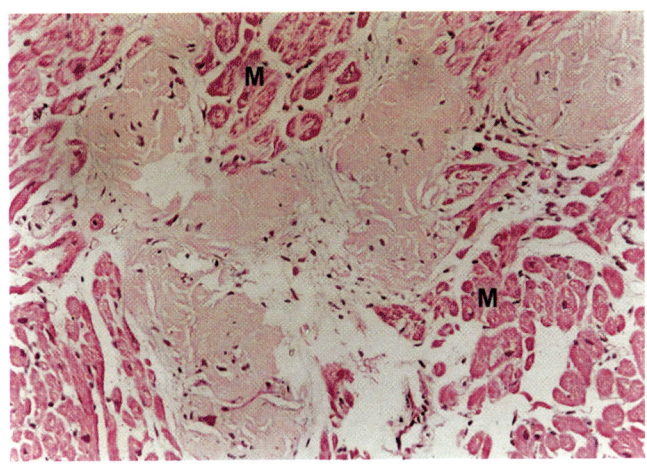

Fig. 9.37: Cardiac amyloidosis. Nodular perivascular aggregates of amyloid are seen. Myocardium (M) is unremarkable

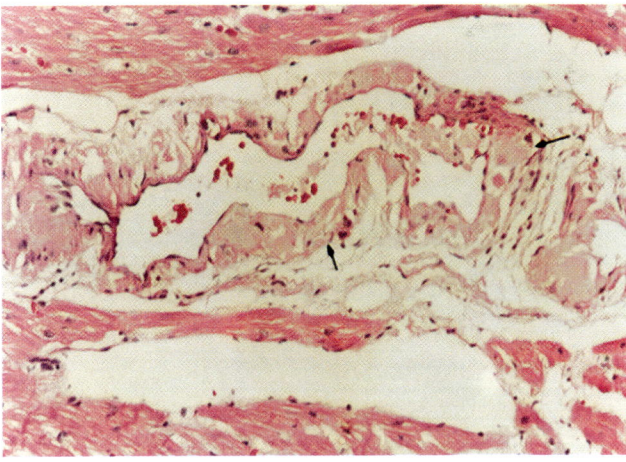

Fig. 9.38: Cardiac amyloidosis. Amyloid deposition (arrow) is seen in the wall of the blood vessel

Myocardial Storage Disorders

Hemochromatosis and hemosiderosis
Hemochromatosis is characterised by excessive deposition of iron in heart and several other parenchymal tissues. It may be present in various forms:
1. Familial or idiopathic disorder,
2. In association with ineffective erythropoiesis,
3. With excessive iron intake for a long duration and
4. In chronic liver disease.

Cardiac involvement may present with features of dilated or restrictive cardiomyopathy (Figs 9.39 and 9.40).

Fabry disease
Fabry disease is an X-linked disorder of glycosphingolipid metabolism due to the deficiency of the enzyme ceramide trihexosidase. Besides myocardium, skin, kidney, peripheral nerves and central nervous system are the seats of accumulation of the abnormal metabolic product. Latter is deposited within the lysosomes. Involvement of myocardium, endothelium, conduction tissues and cardiac valves, most commonly the mitral valve occurs. Clinical manifestations include systemic and renal hypertension, mitral valve prolapse and congestive heart failure. Left ventricular wall thickness often disproportionate simulates hypertrophic cardiomyopathy. Histologically, hypertrophied myocytes, myofiber disarray and vacuolisation of myocytes is seen and the picture may be indistinguishable from hypertrophic cardiomyopathy. Electron microscopy is diagnostic and shows concentric lamellae within myocytes.

Glycogen storage disease
The heart is involved prominently in type II (Pompe's disease) glycogen storage disease which results from a deficiency of a lysosomal enzyme, alpha-1, 4-glycosidase. It is a hereditary disorder transmitted through autosomal recessive gene on chromosome 17. Heart is enlarged and hypertrophied. The ventricular septum may be disproportionately thickened. Microscopically, marked hypertrophy of myocytes is noted. The latter appearance is due to accumulation of large amounts of glycogen both within lysosomes and free in the cytoplasm. Clinically, hypertrophic and/or restrictive hemodynamics are present. Pompe's disease is fatal usually within the first year of life. Diagnosis can be made in life by demonstration of enzyme deficiency in lymphocytes, skeletal muscle or liver. Skeletal muscle biopsy also shows evidence of glycogen accumulation.

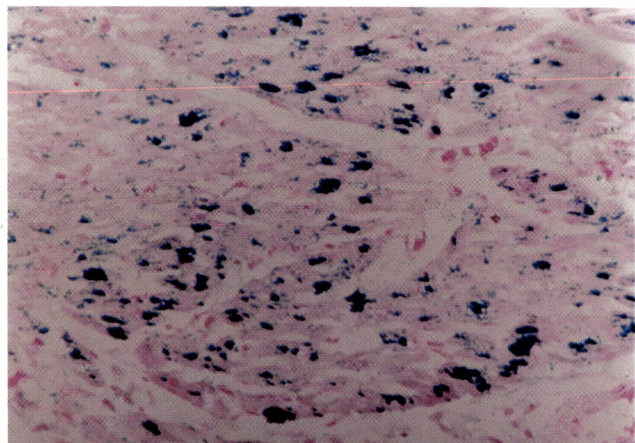

Fig. 9.39: Hemochromatosis heart. Prussian blue reaction to demonstrate abundant hemosiderin pigment in cytoplasm of myofibers

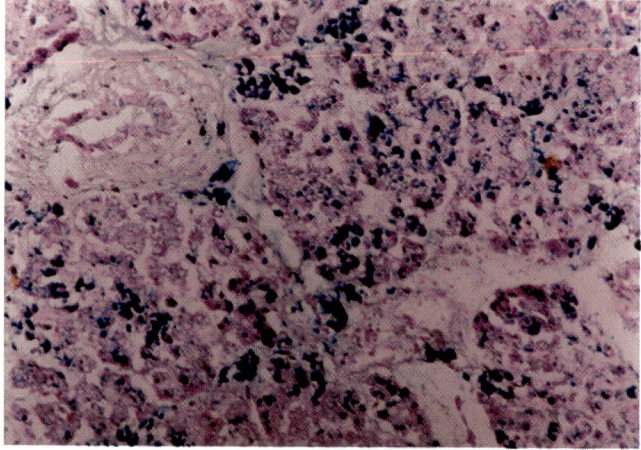

Fig. 9.40: Hemochromatosis pancreas of the same case as illustrated in Figure 9.39. Hemosiderin deposits are present within the exocrine pancreas

Note: This was a case of "bronze diabetes". Extensive hemosiderin deposits were noted in several organs

Hypertrophic Cardiomyopathy

Hypertrophic cardiomyopathy (HCM) also designated as hypertrophic obstructive cardiomyopathy (HOCM), asymmetric septal hypertrophy (ASH) and idiopathic hypertrophic subaortic stenosis (IHSS), is a type of cardiomyopathy which is characterized by impairment in the relaxation of the ventricular muscle and normal systolic function. It may manifest at any age. Common symptomatology includes angina pectoris, palpitations, syncope and dyspnea on exertion. While same cases may be asymptomatic others may manifest for the first time as sudden death. Severity of disease is more in young and familial cases.

Gross examination yields oversized and overweight hearts. The left vertricular wall thickness is increased and often exceeds 2.0 cm. The hypertrophic wall encroaches on the left ventricular cavity which consequently is distorted and diminished in size. Left ventricular hypertrophy may be symmetric or asymmetric. Asymmetric septal hypertrophy (ASH) is commoner and is characterized by disproportionate septal hypertrophy with a ratio of septum to posterior wall thickness being 1.3 or greater. Septal hypertrophy may involve either the entire septum or be localised to subaortic (when it is designated as IHSS), midventricular or apical region. Due to systolic motion of the anterior leaflet of mitral valve (SAM) it strikes with the septum where a "mirror image" imprint is formed. This is manifest by endocardial fibrosis. The corresponding mitral leaflet is also thickened. Right ventricle may be involved in some cases. **Microscopically,** myofiber disarray is a characteriztic feature (but not diagnostic). This is recognized by bizarre appearance of myocytes that are short, thick and branching and appear as whorling or woven patterns around areas of fibrosis (Figs 9.41 to 9.43). Ultrastructurally, myofibrillar disorganization is observed. Intramyocardial blood vessels show thickening of their wall. Prominent myocardial hypertrophy is present often with perinuclear vacuolation (Figs 9.42 and 9.43). Endocardium particularly in the subaortic region is thickened by fibrocollagen tissue. Granulation tissue with a few inflammatory cells may be observed in some cases.

It is important to remember that myofiber disarray is not pathognomonic of HCM. Small foci

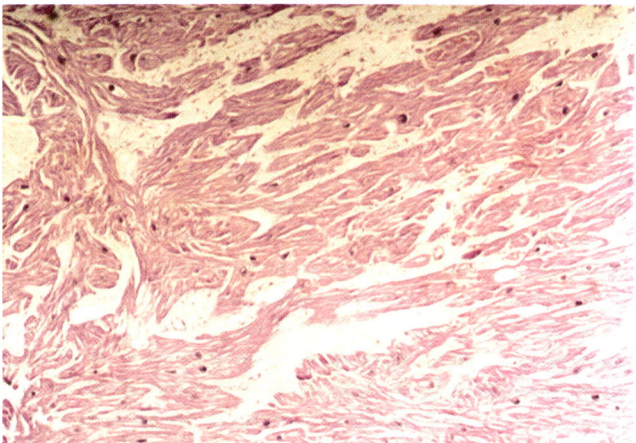

Fig. 9.41: Hypertrophic cardiomyopathy. Myofibers are short and hypertrophic and reveal disarray. Interstitial fibrosis is also present

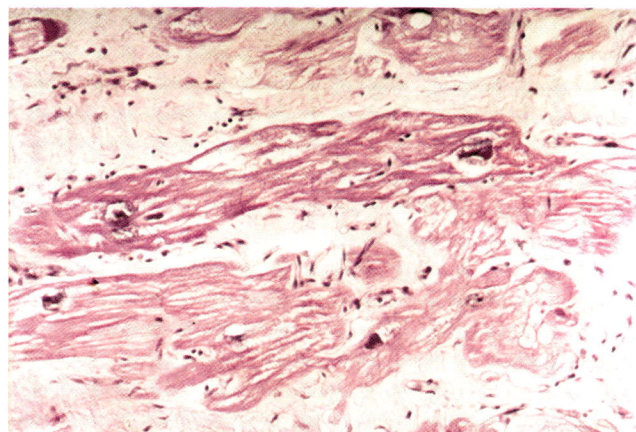

Fig. 9.42: Hypertrophic cardiomyopathy. Hypertrophic myofibers show anisonucleosis and prominent cytoplasmic and perinuclear vacuolation. Interstitial fibrosis is seen

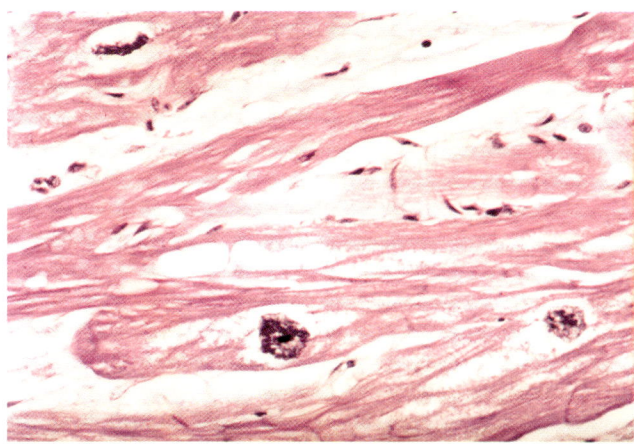

Fig. 9.43: Hypertrophic cardiomyopathy. Myofibers show anisonucleosis and striking perinuclear vacuolation

of disarray have been observed in ventricular septum in some acquired and congenital heart diseases and in normal infants. In HCM, therefore the extent of disorganized myocytes is more than the other situations where it is only focal.

Etiology of HCM is ill-understood. However several important observations regarding etiopathogenesis have been made. In over 50% cases the disease is **familial** with an **autosomal dominant** pattern. Remainder of the cases are sporadic. **Genetic** abnormalities of beta heavy chain cardiac myosin have been identified in familial cases. Missense mutations and deletions in the DNA coding the beta heavy chain myosin gene on chromosome 14 have also been demonstrated.

Arrhythmogenic Right Ventricular Dysplasia (ARVD)

Arrhythmogenic right ventricular dysplasia has been identified as a form of cardiomyopathy. It is characterized by fibro fatty infiltration of myocytes affecting the right ventricle mostly resulting in thinning of the ventricle. ARVD is recognized clinically by ventricular fibrillation, ventricular extrasystoles, supraventricular tachycardia, right ventricular failure and sudden death in young persons in some cases. The disease usually presents in adolescence and adulthood though a few cases have been reported in the pediatric age group.

Gross examination of the heart in ARVD reveals myocardial thinning and dilatation of the right ventricle. Ventricular wall shows adipose and/or fibroadipose tissue in varying proportions. The entire thickness of myocardium may be replaced with predilection of right ventricular outflow tract and the anterior wall of the right ventricle. Right ventricular aneurysm formation may occur. Involvement of the left ventricle and interventricular septum in some cases has also been described. **Microscopic examination** reveals transmural fibrofatty replacement of the myocardium with myocyte atrophy of the remnant fibers. Myocardial fat infiltration is seen in the right ventricle most extensive in the right ventricular outflow tract and lateral apex. Lymphocytic myocarditis is observed in a high proportion of cases (Figs 9.44 to 9.47).

Pathogenesis of ARVD is unclear. Familial occurrence and autosomal dominant inheritance is well-documented. It has been linked to a gene located in chromosome 14q, 23q, 24q. Presence of inflammatory cells in some cases may indicate involvement of infections possibly viral and/or immune factors.

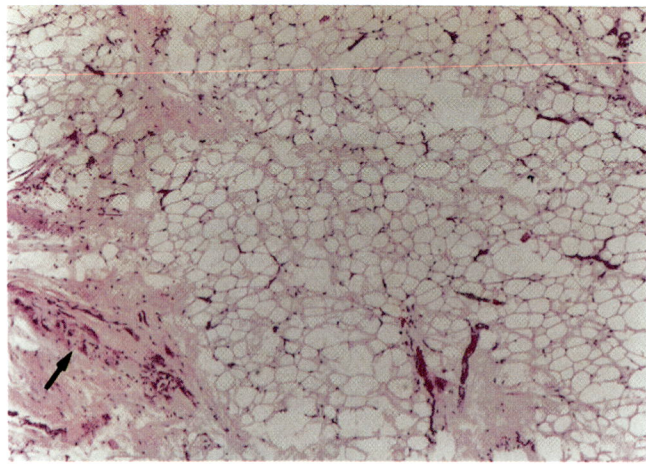

Fig. 9.44: Arrhythmogenic right ventricular dysplasia. Endomyocardial biopsy of anterior wall of right ventricle. The myocardium is replaced by sheets of adipose tissue. Only few remnant myofibers are recognised in lower left hand corner of the picture (arrow)

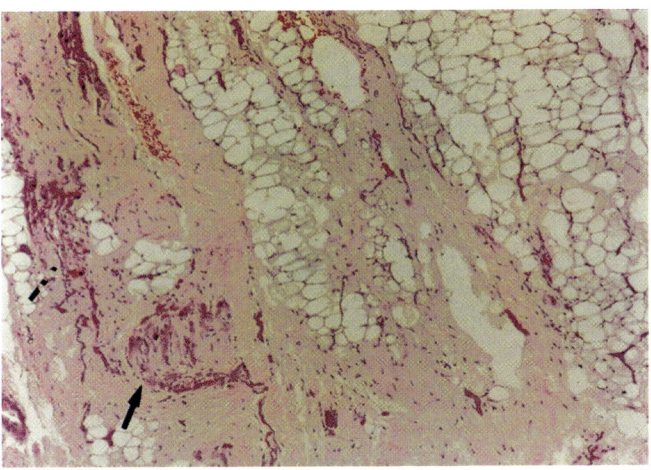

Fig. 9.45: Arrhythmogenic right ventricular dysplasia. The ventricular wall is comprised of adipose tissue and bands of fibroconnective tissue. Tiny islands of the myocardium are also seen (arrow)

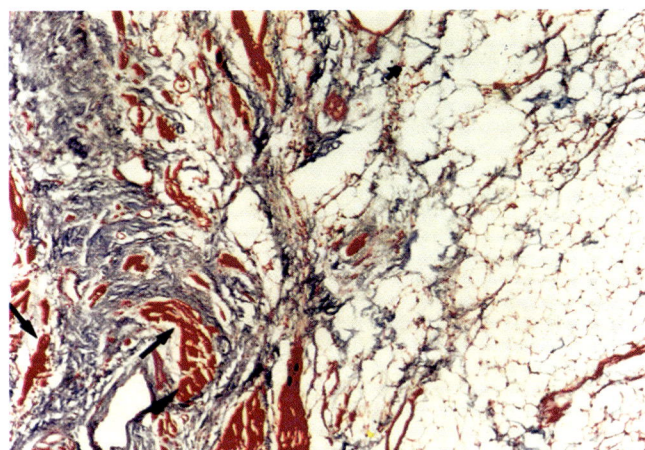

Fig. 9.46: Arrhythmogenic right ventricular dysplasia. Masson trichrome stain to demonstrate fibroconnective and adipose tissue infiltrating and replacing the myocardium. Only small islands of myocardium (arrow) remain

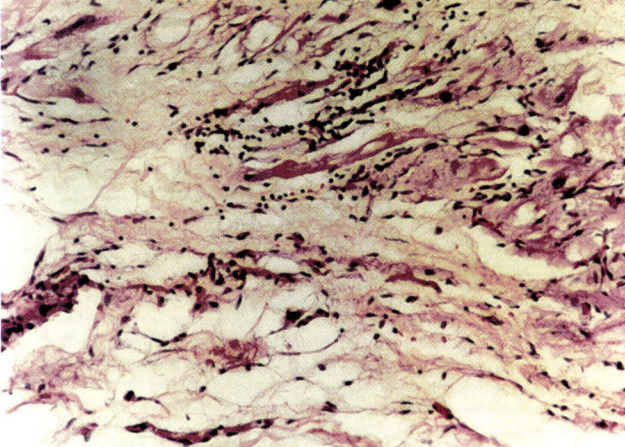

Fig. 9.47: Arrhythmogenic right ventricular dysplasia. Fibro-adipose tissue along with few myofibers are recognised. Additionally, lymphocytic infiltration is noted

SUGGESTED READING

1. Angelini A, Calzolari V, Thiene G, Boffa GM, Valente M, Daliento L, Basso C, Calabrese F, Razzolini R, Livi U, Chioin R: Morphologic spectrum of primary restrictive cardiomyopathy. *Am J Cardiol* **15; 80(8)**: 1046-60, 1997.

2. Arbustini E, Diegoli M, Morbini P, Dal Bello B, Banchieri N, Pilotto A, Magani F, Grasso M, Narula J, Gavazzi J, Gavazzi A, Vigano M, Tavazzi L: Prevalence and characteristics of dystrophin defects in adult male patients with dilated cardiomyopathy. A *Am Coll Cardiol* **35(7)**: 1760-68, 2000.

3. Basso C, Thiene G, Nava A, Dalla Volta S: Arrhythmogenic right ventricular cardiomyopathy: A survey of the investigations at the university of Padua. *Clin Cardiol* **20(4)**: 333-36, 1997.

4. Blankenberg F, Narula J, Strauss HW: *In vivo* detection of apoptotic cell death: A necessary measurement for evaluating therapy for myocarditis, ischemia, and heart failure. *J Nucl Cardiol* **6(5)**: 531-39, 1999.

5. Boura P, Lefkos N, Boudonas G, Kountouras J, Zacharioudaki E, Efthimiadis A, Tsapas G: Antigenic stimulation in T cell cultures in Cardiomyopathies: differences in cytokine profiles. *Eur J Immunogenet* **26(4)**: 285-91, 1999.

6. Brown CS, Bertolet BD: Peripartum cardiomyopathy: A comprehensive review. *Am J Obstet Gynecol* **178 (2)**: 409-14, 1998.

7. Chopra P: Pathology of cardiomyopathies: An autopsy analysis of 25 cases. *Acta Cardiologica* **32**: 1-15, 1977.

8. Corrado D, Fontaine G, Marcus FI, McKena WJ, Nava A, Thiene G, Wichter T: Arrhythmogenic right ventricular dysplasia/cardiomyopathy: need for an international registry. Study Group on Arrhythmogenic Right Ventricular Dysplasia/Cardiomyopathy of the Working Groups on Myocardial and Pericardial Disease and Arrhythmias of the European Society of Cardiology and of the Scientific Council on Cardiomyopathies of the World Heart Federation. *Circulation*. **101(11)**: E101-06, 2000.

9. Cuspidi C, Sampieri L, Pelizzoli S, Pontiggia G, Zanchetti A, Nappo A, Caputo V, Matturri L: Obstructive hypertrophic cardiomyopathy in type III glycogen storage disease. *Acta Cardiol* **52(2)**: 117-23, 1997.

10. Davies MJ: The cardiomyopathies: An overview. *Heart* **83(4)**: 469-74, 2000.

11. Felker GM, Hu W, Hare JM, Hruban RH, Baughman KL, Kasper EK: The spectrum of dilated cardiomyopathy. The Johns Hopkins experience with 1,278 patients. *Medicine Baltimore*. **78 (4)**: 270-83, 1999.

12. Fontaine G, Fontaliran F, Hebert JL, Chemla D, Zenati O, Lecarpentier Y, Frank R: Arrhythmogenic right ventricular dysplasia. *Annu Rev Med* **50**: 17-35, 1999.

13. Hayashi T, Shimomura H, Terasaki F, *et al*: Myocardial DNA strand breaks are detected in biopsy tissues from patients with dilated cardiomyopathy. *Clin Cardiol* **21**: 591-96, 1998.

14. Hayashi T, Shimomura H, Terasaki F, Toko H, Okabe M, Deguchi H, Hirota Y, Kitaura Y, Kawamura K: Collagen subtypes and matrix metalloproteinase in idiopathic restrictive cardiomyopathy. *Int J Cardiol*. **64(2)**: 109-16, 1998.

15. Kanodlf R, Sauter M, Aepinus C, Schnorr JJ, Selinka HC, Klingel K: Mechanisms and consequences of enterovirus persistence in cardiac myocytes and cells of the immune system. *Virus Res* **62(2)**: 149-58, 1999.

16. Katritsis D, Wilmhurst PT, Wendon JA, *et al*: Primary restrictive cardiomyopathy: clinical and pathologic characteristics. *J Am Coll Cardiol* **18**: 1230-35, 1991.

17. Kawai C: From myocarditis to cardiomyopathy: mechanisms of inflammation and cell death: learning from the past for the future. *Circulation* **99(8)**: 1091-100, 1999.

18. Koenen F, Vanderhallen H, Castryck F, Miry C: Epidemiologic, pathogenic and molecular analysis of recent encephalomyocarditis outbreaks in Belgium. *Zentralbl Veterinarmed B* **46(4)**: 217-31, 1999.

19. Kushwaha SS, Fallon JT, Fuster V. Restrictive cardiomyopathy. *NEJM* **336**: 267-76, 1997.

20. Maisch B, Portig I, Ristic A, Hufnagel G, Pankuweit S: Definition of inflammatory cardiomyopathy (myocarditis): On the way to consensus. A status report. *Herz* **25(3)**: 200-09, 2000.

21. Mestroni L, Rocco C, Gregori D, Sinagra G, Di Lenarda A, Miocic S, Vatta M, Pinamonti B, Muntoni F, Caforio AL, Mckenna WJ, Falaschi A, Giacca M, Camerini: Familial dilated cardiomyopathy: evidence for genetic and phenotypic heterogeneity. Heart Muscle Disease Study Group. *J Am Coll Cardiol* **34(1)**: 181-90, 1991.

22. Nishikawa T, Ishiyama S, Nagata M, Sakomura Y, Nakazawa M, Momma K, Hiroe M, Kasajima T: Programmed cell death in the myocardium of arrhythmogenic right ventricular cardiomyopathy in children and adults. *Cardiovasc Pathol* **8(4)**: 185-89, 1999.

23. Saffitz JE: Toward a clearer understanding of the link between viral infection of the heart and dilated cardiomyopathy. *Adv Anat Pathol* **6(3)**: 154-60, 1999.
24. Seki Y, Kai H, Kai M, Muraishi A, Adachi K, Tmaizumi T: Myocardial DNA strand breaks are detected in biopsy tissues from patients with dilated cardiomyopathy. *Clin Cardiol* **21(8)**: 591-96, 1998.
25. Shah G, Roberts R: Molecular genetics of cardiomyopathies. *J Nucl Cardiol* **7(2)**: 150-70, 2000.
26. Zachara E, Bertini E, Lioy E, Boldrini R, Prati PL, Bosman C: Restrictive cardiomyopathy due to desmin accumulation in a family with evidence of autosomal dominant inheritance. *G Ibal Cardiol* **27 (5)**: 436-42, 1997.

10. Cardiac Transplantation

Cardiac transplantation is an established therapeutic modality for end stage heart disease. Over 36,000 cardiac transplants had been performed worldwide between 1967 and 2000. With refinement of techniques of surgery, postoperative care, selection criteria of donors, care in transportation of hearts, revolution in immunosuppressive therapy and most importantly use of endomyocardial biopsy has provided improved survivals. Survival figures of 85%, 65% and 43% at 1,5 and 10 years respectively have been achieved in large centers. The recipients lead an appreciably better quality of life. The major limitation of cardiac transplantation programme is the donor pool. To overcome this much research is ongoing to examine the possibility of alternates to allograft transplantation of which xenotransplantation (cross-species transplantation) is being extensively researched upon.

In India, interest in cardiac transplantation was propogated through media with an aim to create public awareness. Following several public discussions and major meetings the "Transplantation of Human Organs Bill" received the Presidential assent in July 1994 following which India's first heart transplant was done at the Cardio-thoracic Center of the All India Institute of Medical Sciences, New Delhi in August 1994.

Table 10.1: Indications and contraindications of orthotopic cardiac transplantation

Indications	Contraindications
• Cardiomyopathy	• Advanced age > 70 years
• Ischemic heart disease	• Increased pulmonary vascular resistance
• Valvular disease	• Cytotoxic crossmatch between donor and recipient
• Congenital heart disease	• Generalised peripheral and cerebral vascular disease
• Retransplantation	• Irreversible hepatic damage or renal dysfunction
	• Active peptic ulcer
Donor heart exclusion criteria	• Drug addiction, including alcohol
	• Systemic illnesses that may limit life expectancy or
• Malignancy with metastatic potential	compromise recovery from transplantation
• Systemic sepsis or endocarditis	• Chronic obstructive/restrictive airway disease
• Significant coronary artery disease	• Active infection
• Anatomic heart disease	• Psychosocial instability
• Poor ventricular function	• Insulin-dependent diabetes mellitus

Indications of cardiac transplantation include cardiomyopathy (Figs 10.1 to 10.5), ischemic heart disease (Figs 10.6 to 10.8), valvular disease, congenital heart disease and retransplantation. Major indications, contraindications and donor exclusion criteria are indicated in Table 10.1. **Endomyocardial biopsy** has contributed importantly to the success of the cardiac transplantation programme. Sequential biopsies can be performed with ease and safety and provide the basis for diagnosis and monitoring of allograft rejection (Table 10.2). Pre-transplantation biopsies are done in all cases and evaluated. The patient's native heart is also carefully examined and changes noted in relation to myocardium including interstitium, endocardium, pericardium, valves and coronary arteries. Additionally, conditions known to recur in the donor heart can be recognised. Diseases documented to have **recurred from the recipient** in the allograft include amyloidosis, giant-cell myocarditis and Chaga's disease. Melanoma, HIV, toxoplasma and cytomegalovirus have been known to **recur from the donor.**

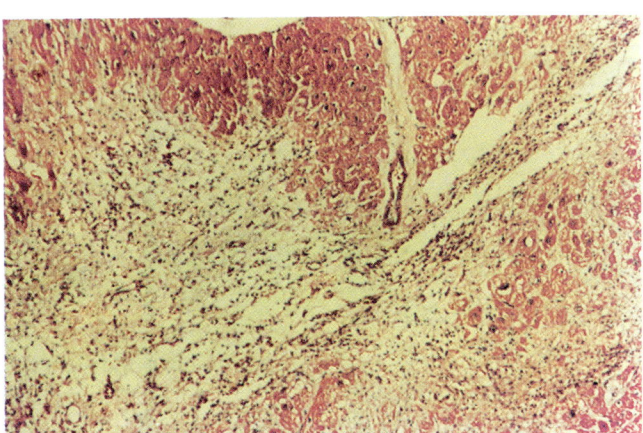

Fig. 10.1: Photomicrograph of explanted heart-from a case of dilated cardiomyopathy. On microscopic examination, multifocal microinfarcts with prominent myofiber dropout is a striking feature. Viable myofibers are seen at the periphery. These show prominent anisonucleosis. Coronary arteries were normal

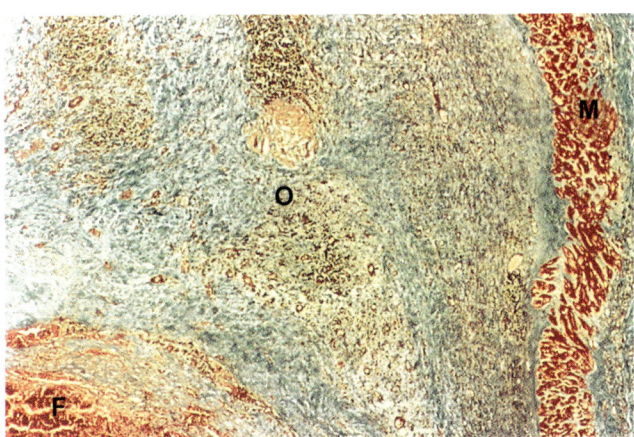

Fig. 10.2: Photomicrograph of explanted heart, from a case of dilated cardiomyopathy. Section shows fresh (F) and organised (O) thrombus overlying the apical myocardium (M) in the left ventricle (Masson trichrome stain)

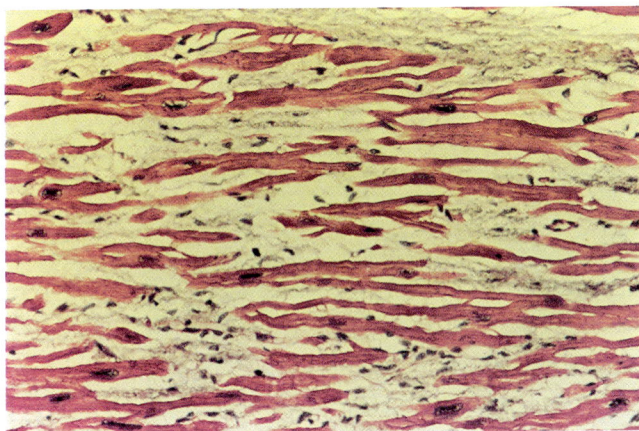

Fig. 10.3: Photomicrograph of explanted heart from a case of dilated cardiomyopathy. The picture shows attenuated myofibers admixed with hypertrophic ones. Notice the prominent nucleomegaly

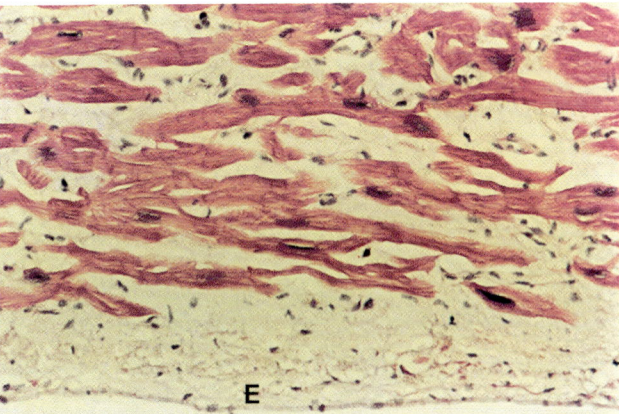

Fig. 10.4: Dilated cardiomyopathy. Photomicrograph highlights myocyte hypertrophy with prominent nucleomegaly. Endocardium (E) is unremarkable

Complications

Rejection and **infection** are the major complications of cardiac transplantation. Others are toxicity of immunosuppressive agents and late complications namely graft vascular disease, and post-transplantation B lymphoproliferative disorders (PTLD).

Graft Rejection

This may occur at different time intervals following transplantation. Various types of rejection are: (1) acute cellular rejection, (2) late or chronic rejection, (3) hyperacute rejection and (4) humoral or vascular rejection.

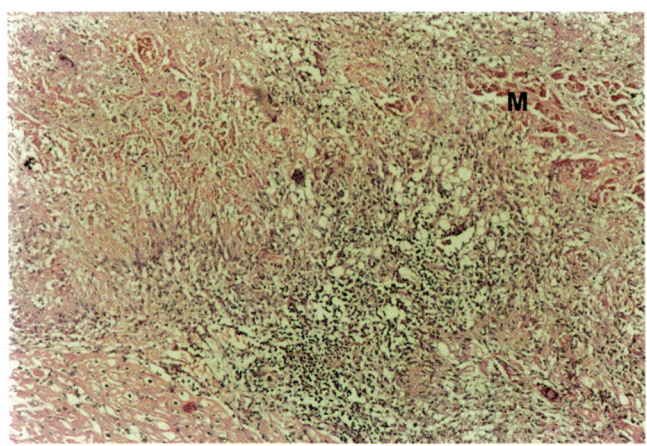

Fig. 10.5a: Explanted heart from a case of dilated cardiomyopathy. The picture shows extensive inflammation with giant cells and destruction of the myocardium. Necrotic myofibers (M) are observed

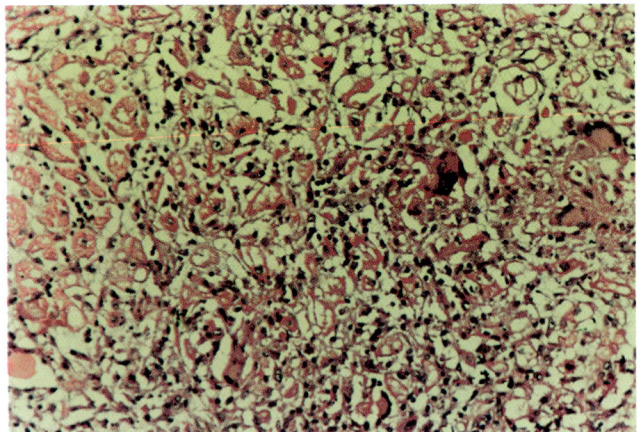

Fig. 10.5b: Explanted heart from a case of dilated cardiomyopathy (same case as above). The picture shows mixed inflammatory cell infiltrate, numerous giant cells and necrotic myofibers

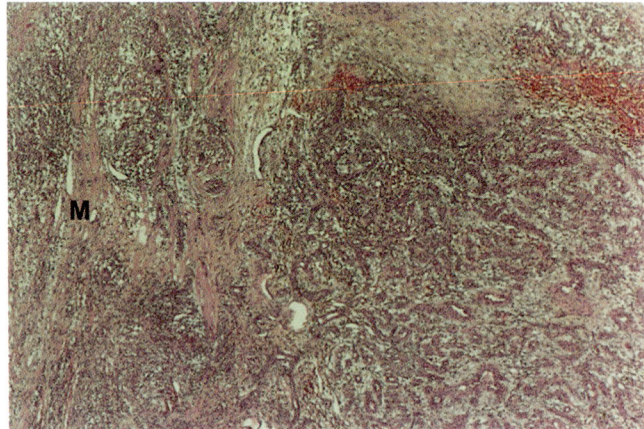

Fig. 10.5c: Explanted heart from a case of dilated cardiomyopathy. An organised thrombus is present in the right ventricle. Necrotic muscle (M) with giant cell myocarditis is also seen in left hand of picture

Note: Explanted heart from a clinically diagnosed case of dilated cardiomyopathy showed histological features of giant cell myocarditis. Figures 10.5a to c are from the same case

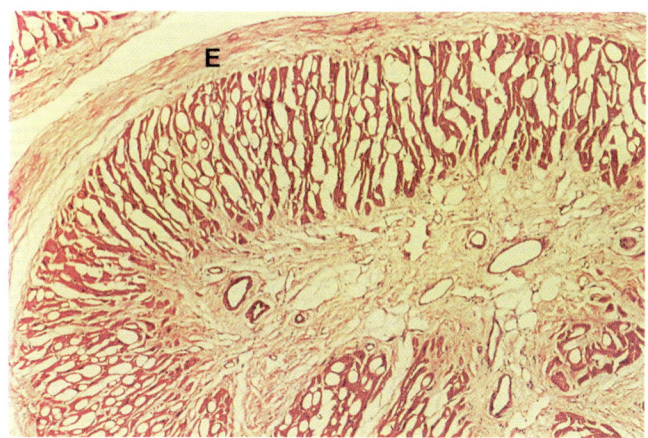

Fig. 10.6a: Explanted heart from a case of ischemic heart disease. Photomicrograph demonstrates uniform glycogen depletion (myocytolysis) of the subendocardial (E) myocytes

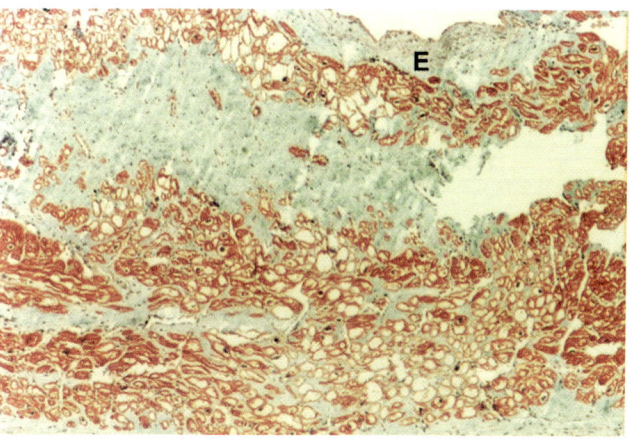

Fig. 10.6b: Explanted heart from a case of ischemic heart disease. Masson trichrome stain demonstrates replacement fibrosis of the myocardium. Prominent sarcoplasmic vacuolation of myocytes is observed. E–Endocardium

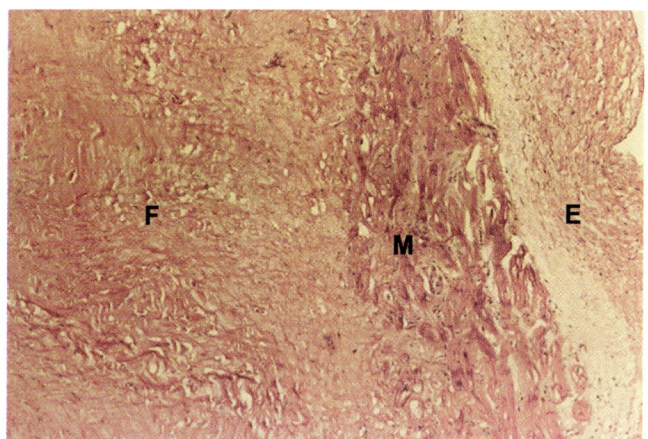

Fig. 10.7a: Explanted heart from a case of ischemic heart disease. Dense replacement fibrosis (F) of the myocardium, hypertrophy of the surviving myocardium (M) and thickened endocardium (E) is seen

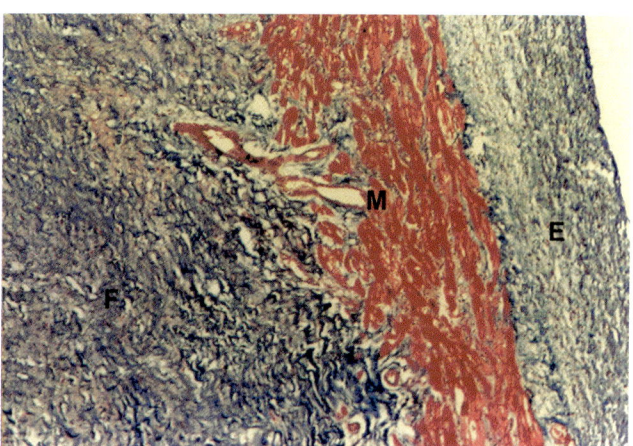

Fig. 10.7b: Explanted heart of a case of ischemic heart disease. Masson trichrome stain highlights myocardial (M) and endocardial (E) fibrosis. Large part of the myocardium shows replacement fibrosis (F)

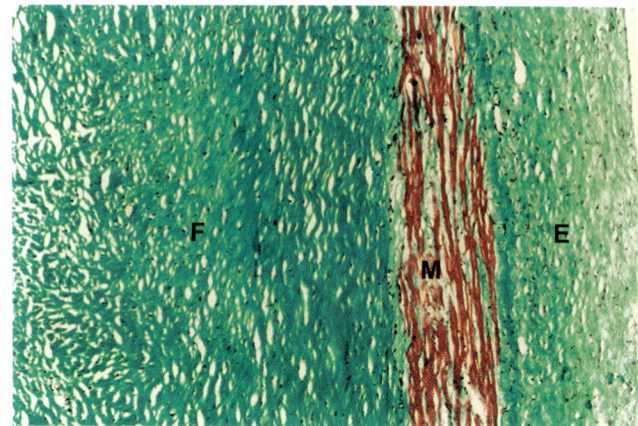

Fig. 10.8a: Explanted heart from a case of ischemic heart disease. Left ventricular aneurysm was present. The picture shows marked thinning and attenuation of the surviving myofibers (M) with dense replacement fibrosis (F) of the myocardium. Endocardium (E) is also thickened (Masson Trichrome stain)

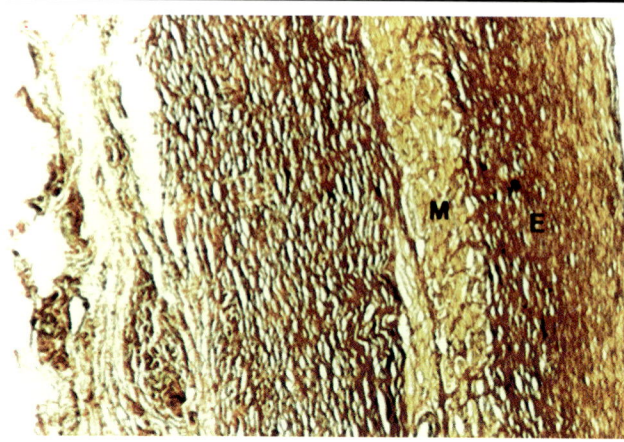

Fig. 10.8b: Photomicrograph of the same case as in figure 10.8a to show few elastic fibers in the thickened endocardium (E). Surviving thinned myocardial muscle (M) is also seen (Verhoeff-van Gieson stain)

Acute cellular rejection (Figs 10.9 to 10.12) This is the most common type of rejection experienced by nearly all patients. It is most common within the first three months but may occur at any time. Sequential endomyocardial biopsies are performed to monitor cardiac allografts. An international protocol devised by the International Society for Heart and Lung Transplantation (ISHLT) is used for diagnosing the various grades of rejection (Table 10.2). If changes of grade 3 and 4 rejection are seen in the biopsy, the patient needs to be treated. Grade 1 and 2 changes do not require extra therapy.

Table 10.2: Working formulation for acute cardiac rejection by the International Society for Heart and Lung Transplantation (ISHLT)

Grade 0: (ISHLT) No rejection	The myocardium is normal. No inflammatory infiltrate or myocyte damage is seen.
Grade 1A: (ISHLT) Mild rejection focal	This is a form of mild rejection. The myocardium shows one or more focal, perivascular infiltrates of activated lymphocytes. No myocyte damage is seen.
Grade 1B: (ISHLT) Mild rejection diffuse	This is also categorised as mild rejection and differs from grade 1A in that the inflammatory infiltrates extend into the surrounding myocardium.
Grade 2: (ISHLT) Moderate rejection unifocal	It is also known as focal moderate rejection and comprises a single focus. Myocyte damage is usually absent.
Grade 3A: (ISHLT) Moderate rejection multifocal	Also known as "low" moderate rejection. It is characterised by multifocal infiltrates which may be seen in the perivascular, endocardial or interstitial locations. Myocyte damage is prominent.
Grade 3B: (ISHLT) Moderate rejection diffuse	The infiltrate is diffuse and extensive and of a polymorphous nature-lymphocytes, eosinophils and neutrophils. Myocyte damage is prominent.
Grade 4: (ISHLT) Severe rejection	It is a severe form of rejection marked by diffuse and extensive hemorrhage, edema, myocyte damage and marked infiltration by lymphocytes and polymorphs. Vasculitis is often present.

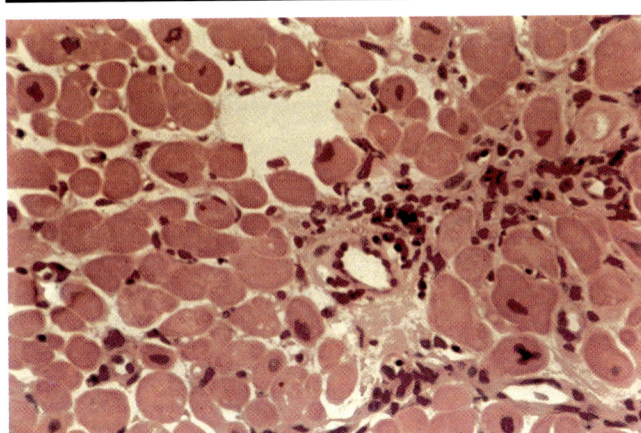

Fig. 10.9a: Post-transplant endomyocardial biopsy done 4 weeks after transplantation showing features of acute cellular rejection grade 1A (ISHLT). Perivascular lymphocytic cell infiltration is observed. The myocytes reveal hypertrophy as evident by nucleomegaly

Note: Myocyte hypertrophy is a common observation in cardiac allografts and can be seen as early as 1 to 2 months post-transplantation

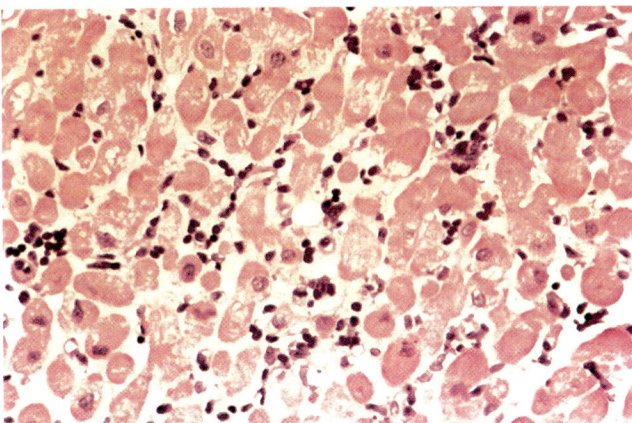

Fig. 10.9b: Post-transplant endomyocardial biopsy showing features of acute cellular rejection Grade 1B (ISHLT). This picture shows a sparse, diffuse interstitial lymphocytic infiltrate without myonecrosis

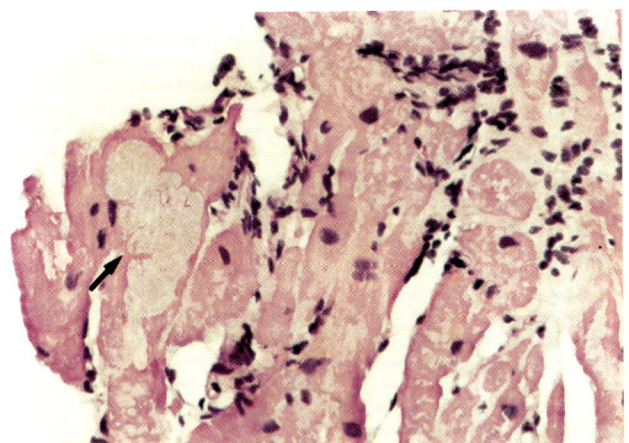

Fig. 10.9c: Post-transplantation endomyocardial biopsy. In the right hand side of the picture, the myofibers show basophilic degeneration (arrow). Diffuse lymphocytic infiltrate is present in the interstitium. The rest of the biopsy showed similar interstitial infiltrate and was diagnosed as acute cellular rejection Grade 1B (ISHLT)

Note: Basophilic degeneration is a non-specific accumulation of glycoprotein that is amphophilic on hematoxylin and eosin staining

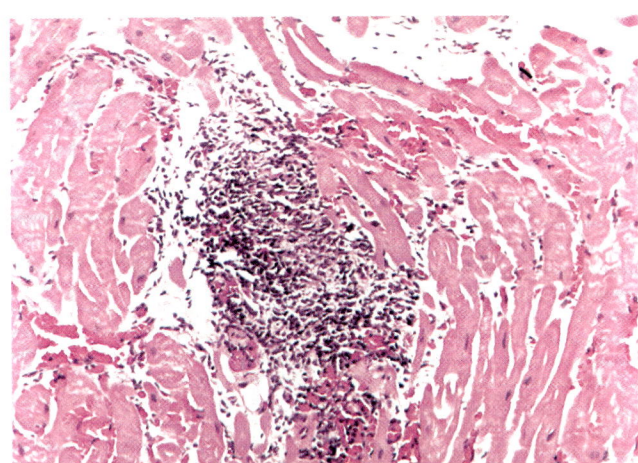

Fig. 10.10: Cardiac allograft rejection Grade 2 (ISHLT). A single focus of inflammatory infiltrate along with myonecrosis is seen. This was the only focus of inflammation in the four biopsy pieces

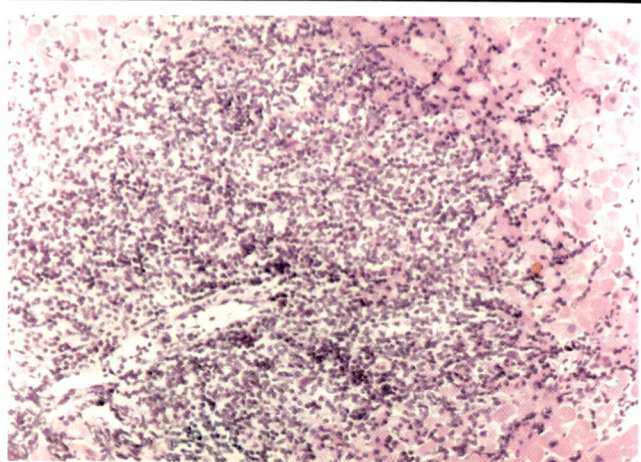

Fig. 10.11: Cardiac allograft rejection Grade 3A (ISHLT). Multifocal lymphocytic infiltrates were observed. In one of the biopsy fragments a large focus of interstitial infiltrate along with myonecrosis is seen

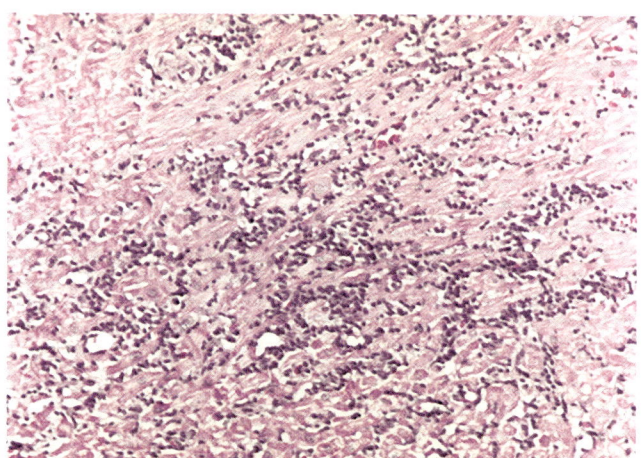

Fig. 10.12a: Cardiac allograft rejection Grade 3B (ISHLT). Diffuse and extensive infiltrate is present in the interstitium. Foci of myocyte necrosis are also seen

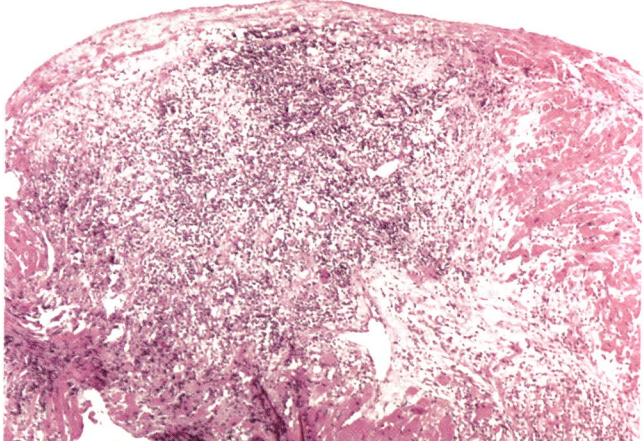

Fig. 10.12b: Cardiac allograft rejection Grade 3B (ISHLT). Extensive diffuse infiltrate with widespread replacement of the myofibers is seen. Other biopsy fragments also showed a diffuse infiltrate

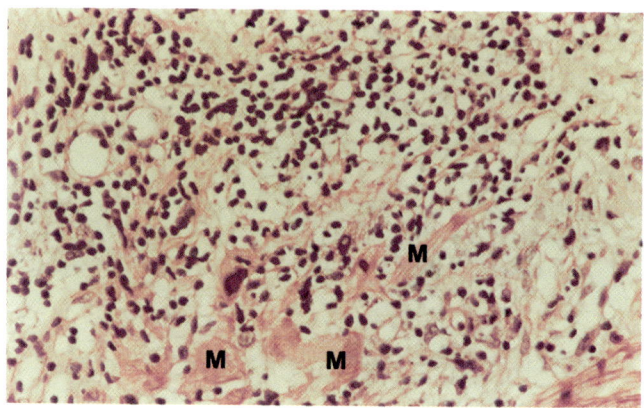

Fig. 10.12c: Higher magnification of Figure 10.12b to illustrate myonecrosis. Remnants of degenerated and necrotic myofibers (M) are seen amidst cellular infiltrates

Late complications of cardiac allograft These may occur any time beyond one year of transplantation but may develop earlier also. The major threat is graft vascular disease.

Hyperacute rejection This type of reaction is extremely rare and occurs within 1-24 hours of transplantation. It seems to be related to major blood group incompatibility or major histocompatibility differences and presence of pre-formed antibodies in the recipient. Retransplantation has to be performed in such cases.

Humoral rejection When patients have features of graft dysfunction in the absence of features of acute cellular rejection in the biopsy, the possibility of antibody mediated rejection must be considered. Microvasculature is affected which is best appreciated by demonstration of immune complexes either by immunofluorescence or immunohistochemistry. Light microscopically, endothelialitis and/or vasculitis may be demonstrated.

Infections The two most common types of infection encountered after cardiac transplantation are **cytomegalovirus** (Fig. 10.13) and **Toxoplasma gondii**. These may be picked up on routine hematoxylin and eosin stained sections with diligent search. *In situ* hybridisation and immunohistochemistry facilitate recognition. Inflammatory infiltrate in infections may at times pose a difficulty in interpretation of rejection. When both co-exist special techniques and laboratory parameters have to be evaluated critically. It is mandatory to distinguish rejection from infection as augmentation of antirejection therapy will enhance the infection.

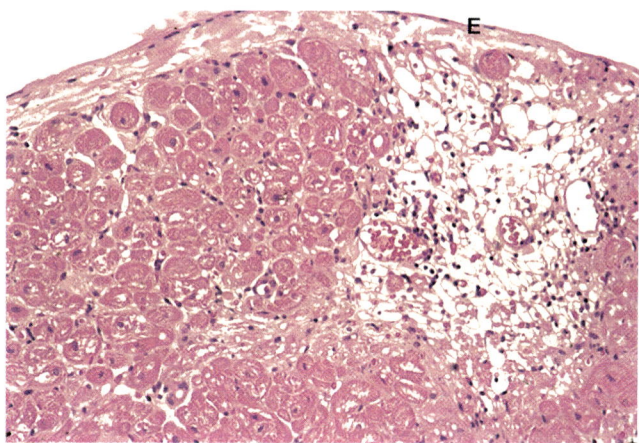

Fig. 10.13a: Post-transplant endomyocardial biopsy. Multiple foci of ischemia were seen evident as myocardial cell drop put, infiltration by lymphocytes, vascularisation and hemosiderin laden macrophages. In addition, intranuclear inclusions suggestive of cytomegalovirus (CMV) are seen. E–Endocardium

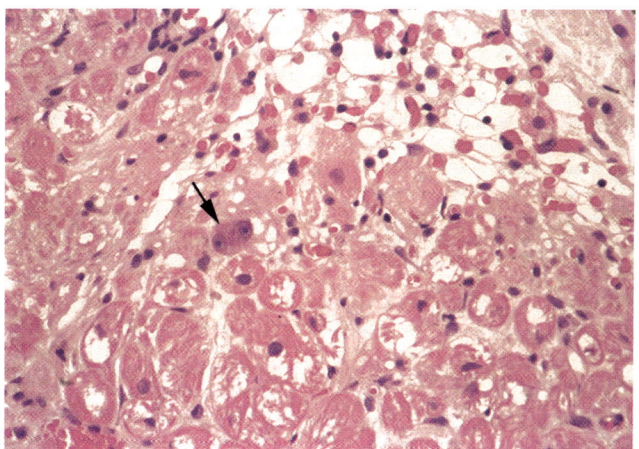

Fig. 10.13b: Higher magnification of Figure 10.13a to highlight the ischemic change and CMV (arrow)

Graft vascular disease (GVD) *(Fig. 10.14)* poses a major threat to long time survival of the graft. It affects infants, children and adults. Its incidence varies from 34.5% after one year and about 90% after 5 years of transplantation. The only remedy of GVD is retransplantation. GVD has several features common with atherosclerosis, however, there are some distinct differences. In contrast with atherosclerosis, GVD affects both large epicardial arteries and intramyocardial branches and the changes involve the entire length of the vessel as opposed to the focal lesions in atherosclerosis. Necrotic atheromas, calcification and lipid is scarce in GVD when compared with conventional atherosclerosis. Importantly, lesions in GVD develop rapidly while atherosclerosis is a slowly progressive process. Microscopically GVD reveals concentric intimal proliferation. Intima in the early stages may show smooth muscle cells, lipid filled macrophages and lymphocytes (Table 10.3). Etiology of GVD is ill-understood and considered to be multifactorial. Some of the factors implicated are HLA mismatches, CMV infection and repititive immune mediated insults to the endothelium.

Table 10.3: Comparison of histopathologic features of graft coronary artery disease versus conventional atherosclerosis

Graft coronary artery disease	*Conventional atherosclerosis*
Concentric intimal lesion common	Eccentric intimal lesion common
Elastica mostly intact	Elastica damaged
Diffuse	Focal
Branches involved	Spares branches
Intramyocardial arteries involved	Spares intramyocardial vessels
Calcification not extensive	Calcification frequent
Necrotic atheroma rare	Atheroma frequent
Lipid less prominent	Lipid more prominent
Develops rapidly	Develops slowly

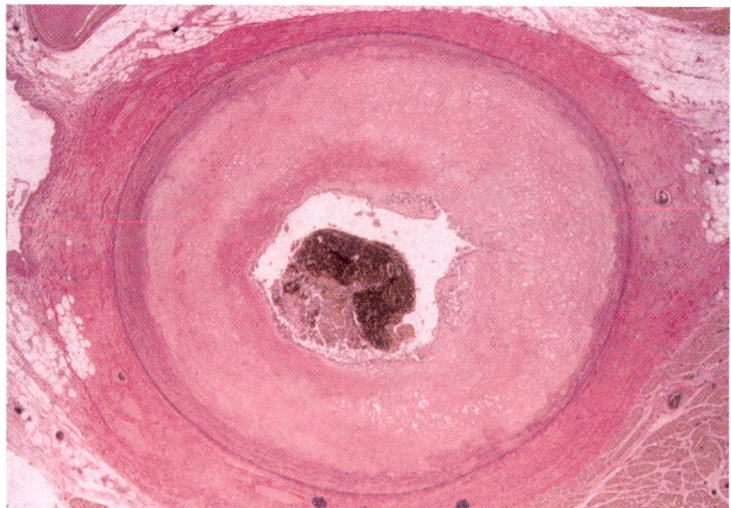

Fig. 10.14: Graft vascular disease. Marked concentric thickening of the intima is observed

Malignancy *(Fig. 10.15)* Association between **Post-transplantation lymphoproliferative disorders (PTLD)** and Epstein-Barr virus is well-established. Postgraft PTLD which is most commonly of B cell type range from benign reactive hyperplasia to malignant proliferations with aggressive behavior. These can be recognised and characterised on biopsy material. Management is by reduction of immunosuppressive therapy and treatment with antiviral agents. The other types of malignancy related to immunosuppressive therapy include squamous cell carcinoma of the skin, lip, vulva, cervix, perineum and Kaposi's sarcoma.

Non-rejection Pathology

Some of the transplantation associated changes will be encountered in sequential biopsies and need to be kept in mind during evaluation of the biopsy for rejection and other changes. These include: (1) ischemic injury, (2) quilty effect, (3) previous biopsy site.

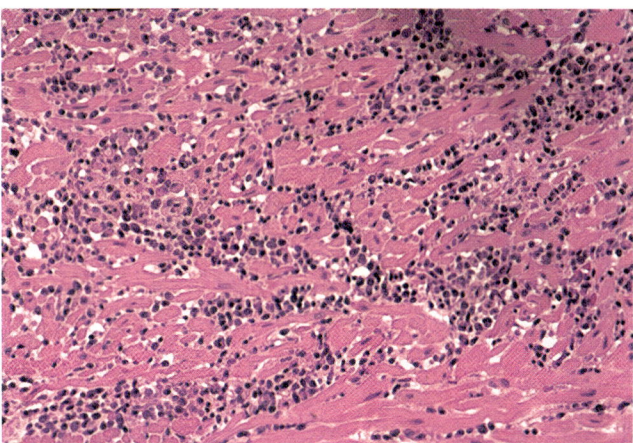

Fig. 10.15a: Follow up endomyocardial biopsy from a case of cardiac transplantation. Post-transplant lymphoproliferative disease (PTLD). Extensive diffuse, mononuclear cell infiltrates are present in the interstitium of the myocardium. The cells show mild to moderate pleomorphism

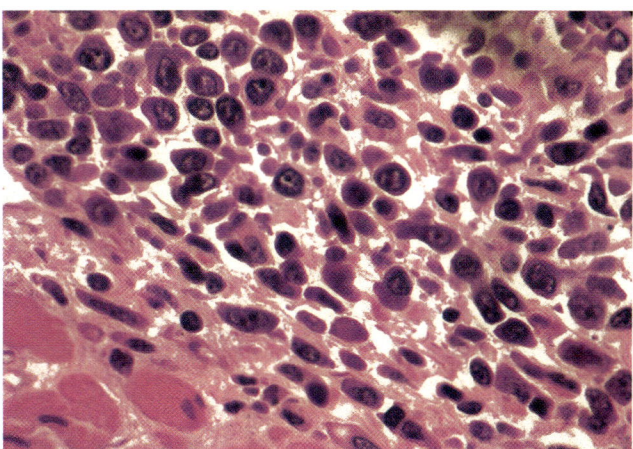

Fig. 10.15b: Higher magnification of the infiltrate (Fig. 10.15a) to demonstrate cellular pleomorphism. The nuclei are vesicular. The cells have moderate amount of eosinophilic cytoplasm. Some cells appear plasmacytoid in nature

Ischemic injury (Figs 10.13, 10.16, 10.17, 7.1 and 7.2) Endomyocardial biopsies performed within the first few weeks after transplantation may reveal ischemic changes which are located mostly in the subendocardium. These could be due to delay in the transplantation time, use of inotropic drugs and occurrence of small air emboli intraoperatively. Ischemic myofibers are well-appreciated on Masson trichrome stain where they appear greyish blue contrasted with the reddish appearane of viable fibers. Healing shows granulation tissue, hemosiderin laden macrophages and inflammatory cells. If evaluated carefully, these changes are distinct from rejection.

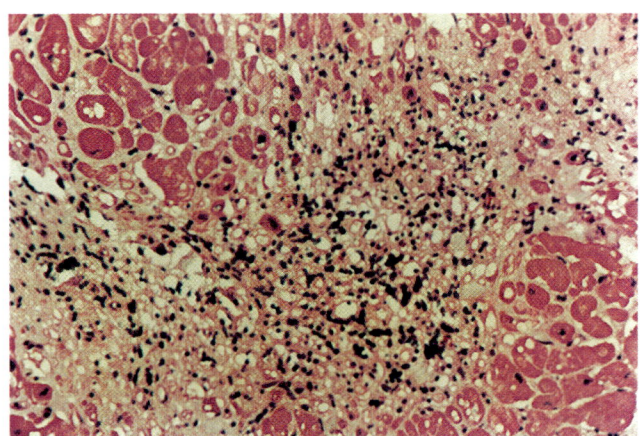

Fig. 10.16a: Post-transplant endomyocardial biopsy at four years. This patient had several episodes of rejection. The immediate previous biopsy revealed acute cellular rejection Grade 3A (ISHLT) which was treated appropriately. Photomicrograph of biopsy repeated a week later shows large areas of myocyte drop out with lymphomononuclear cell infiltrate. These changes can be attributed either to ischemia or a sequelae to resolving rejection. The graft coronary arteries were normal

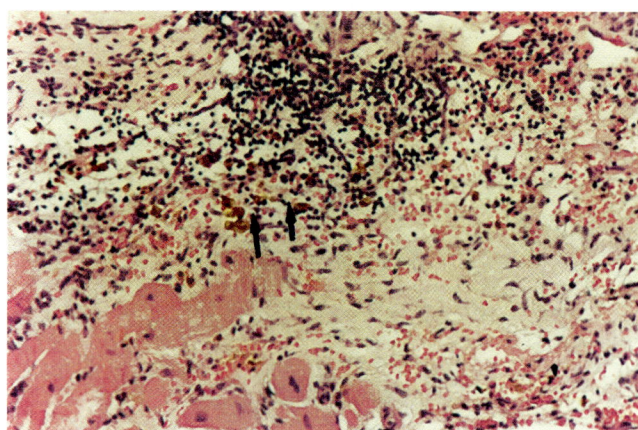

Fig. 10.16b: Post-transplant endomyocardial biopsy of the same case as in Figure 10.16a at 4 years. This biopsy was repeated a week later as there was clinical suspicion of recurrence of rejection. The photomicrograph shows numerous siderophages (arrows), fibroblasts, edema, extravasation of red blood cells and lymphocytic infiltrates. This lesion was subendocardial in location overlying which fibrin was also noted. These changes are reparative in nature and represent the previous biopsy site. Ischemic injury cannot be ruled out

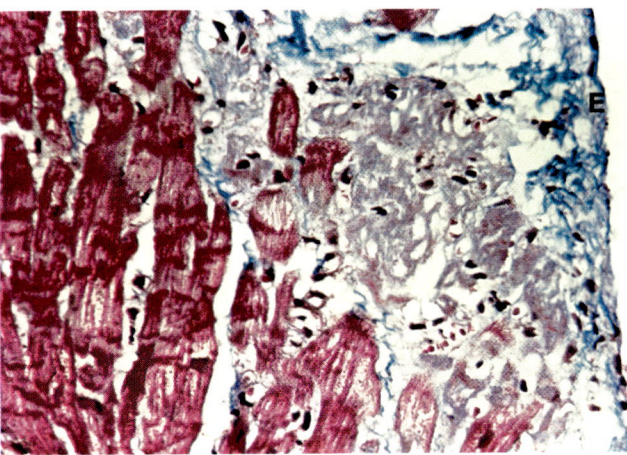

Fig. 10.16c: Post-transplant endomyocardial biopsy. Myofibers in subendocardial location show ischemic changes. With Masson trichrome stain these myofibers appear greyish blue as contrasted with the viable ones which stain red

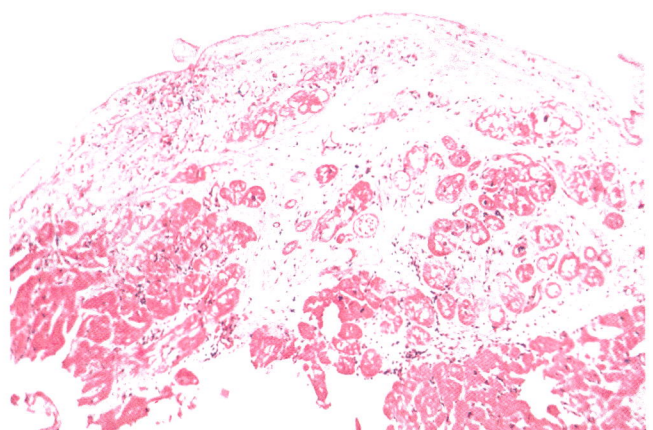

Fig. 10.17a: Post-transplant endomyocardial biopsy at 4 years. Extensive replacement fibrosis of the myocardium is observed. The remaining myofibers show features of hypertrophy. The patient was on cyclosporine therapy

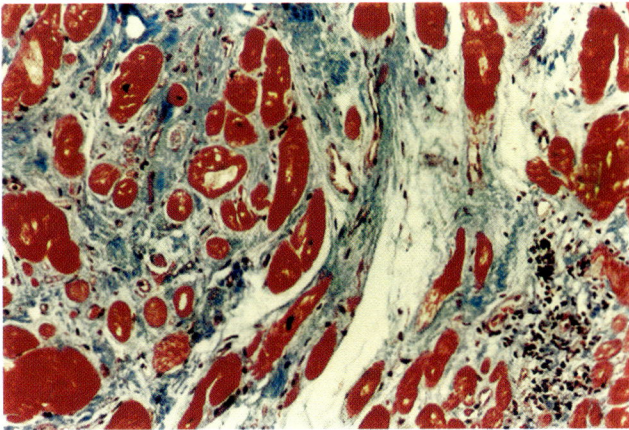

Fig. 10.17b: Post-transplantation endomyocardial biopsy taken at 4 years. Another area from the case illustrated in Figure 10.17a shows diffuse perimyocytic fibrosis. This patient was on cyclosporine therapy. Lower right hand corner shows focal interstitial lymphocytic infiltrates (Masson trichrome stain)

Quilty effect *(Fig. 10.18)* This is a change observed in cases of cardiac transplantation on cyclosporine therapy. Endocardial infiltration comprising a mixture of T and B lymphocytes and macrophages are seen. Characteristically thin walled vascular channels are interspersed within the infiltrate. Infiltrate when limited to the endocardium is designated as Quilty A. Extension into the myocardium qualifies for a Quilty B change. At times Quilty B change may closely simulate rejection changes and interpretation may cause difficulties. Though Quilty change and rejection can co-exist, Quilty change when present by itself needs to be differentiated from rejection.

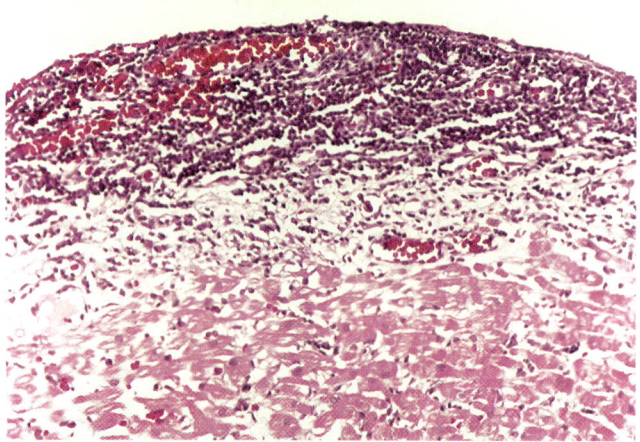

Fig. 10.18a: Quilty A effect in a cardiac allograft. A well-defined lymphocytic infiltrate is present confined to the endocardium. Numerous thin walled vascular channels are seen amidst the infiltrate

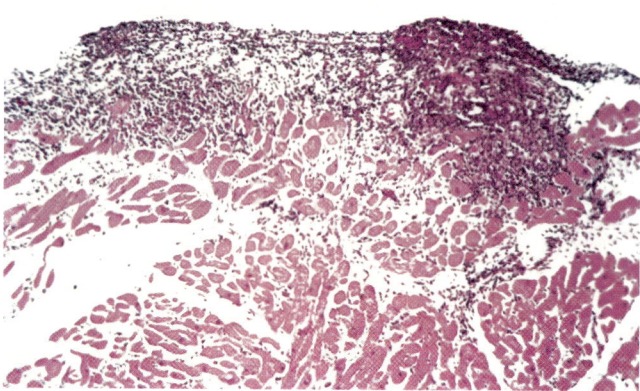

Fig. 10.18b: Post-transplant endomyocardial biopsy showing Quilty B effect. Endocardial infiltrate is seen to extend into the underlying myocardium

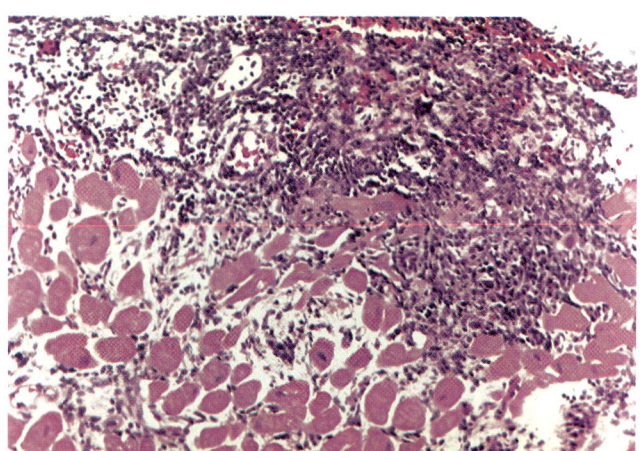

Fig. 10.18c: Post-transplant endomyocardial biopsy showing. Quilty B effect. Higher magnification of Figure 10.18b to show lymphocytic infiltrate, thin walled blood vessels and its extension into the myocardium

Note: Myocardial extension of Quilty B at times may pose problems. To distinguish it from rejection one must be aware of such a problem and in these cases serial step sections and a detailed clinicopathological evaluation may help in settling the issue

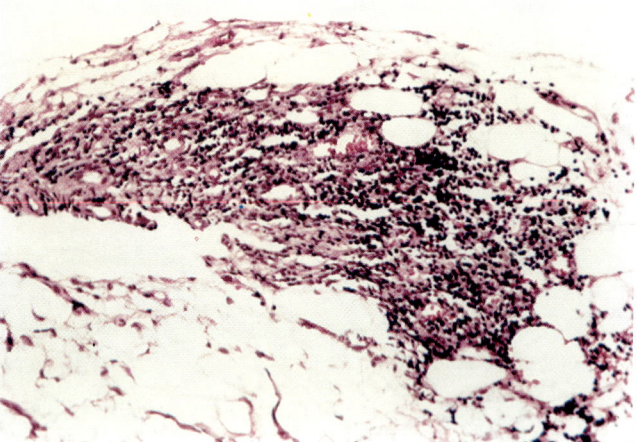

Fig. 10.18d: Post-transplant endomyocardial biopsy of a cardiac allograft showing an epicardial infiltrate comprising of dense lymphocytic aggregates. There are several blood vessels admixed with this cellular infiltrate

Note: This lesion is morphologically similar to the endocardial infiltrate of Quilty effect and can occasionally be seen in post-transplant endomyocardial biopsy specimens

Cardiac Transplantation

Previous biopsy site *(Figs 10.16b and 10.19)* This is commonly encountered as multiple sequential biopsies need to be performed. The bioptome is so designed that it slips to the previously biopsied area. The biopsy site is located in the subendocardial region. Recent biopsy site may yield a fresh thrombus. Healed biopsy site reveals fibrosis, inflammatory granulation tissue and characteristic myofiber disarray. These changes therefore should be interpreted in the right perspective.

Hypertrophy and myocardial fibrosis (Fig. 10.17) is invariably seen in transplanted hearts. Myocardial fibrosis is due to several reasons namely ischemia, adaptation, drug induced injury (cyclosporine), etc.

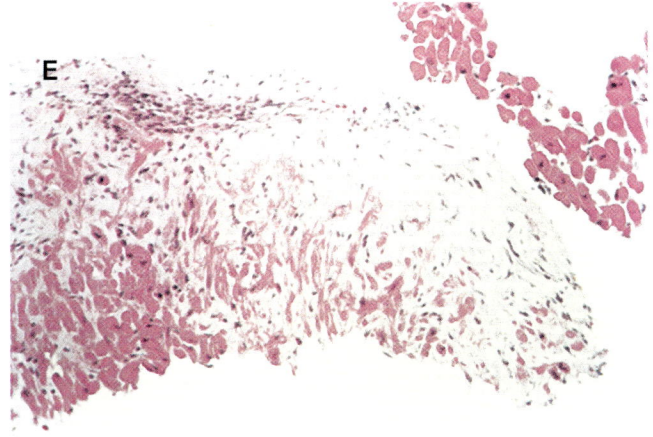

Fig. 10.19a: Post-transplant endomyocardial biopsy shows a thickened endocardium, with fibrosis and few trapped lymphocytes. The surrounding myocytes in the right side of the figure shows disarray, a feature which is often seen in a healed biopsy site

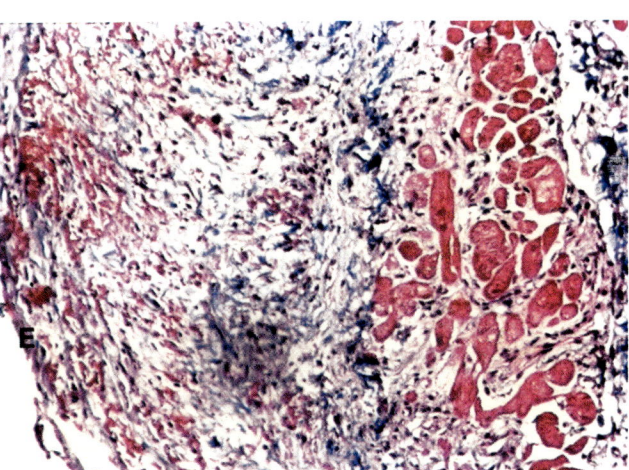

Fig. 10.19b: Post-transplant endomyocardial biopsy from a cardiac allograft to show a previous biopsy site. Masson trichrome stain shows thickened endocardium with fibrin deposition on the surface of endocardium (E). Organisation is seen at the base. Myocardium is seen in the right third of the picture

Cardiac transplantation is indicated in end stage cardiac diseases. The one year survival figures, range from 85% to 90% in the major centers. The major setback to the cardiac transplantation is the limited donor pool. Various efforts are being made to increase the donor pool by exploitation of "presumed" consent where removal of an organ for transplantation is allowed from somebody who has been declared brain dead (strong presumed consent). Alternatively, it is presumed that everyone is willing to donate their organs unless they have wished otherwise during their life time (weak presumed consent). This type of consent is obviously not quite acceptable by most countries. However, if the legislation is modified and made flexible it will signficantly increase donor availability. **Xenotransplantation-**(cross-species transplantation) is under active research scrutiny for use in human cardiac transplantation. The selection of an animal donor requires that the animal must be available readily and in large numbers. They must be free of transmissible disease, be available in sizes matching with humans, have cardiac physiology like that in man and ideally be ABO compatible.

Importantly, the species chosen must not be an endangered one. Due to various ethical considerations use of non-human primates is virtually abandoned. There is much enthusiam regarding use of domesticated animals, e.g. pigs as donors for humans. Rejection in xenotransplant occurs predominantly due to vascular damage, which is both antibody and complement mediated. Latter can be overcome by removing antibodies by absorption and decomplementation of the recipient or transplantation of graft endothelium with molecules that protect against complement-mediated damage. T cell mediated response is not a major problem as the vascular damage. Human T cell receptor binds human MHC molecule; it is likely that human T cell receptor do not recognise xenogenic MHC molecules very well. Thus T cells activation could be countered by immunosuppression.

The other ongoing efforts to further increase the allograft survival are new improved immunosuppression protocols, induction of specific graft tolerance and permanent left ventricular assist devices.

SUGGESTED READING

1. Balk AH, Zondervan PE, Van der Meer P, Van Gelder T, Mochtar B, Simoons MLL, Weimar W: Effect of adopting a new histological grading system of acute rejection after heart transplantation. *Heart* **78(6)**: 603-07, 1997.

2. Beltrami CA, Di Loreto C, Finato N, Rocco M, Artico D, Cigola E, Gambert SR, Olivetti G, Kajstura J, Anversa P: Proliferating cell nuclear antigen (PCNA), DNA synthesis and mitosis in myocytes following cardiac transplantation in man. *J Mol Cell Cardiol* **29(10)**: 2789-802, 1997.

3. Chopra P, Joshi A, Talwar KK, Airan B, Srivastava S, Venugopal P: Pathology of cardiac transplantation the initial AIIMS experience. *Nat Med J India* **10/6**: 264-69, 1997.

4. Curtil A, Robin J, Tronc F, Ninet J, Boissonnat P, Champsaur G: Malignant neoplasm following cardiac transplantation. *Eur J Cardiothrac Surg* **12 (1)**: 101-06, 1997.

5. Deng MC, Erren M, Roeder N, Dreimann V, Gunther F, Kerber S, Baba HA, Schmidt C, Breithardt G, Scheld HH: T-cell and monocyte subsets, inflammatory molecules, rejection, and hemodynamics early after cardiac transplantation. *Transplantation* **65(9)**: 1255-61, 1998.

6. Dong C, Winters GL, Wilson JE, McManus BM: Enhanced lymphocyte longevity and absence of proliferation and lymphocyte apoptosis in Quilty effects of human heart allografts. *Am J Pathol* **151(1)**: 121-30, 1997.

7. Frigerio M, Bonacina E, Gronda E, Andreuzzi B, Anjos MC, De Vila C, Manngiavacchi M, Masciocco C, Oliva F, Dellegrini A. A semiquantitative approach to the evaluation of acute cardiac allograft rejection at endomyocardial biopsy. *J Heart Lung Transplant* **16(12)**: 1248-54, 1997.

8. Grandss AM, Minzioni G, Martinelli L, Campana C, Rinaldi M, D'Armini AM, Ragni T, Pederzolli C, Ardemagni E, Pederzolli N, De Pieri G, Casliglione N, Vigano M. Echo-controlled endomyocardial biopsy in orthotopic heart transplantation with bicaval anastomosis. *G Ital Cardiol.* **27(9)**: 877-80, 1997.

9. Guy TS: Evolution and current status of the total artificial heart: the search continues. *Asaio J* **44(1)**: 28-33, 1998.

10. John R, Chen JM, Weinberg A, Oz MC, Manchini D, Itescu S, Galantowicz ME, Smith CR, Rose EA, Edwards NM: Long-term survival after cardiac retransplantation: a twenty-year single-center experience. *J Thorac Cardiovasc Surg* **117(3)**: 543-55, 1999.

11. Lin Y, Soares MP, Sato K, Takigami K, Csizmadia E, Anrather J, Bach FH: Rejection of cardiac xenografts by $CD4^+$ or $CD8^+$ T cells. *J Immunol* **162(2)**: 1206-14, 1999.

12. McCarthy JF, Cook DJ, Smeditra NG, O'Malley KJ, Massad MG, Sano Y, Young JB, Starling RCl, Ratliff NB, McCarthy PM: Vascular rejection in cardiac transplantation. *Transplant Proc* **31(1-2)**: 160, 1999.

13. Mindan JP, Paniizo A: Pathology of heart transplant. *Curr Top Pathol* **92**: 137-65, 1999.

14. Mills RM, Naftel DC, Kirklin JK, Van Bakel AB, Jaski BE, Massin EK, Eisen HJ, Lee FA, Fishbelin DP, Bourge RC: Heart transplant rejection with hemodynamic compromise: a multiinstitutional study of the role of endomyocardial cellular infiltrate. Cardiac Transplant Research Dalabase. *J Heart Lung Transplant* **16(8)**: 813-21, 1997.

15. Olivari MT: Cardiac transplantation: A review of indications and results. *Cardiologia* **43(5)**: 459-63, 1998.

16. Orbaek Andersen H: Heart allograft vascular disease: An obliterative vascular disease in transplanted hearts. *Atherosclerosis* **142(2)**: 243-63, 1999.

17. Platt JL: Prospects for xenotransplantation. *Pediatr Transplant* **3(3)**: 193-200, 1999.

18. Sambiase NV, Higuchi ML, Nuovo G, Gutierrez PS, Ffiorelli AI, Uip DE, Ramires JA: CMV and transplant-related coronary atherosclerosis: An immunohistochemical, in situ hybridization, and polymerase chain reaction in situ study. *Mod Pathol* **13(2)**: 173-79, 2000.

19. Winters GL. The challenge of endomyocardial biopsy interpretation in assessing cardiac allograft rejection. *Curr Opin Cardiol* **12(2)**: 146-52, 1997.

11 The Pericardium

Heart is encased by the pericardium which has a visceral layer closely apposed to the heart and the parietal layer. In normal states it is thin, transparent and the myocardium can be seen through it. It shows a lining of flattened to cuboidal mesothelial cells.

Serous effusion The normal pericardial cavity contains from 30 to 50 ml of clear fluid. Collection of excess amounts of fluid is termed as **pericardial effusion**. This may be either inflammatory or non-inflammatory in nature. Effusion is commonly referred to as per its appearance, e.g. serous, serosanguinous, hemorrhagic, purulent, caseous, chylous, cholesterol, etc.

Investigative Procedures

Pericardial tap examination of the pericardial aspirate can provide useful diagnostic information. Pericardial fluid cytology can be helpful in the diagnosis of pericardial tuberculosis (Fig. 11.1) and pericardial tumors in particular mesothelioma. A great deal of difficulty can be encountered in distinguishing reactive mesothelial cell (Figs 11.2, 11.14a and b) from cells shed from a mesothelioma (Figs 11.3a to g) and carcinoma. A final diagnosis in most of the cases rests on a combined evaluation of histological, histochemical and immunocytochemical findings (Table 11.1) in addition to clinical features of the thickened pericardium.

Pericardiectomy Surgically excised thickened pericardium is evaluated in cases of constrictive pericarditis (Figs 11.4 and 11.5). While tuberculosis is encountered in a large majority of cases (Figs 11.6 to 11.8), non-specific thickening of the pericardium is also observed in a fair number of cases (Fig. 11.9). The latter diagnosis is given only after extensive

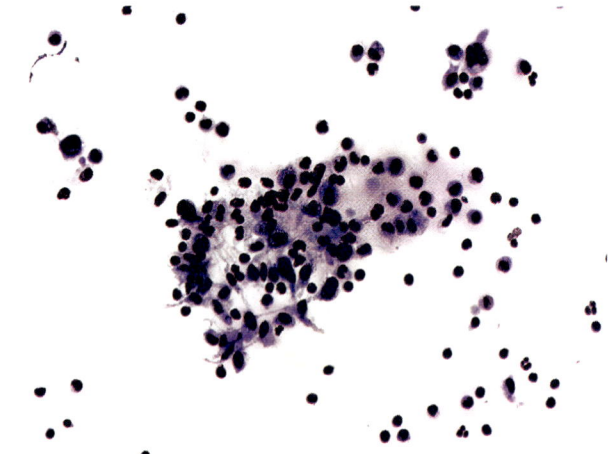

Fig. 11.1: Tuberculous pericarditis. Aspirate from pericardial effusion. Numerous lymphocytes are present. Few ill-formed epithelioid granulomas are also observed

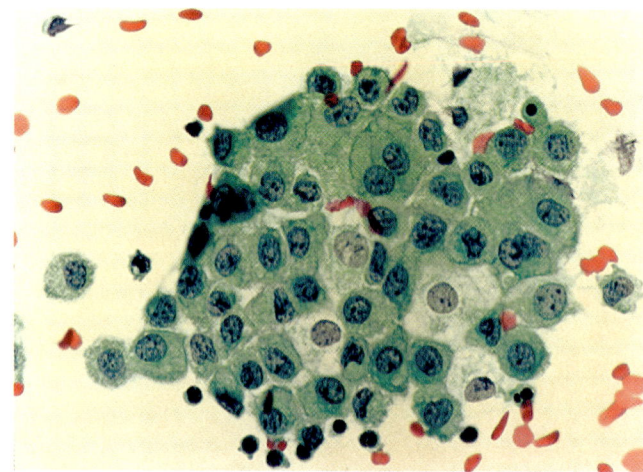

Fig. 11.2: Pericardial effusion. Aspirate shows groups of reactive mesothelial cells with intercellular windows. The nuclei are small, round and uniform and show only mild variation in size and shape. Cytoplasm has fine vacuolations

The Pericardium

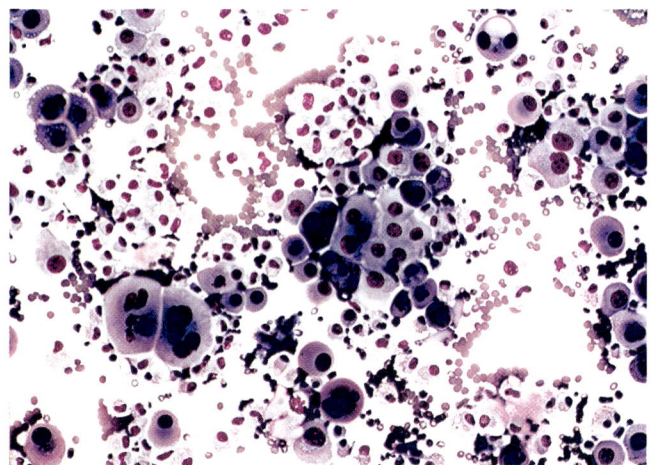

Fig. 11.3a: Mesothelioma of the pericardium. Cells are present in small clusters. They show prominent variation in size. Nuclei exhibit irregularity and hyperchromasia. Also seen interspersed are few smaller mesothelial cells with small, round, uniform nuclei

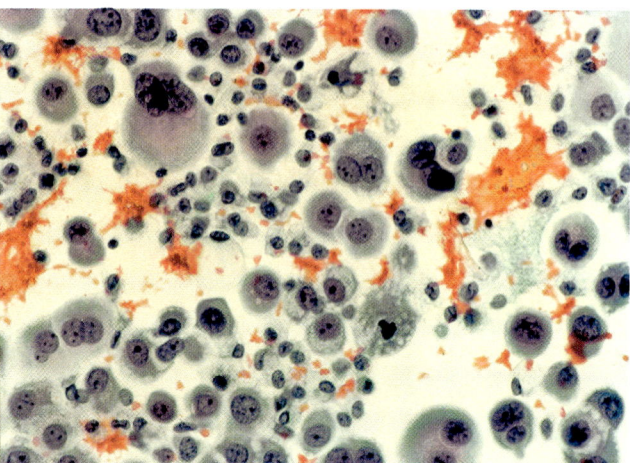

Fig. 11.3b: Mesothelioma of pericardium. Tumor cells are present singly and show hyperchromasia of nuclei, variation in size, binucleation, open chromatin and prominent nucleoli. The cytoplasm is uniform staining and appears dense. Occasional cells show fine vacuolation of the cytoplasm

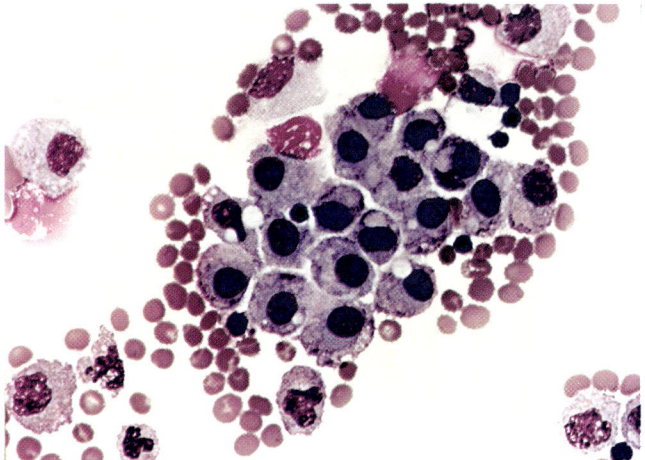

Fig. 11.3c: Mesothelioma of the pericardium. Gaps (windows) are seen in between the cell borders. Cytoplasm shows prominent vacuolation near the cell membrane

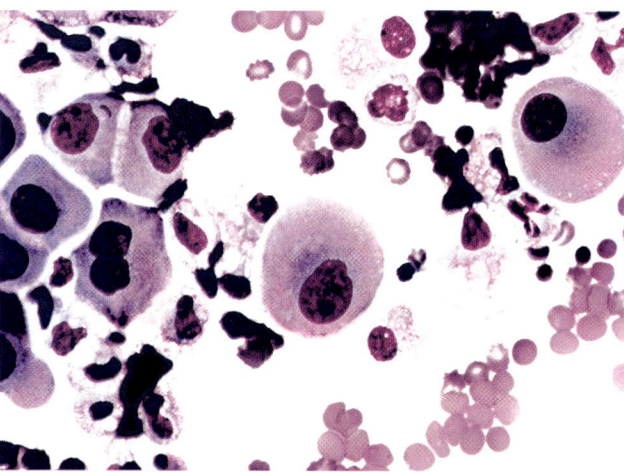

Fig. 11.3d: Mesothelioma. Surface of the tumor cells shows numerous hairy processes (brush border) (This appearance represents microvilli on surface cells seen ultrastructurally)

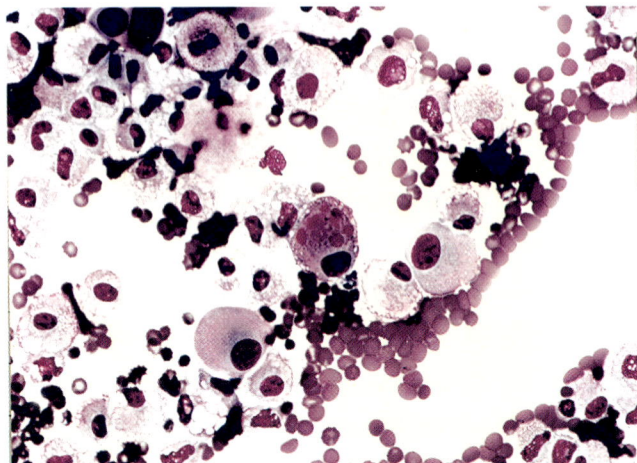

Fig. 11.3e: Mesothelioma of the pericardium. Tumor cells shows intracytoplasmic pink inclusions

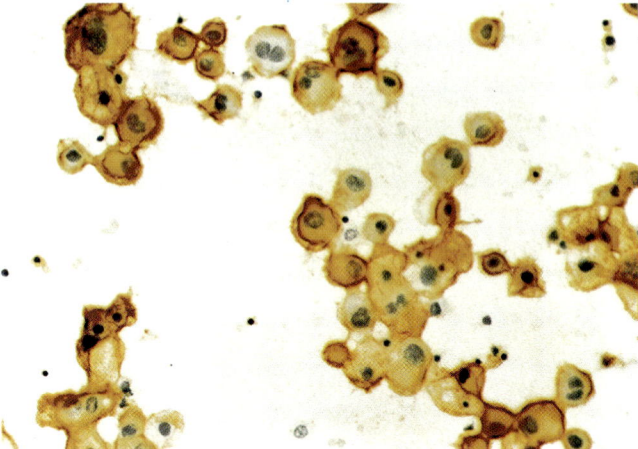

Fig. 11.3f: Mesothelioma of the pericardium stained with antibody to EMA (epithelial membrane antigen). Strong membrane staining of tumor cells is evident

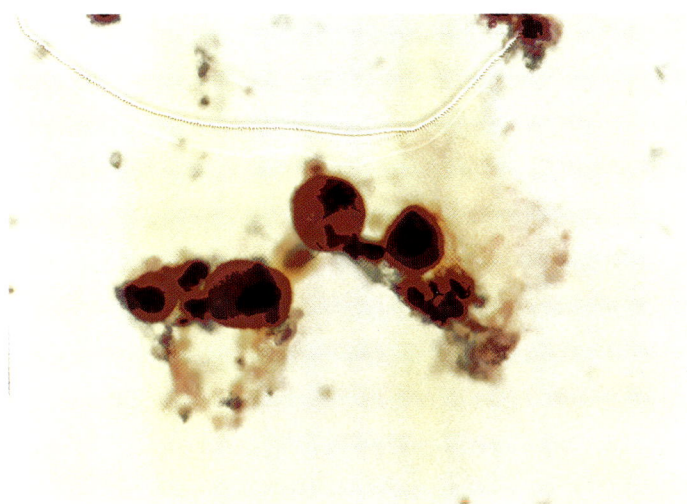

Fig. 11.3g: Mesothelioma of the pericardium. Mucicarmine stain shows mucin within the cytoplasm
Note: Quite often there is a difficulty in distinguishing adenocarcinoma from mesothelioma. Staining for epithelial mucin favors adenocarcinoma. It should be remembered, however, that rarely mesotheliomas may stain for neutral mucin

sampling of the excised pericardium to exclude tuberculosis.

Pericardial biopsy Although pericardial biopsy is indicated in cases of myopericarditis, we have limited experience with this procedure. However, when performed it can be of diagnostic utility (Figs 11.7 and 11.8).

Non-inflammatory Effusion

Serous effusion is accumulation of clear or straw colored fluid in the pericardial cavity. Common causes include congestive heart failure, and hypoproteinemia. Myxedema, rheumatic fever, systemic lupus erythematosis are some of the other causes.

Table 11.1: Morphological features and immunohistochemical reactions in mesothelial hyperplasia, mesothelioma, carcinoma

	Mesothelial hyperplasia	Mesothelioma	Metastatic carcinoma
Morphology			
• Cytologic atypia	–	+	+
• Irregular nucleoli	–	–/+	+
• Necrosis of cells	–	+ (often)	+ (often)
• Intracytoplasmic mucin vacuoles	–	–/+	–/+
• Biphasic growth	–	+	–
• Desmoplasia	–	–/+	–/+
• Hyalinised stroma	–/occasional +	–/+	–
Immunostaining			
• CEA	–	– (Most of the cases)	+ (70-100%)
• EMA	–/weak +	+ (Strong membrane staining)	+ (Strong cytoplasmic staining)
• Leu-M1 (CD15)	–	–/occasional +	+ (60-100%)
• Cytokeratin (Low molecular weight)	–/weak +	+ (patern is perinuclear) useful in distinguishing sarcomatous mesothelioma from sarcoma)	+ (diffuse or beneath cell membrane)
• Cytokeratin (High molecular weight)	–	+ (more often)	– (most cases)
• Human milk fat globule-2 (HMFG-2)	–	+ (Membranous staining)	+ (Prominent cytoplasmic staining)
• B72.3	–	–	–/+
• Thrombomodulin	+	+	–/+ occasional

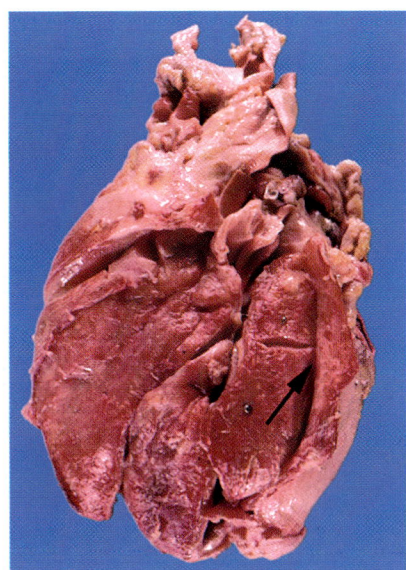

Fig. 11.4: Constrictive pericarditis. The thickened parietal pericardium (arrow) has been reflected to expose the surface of the heart which appears irregular due to adhesions between the visceral and parietal layers of the pericardium

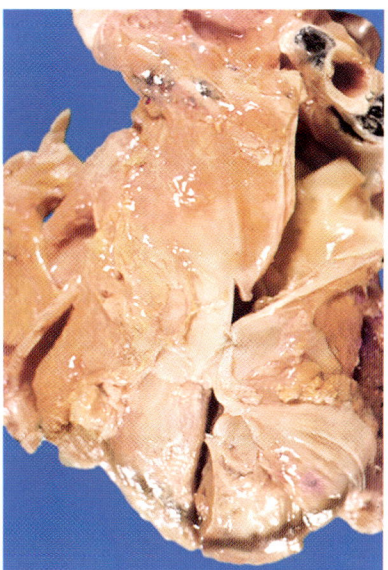

Fig. 11.5: Constrictive pericarditis. The pericardium is markedly thickened and appears to encase the heart. The thickened pericardium has been cut and stripped to show the external surface of the heart which appears opaque and irregular due to adhesions of the pericardium

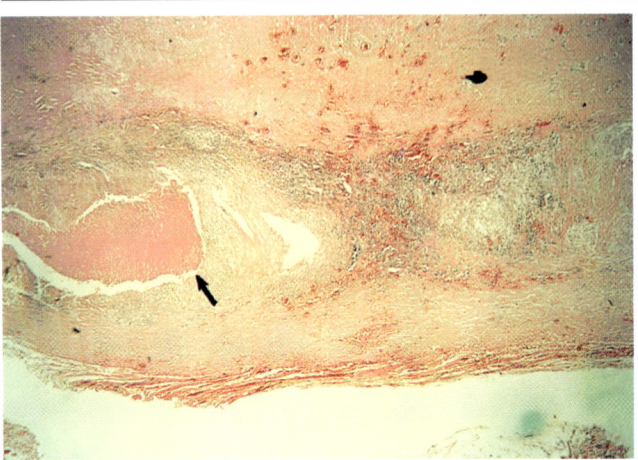

Fig. 11.6a: Pericardiectomy specimen from a case of constrictive pericarditis. Granulomatous inflammation with areas of necrosis (arrow) is seen. The granulomas are bordered by chronic inflammation. The rest of the pericardium is markedly thickened, hyalinised and shows increased vascularity

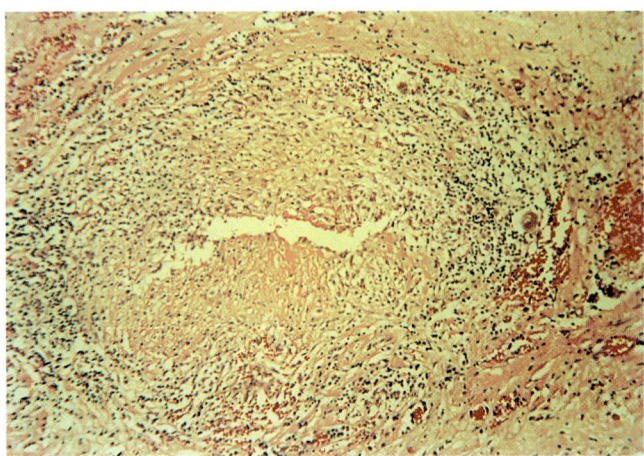

Fig. 11.6b: Tuberculous pericarditis. Granulomatous inflammation with necrosis. Chronic inflammatory cell infiltration and giant cells are also observed

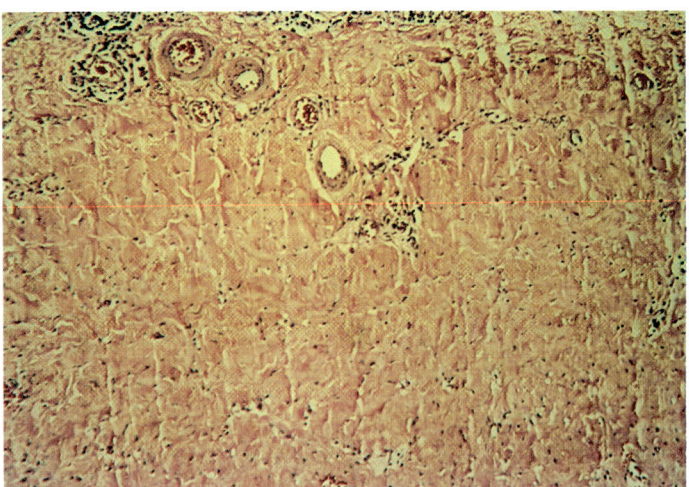

Fig. 11.6c: A case of tuberculous pericarditis. Dense hyalinisation of the pericardium is observed. Granulomatous inflammation with necrosis was seen in other sections.

Note: If pericardiectomy specimen is not sampled adequately, this appearance would be documented as non-specific

The Pericardium

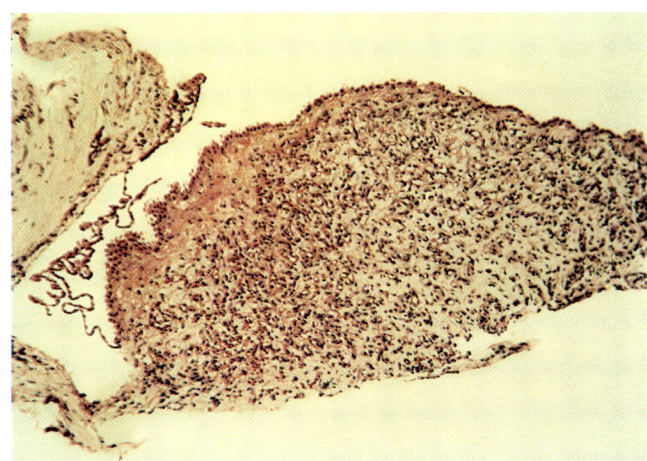

Fig. 11.7a: Pericardial biopsy. Photomicrograph shows prominent mesothelial cells and numerous capillaries within the pericardium. This change was initially interpreted as granulation tissue/hemangioma
Note: 10-year-old boy presented with incapacitating recurrent pericardial effusion which was hemorrhagic in nature. Pericardial biopsy was performed (See Fig. 11.7b for details)

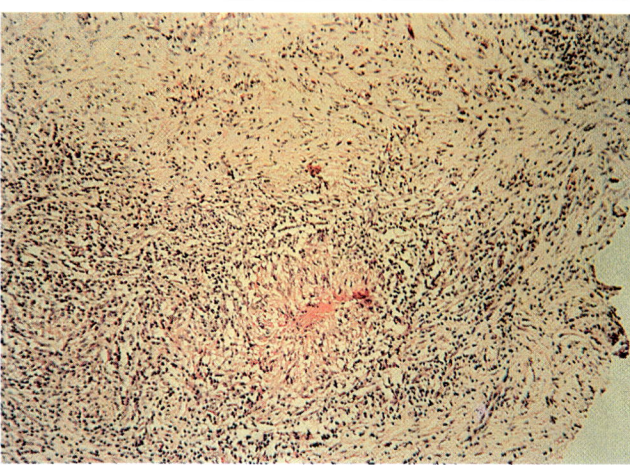

Fig. 11.7b: Granulomatous inflammation with necrosis, pericardium. Large areas of hemorrhage, increased vascularity, hyalinisation and chronic inflammation were seen in other areas
Note: Same case as illustrated in Figure 11.7a. The patient was subjected to pericardiectomy as he had signs and symptoms of constrictive heart disease. At surgery the pericardium was markedly thickened. The pericardial cavity contained large blood clots and the pericardial surfaces appeared irregular and shaggy. The case was finally labelled as tuberculous pericarditis and the increased vascularity as observed on the biopsy (Fig. 11.7a) was part of the exuberant granulation tissue.

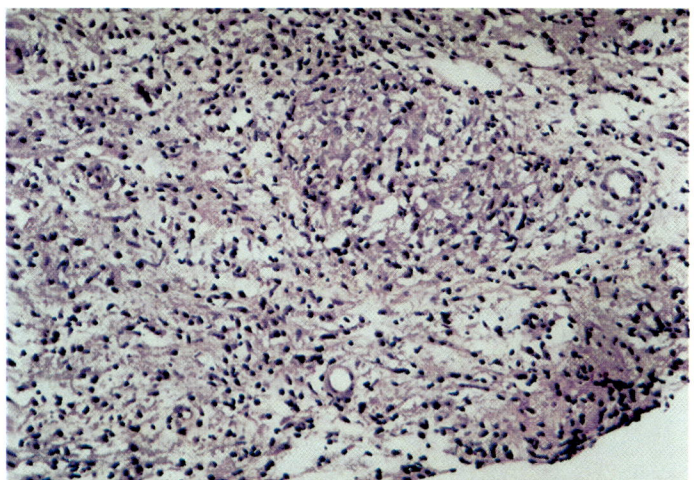

Fig. 11.8: Pericardial biopsy from a case suspected of tuberculous pericarditis. The pericardium shows granulomatous inflammation, increased vascularity and lymphocytic infiltration is also seen in the picture

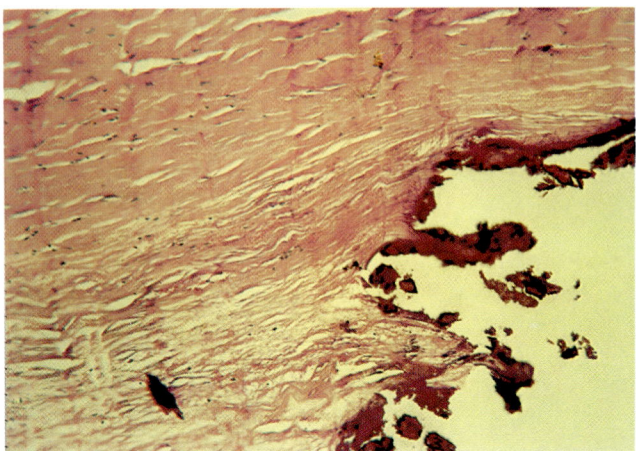

Fig. 11.9a: Pericardiectomy specimen removed from a case of constrictive pericarditis. Non-specific chronic pericarditis, marked hyalinisation of pericardial collagen and focal calcification is seen

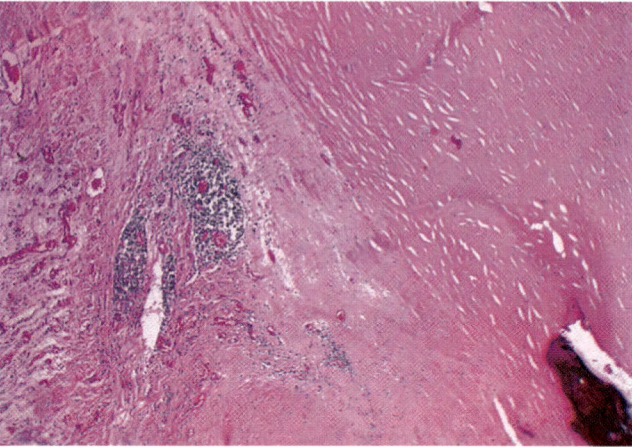

Fig. 11.9b: Chronic nonspecific pericarditis. Pericardiectomy specimen from a case of constrictive pericarditis. The pericardium is thickened by vascular fibrocollagen tissue, focal chronic inflammation and calcification

Hemopericardium As the name indicates there is collection of pure blood in the pericardial sac consequent to penetrating injury to the heart, rupture of the heart due to full thickness myocardial infarction, rupture of thoracic aneurysm of aorta into pericardial cavity, extensive tumor metastasis, bleeding diathesis, etc. The pericardium may appear shaggy, hemorrhagic and irregular (Fig. 11.10).

Chylous Collection of milky fluid (chyle) in the pericardial cavity. This is due to lymphatic obstruction of varied etiology.

Pericarditis

Inflammation of the pericardium commonly due to infective organisms. Non-infective pericarditis may also occur. Common types of pericarditis are discussed.

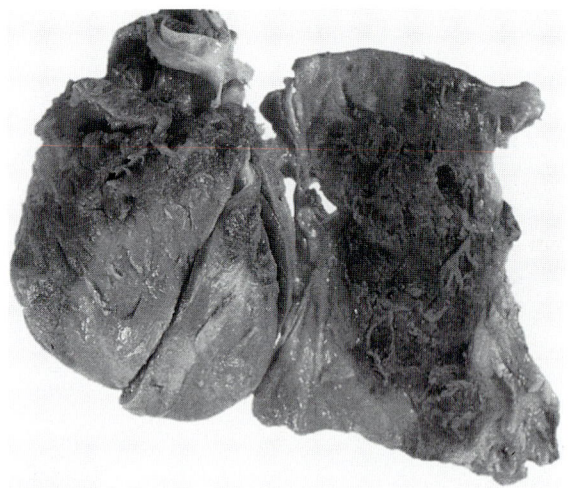

Fig. 11.10a: Fibrous hemorrhagic pericarditis. Picture shows the external surface of the heart and the inner surface of the reflected parietal pericardium. Latter shows hemorrhagic and shaggy areas with fibrous tags

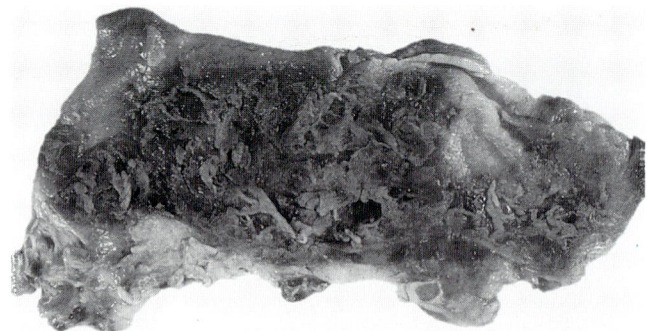

Fig. 11.10b: Fibrous hemorrhagic pericarditis. Inner surface of the parietal pericardium shows an irregular, shaggy hemorrhagic appearance
Note: 16 years male a case of rheumatic heart disease had features of acute rheumatic mitral and tricuspid valvulitis. Serosanguinous pericardial effusion was detected

The Pericardium

Fibrinous/Serofibrinous pericarditis There is fibrin deposition on the surface of the pericardium which may or may not be accompanied by effusion. This is seen in a large number of conditions and is not specific of a particular disease. This reaction occurs in infections namely bacterial, viral and other conditions. It is also seen in acute rheumatic fever, transmural myocardial infarction, uremia etc. **Grossly** the pericardium shows fine, granular deposits on the surface (Figs 11.11 and 11.12) which on **microscopic** examination manifest as fibrin with or without inflammation depending upon the cause and duration of disease (Fig. 11.13). Serofibrinous pericarditis may either resolve or organise. Latter may be significant enough to cause adhesion of the two layers and obliteration of the pericardial space.

The pericardium in acute rheumatic fever characteristically shows fibrinous pericarditis with or without serous effusion (Figs 11.11a and b). The pericardium on gross and microscopic examination shows fibrin deposition, increased vascularity and infiltration by lymphocytes predominantly. In some cases fibrinoid necrosis of the pericardial collagen along with infiltration by histiocytes is seen (Figs 11.13 to 11.16). This change is quite reminiscent of changes seen in subcutaneous nodule of acute rheumatic fever.

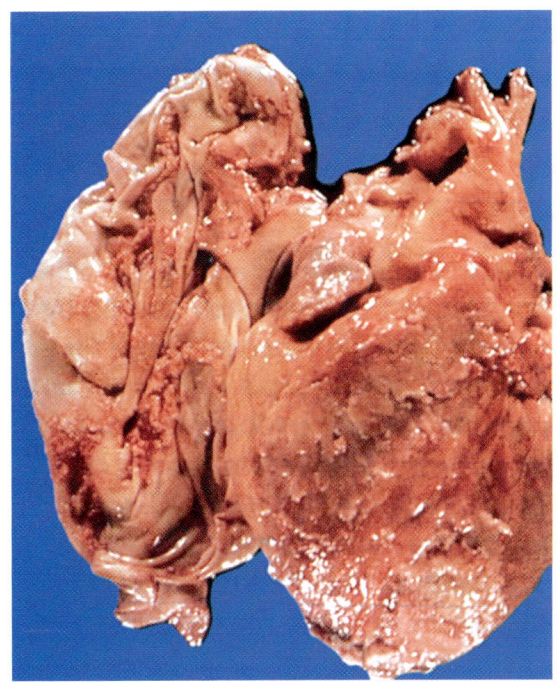

Fig. 11.11a: Acute rheumatic carditis. Both the visceral and parietal pericardium show features of fibrinous pericarditis

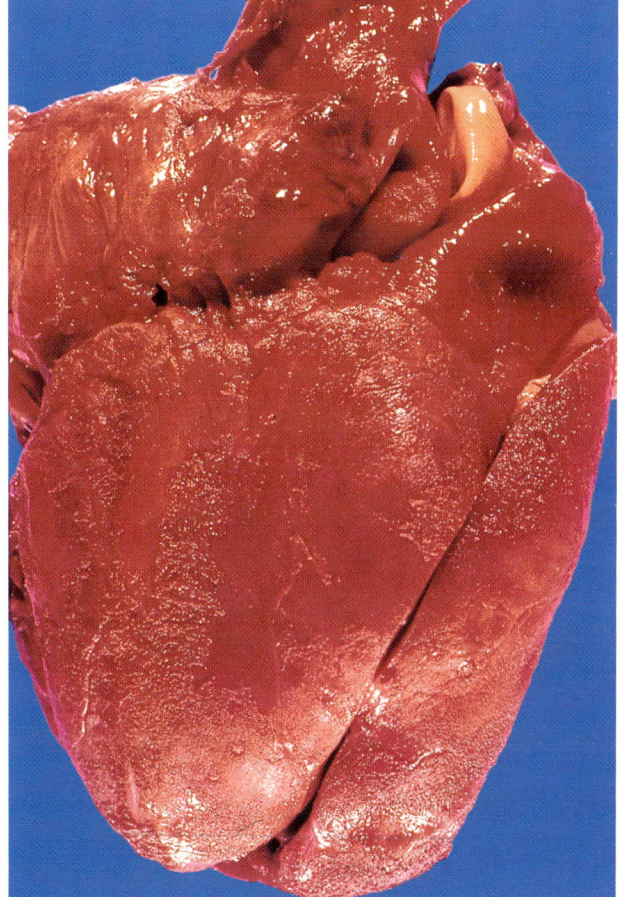

Fig. 11.11b: Fibrinous pericarditis. The external surface of the heart shows fine confluent granularity in large foci over both atria and ventricles

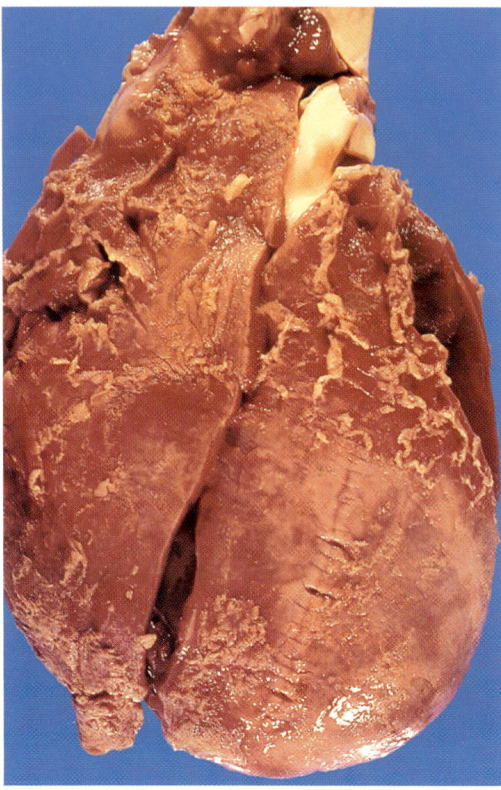

Fig. 11.12: Fibrinous and fibrous pericarditis. The external surface is opaque and shows fine granularity and fibrous tags on the visceral pericardium

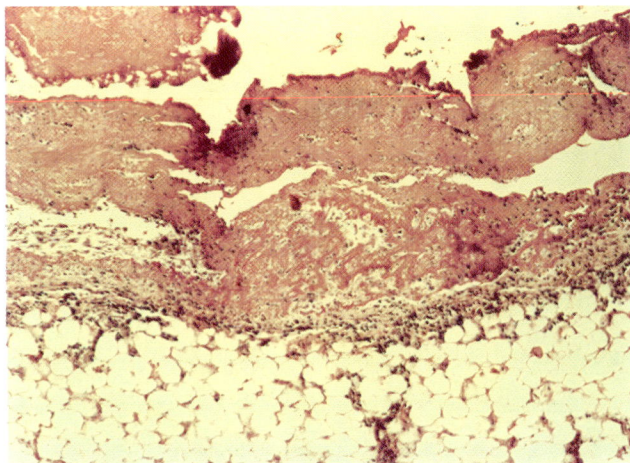

Fig. 11.13a: Fibrinous pericarditis from a case of acute pericarditis possibly of viral etiology (history of breathlessness of short duration). The pericardial surface shows abundant fibrin and few inflammatory cells in the deeper portion

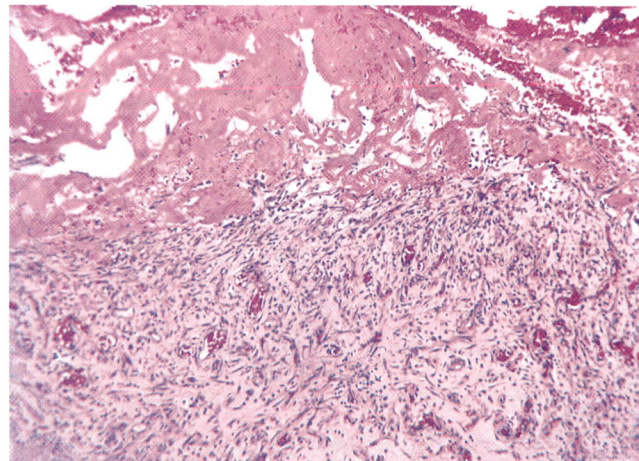

Fig. 11.13b: Fibrinous pericarditis. The surface shows a layer of deep pink smudgy material-fibrin deposition. Inflammatory granulation tissue is seen in the deeper layers

The Pericardium

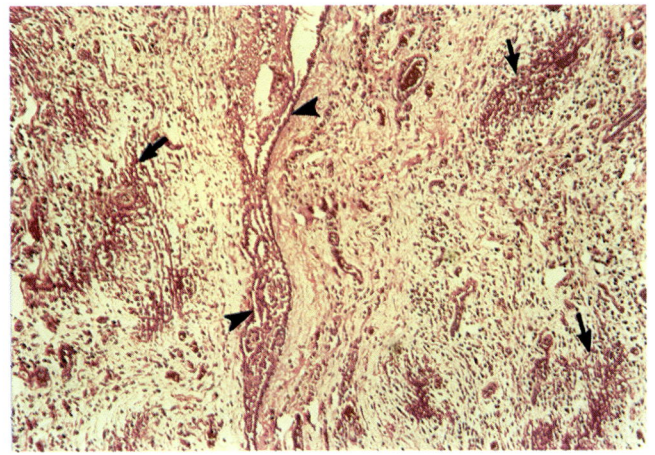

Fig. 11.14a: Acute rheumatic pericarditis. The pericardium shows several foci of necrosis of the collagen evident as deep pink smudgy material (arrows). Edema, chronic inflammatory cell infiltration and increased vascularity are also noted. In addition, marked proliferation of mesothelial cells of the pericardium is seen (arrow heads)

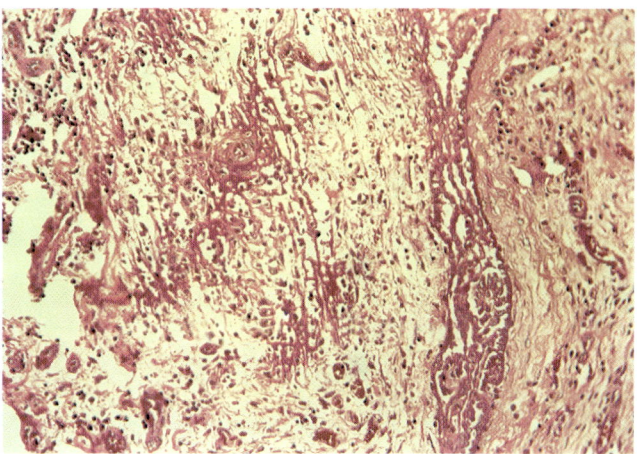

Fig. 11.14b: Acute rheumatic pericarditis. Higher magnification of Figure 11.14a to show fibrinoid necrosis and the reactive mesothelial cells in the pericardium

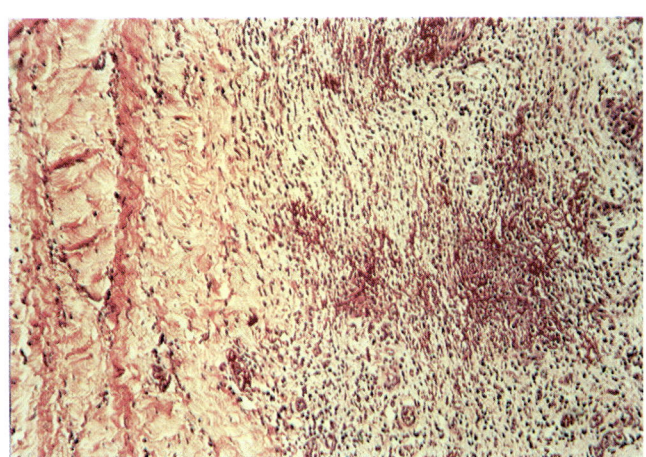

Fig. 11.14c: Acute rheumatic pericarditis. Fibrinoid necrosis is seen as deep pink smudgy material within which and surrounding it a few mononuclear cells are present. Fibrous thickening of the pericardium is seen on left of the picture

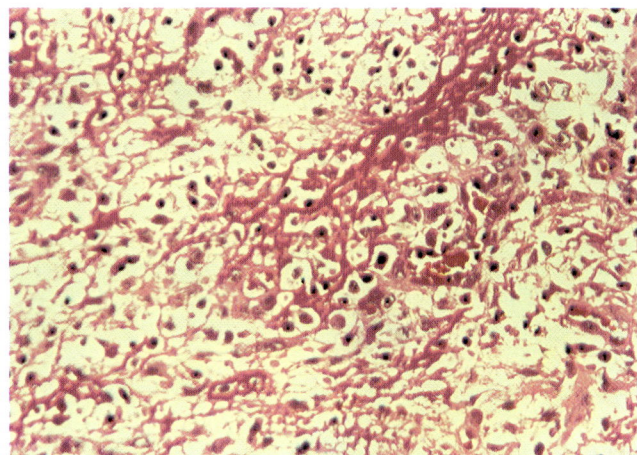

Fig. 11.14d: Acute rheumatic pericarditis. This picture shows details of fibrinoid necrosis of the pericardium. Homogeneous pink material represents fibrinoid necrosis of pericardial collagen. Mononuclear cells are embedded within the smudgy material. This change has a resemblance to subcutaneous nodule of acute rheumatic fever

Note: 15 years male—a case of rheumatic heart disease with recurrence. At autopsy, pancarditis was present. All four valves were involved. Rheumatic vegetations were present on the mitral valve

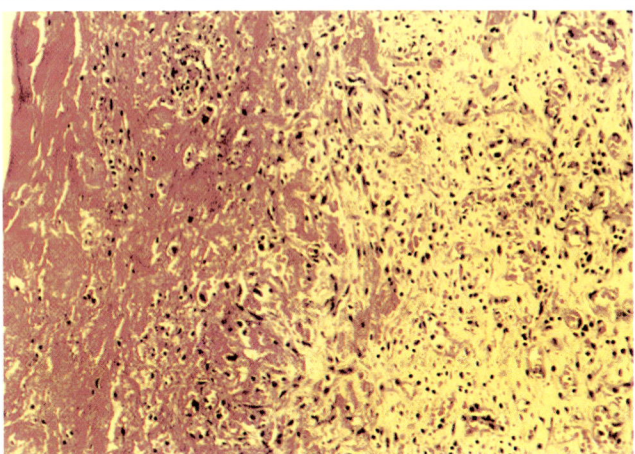

Fig. 11.15: Fibrinous pericarditis in a case of rheumatic heart disease with recurrence. Pancarditis was noted at autopsy. The surface of the pericardium is covered with abundant fibrin (left of picture) beneath which a few mononuclear cells, prominent blood vessels and edema are seen

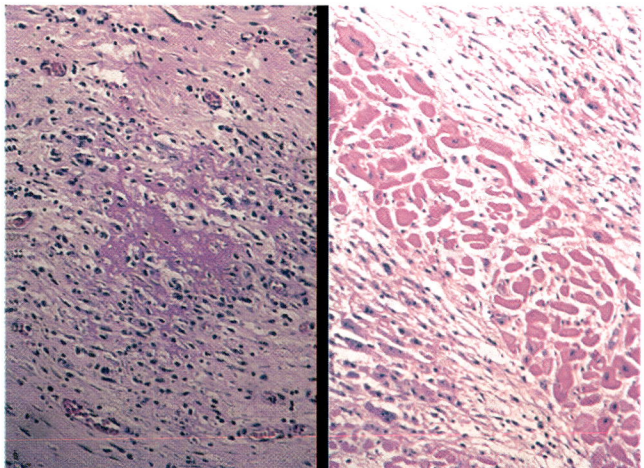

Fig. 11.16: Rheumatic carditis. The left panel of the photomicrograph shows fibrinoid necrosis of the pericardial collagen around which histiocytes and lymphocytic infiltration is seen. The right panel shows typical Aschoff nodules within the myocardium from the same case

Purulent/Suppurative pericarditis (Fig. 11.17) The pericardium may be affected by pus producing organisms which reach the pericardium either by direct extension from adjacent infective foci or the infection may be hematogenous. The process of healing and organisation may lead to adhesions not only within the pericardial cavity and cause adhesive or constrictive pericarditis but also may envelop surrounding structures (mediastinopericarditis).

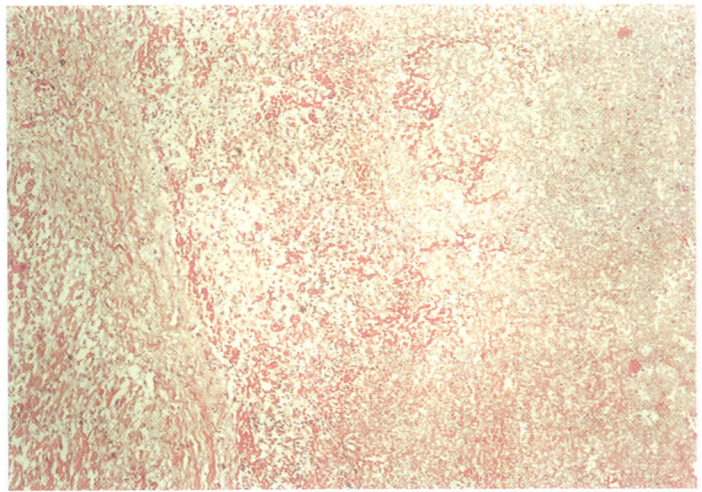

Fig. 11.17a: Purulent pericarditis. The pericardium is markedly thickened, necrotic and shows a few inflammatory cells

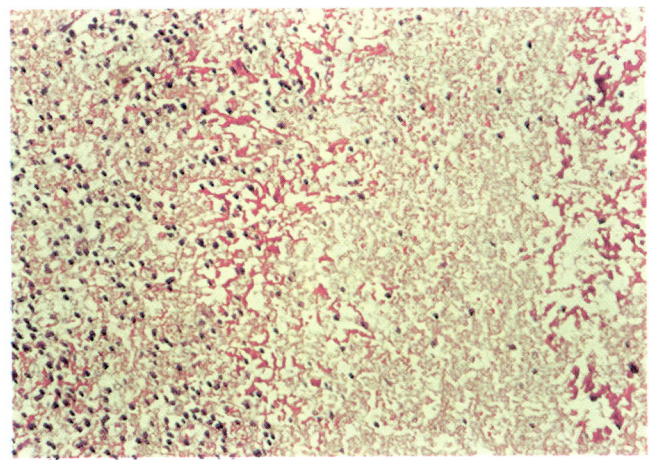

Fig. 11.17b: Purulent pericarditis. Higher magnification of Figure 11.17a to show marked necrosis, fibrin, minimal inflammatory cell infiltration and abundant nuclear debris

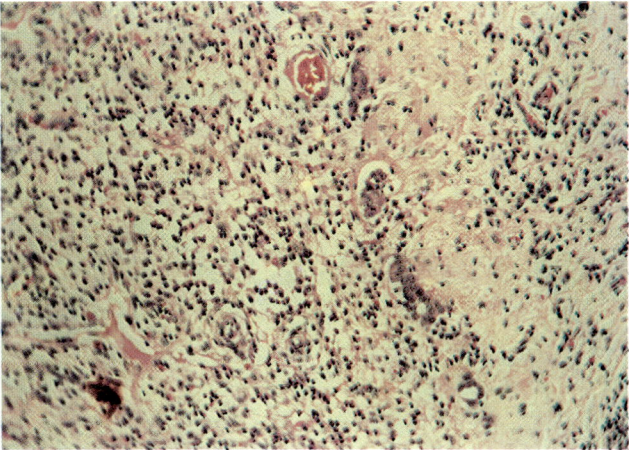

Fig. 11.17c: Purulent pericarditis. The pericardium reveals increased vascularity, numerous polymorphs and groups of reactive mesothelial cells

Tuberculous pericarditis Involvement of the pericardium by tuberculosis continues to be an important cause of cardiac embarrassment (constrictive pericarditis). As in purulent pericarditis, the tuberculous infection of the pericardium is either by direct spread from pulmonary/tuberculous mediastinal lymph nodes or through a hematogenous spread. Naked eye examination shows marked thickening of both layers of pericardium (Figs 11.4 and 11.5). Caseation necrosis may be seen. Microscopically, epithelioid cell granulomas with or without necrosis are observed (Figs 11.6, 11.7b, 11.8 and 11.9). Chronic inflammation, scarring and focal calcification are often encountered. These changes may represent healed tuberculous infection. Healed tuberculous pericardium is a common cause of constrictive pericarditis. Constriction can be successfully relieved by pericardiectomy.

Healed pericarditis Healing of pericarditis leads to obliteration of the pericardial cavity with thickening (**adhesive pericarditis**) (Fig. 11.18). This is generally not associated with clinical symptoms. Marked thickening of the pericardium may result consequent to tuberculous or suppurative pericarditis, the former being more common. This may produce symptoms and signs of constriction of the pericardium. Pericardiectomy is indicated to relieve the symptoms. In **constrictive pericarditis,** the heart may be encased within a thickened coat of pericardium which limits its diastolic expansion. Microscopically, abundant collagen/fibrosis of the pericardium is observed. Calcification is often present (Fig. 11.9).

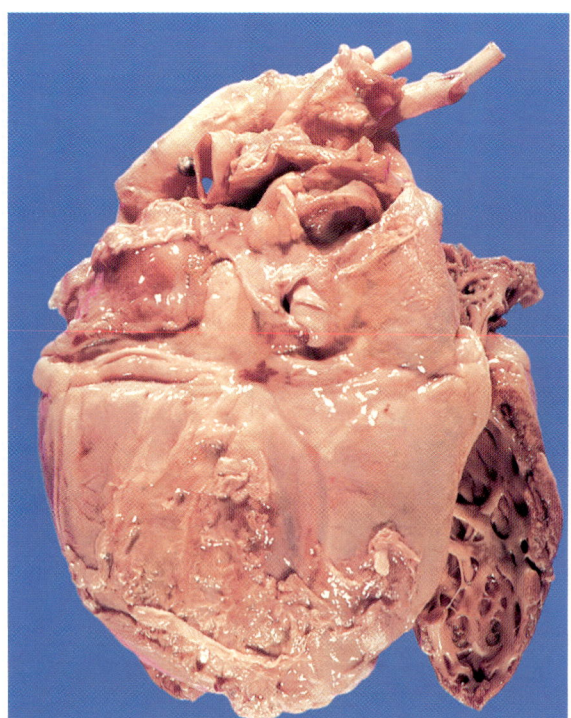

Fig. 11.18a: Fibrous pericarditis. External surface of the inferior surface of the heart shows irregularity of the surface due to focal fibrous thickening of the visceral pericardium. Adhesions were present between the visceral and the parietal layers

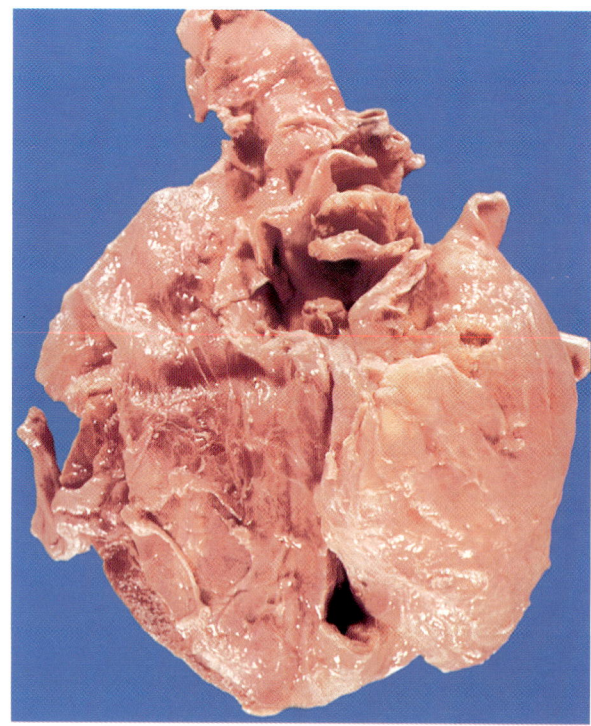

Fig. 11.18b: Adhesive pericarditis. The pericardium is thickened and is adherent to the surface of the heart. The adhesions had to be cut. Adhesions were also present between the heart and mediastinal structures

Tumors of the Pericardium

Primary pericardial tumors are rare. Almost any tumor can involve the pericardium. Benign tumors include mesothelial cysts (most common) angiomas, lymphangiomas, fibroma (Fig. 11.19) teratoma, fibrous histiocytoma (Fig. 11.20) lipoma, mesothelial papillomas, etc. Malignant pericardial tumors may be primary or metastatic. Primary tumors are generally malignant mesothelioma (Figs 11.3 and 11.21) and various sarcomas (Fig. 11.22). Malignant melanoma (Fig. 11.23) leukemic infiltration (Fig. 11.24) lymphoma both Hodgkin's (Fig. 11.25) and non-Hodgkin's (Figs 11.26 and 11.27) can affect the pericardium. Primary cardiac lymphoma of the heart is extremely rare. Cardiac involvement as part of disseminated malignant lymphoma has been observed in 20% cases at autopsy. Cytological examination of pleural fluid is diagnostic in most cases (Fig. 11.27).

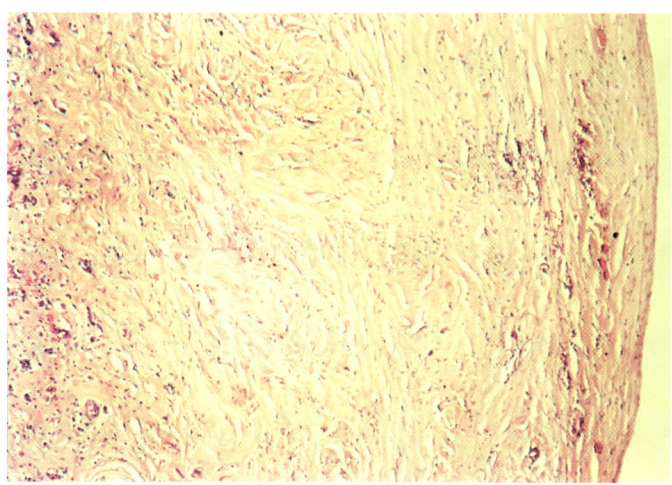

Fig. 11.19a: Pericardial fibroma. The lesion is composed of abundant collagen, few blood vessels and chronic inflammatory cells. This lesion was encountered incidentally during mitral valvotomy which was performed for mitral stenosis of rheumatic etiology. A well circumscribed nodule 2.5 cm in diameter attached to the pericardium was detected within the pericardial sac

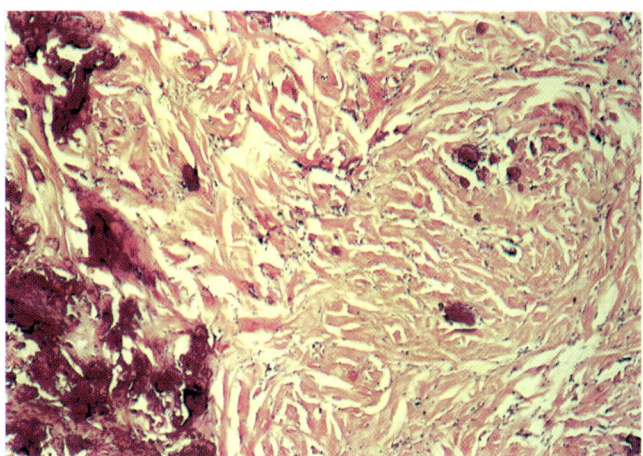

Fig. 11.19b: Another area of pericardial fibroma to show abundant collagen in a whorled arrangement. Focal calcification is also observed

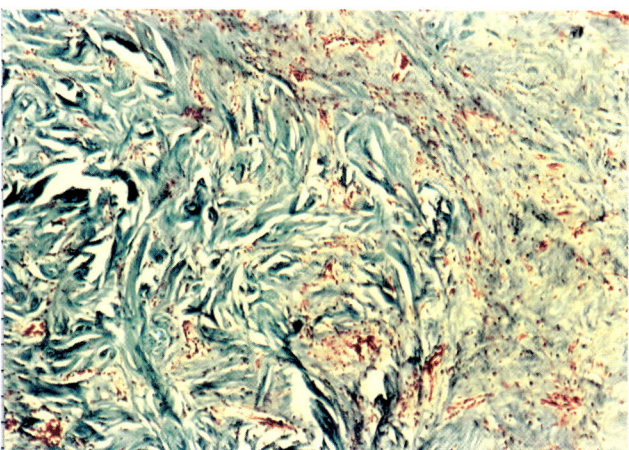

Fig. 11.19c: Masson trichrome stain to highlight the abundant collagen comprising the lesion

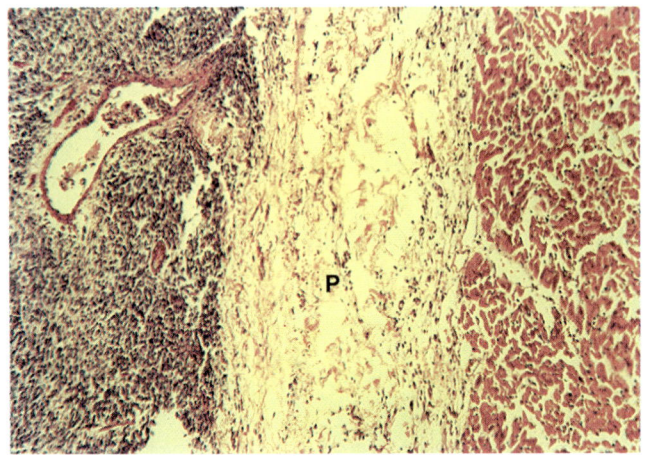

Fig. 11.20a: Fibrous histiocytoma of the pericardium. Tumor is present on the surface. The myocardium is unremarkable. Portion of the pericardium (P) free of tumor is also seen

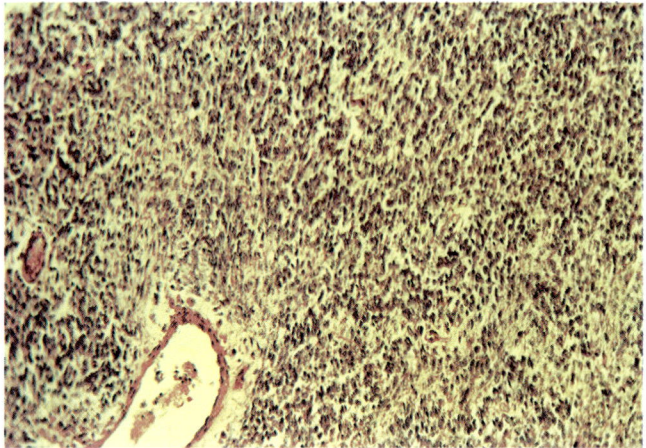

Fig. 11.20b: Fibrous histiocytoma of the pericardium. Higher magnification of Figure 11.20a. Tumor cells are arranged in sheets and show mild pleomorphism and low mitotic activity. Foamy histiocytes were interspersed amidst the spindle shaped cells

Note: A 40 years male presented with pain in the retrosternal and epigastric regions. At autopsy, the pericardial sac was markedly increased in size. A mass measuring 25 cm in largest diameter, weighing 1200 gm was present within the sac

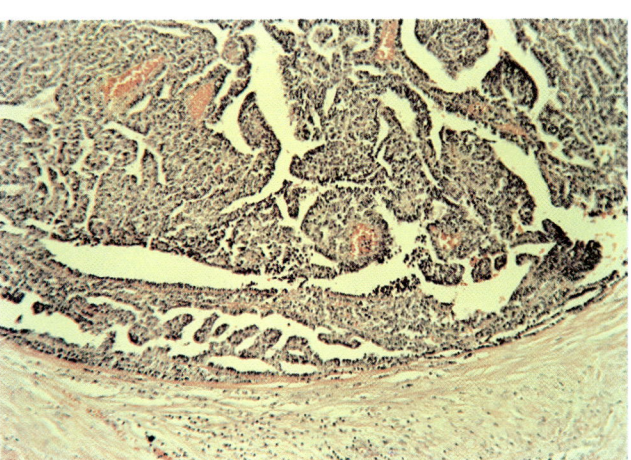

Fig. 11.21a: Malignant mesothelioma of the pericardium. Numerous slit like spaces with interspersed tumor cells arranged in groups and glandular fashion are seen

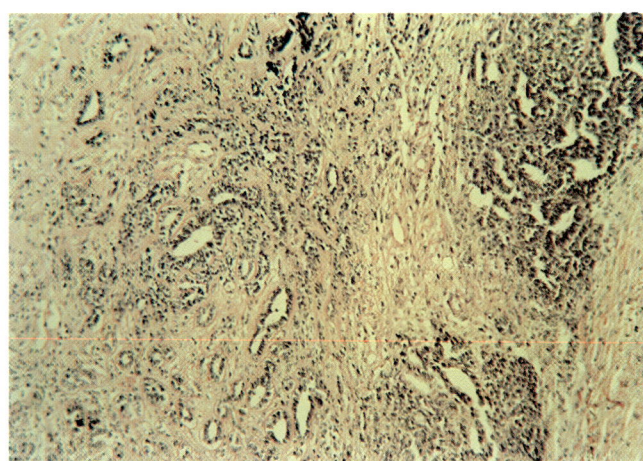

Fig. 11.21b: Malignant mesothelioma of the pericardium. Numerous gland like spaces dispersed within fibrous tissue are seen

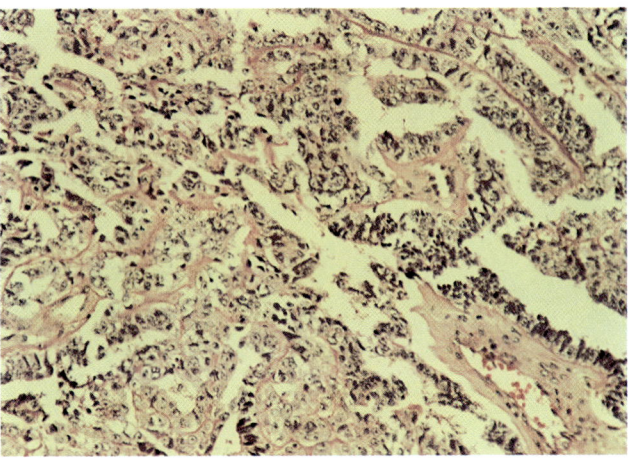

Fig. 11.21c: Malignant mesothelioma of the pericardium. The epithelial component is seen as glandular spaces and in papillary configurations

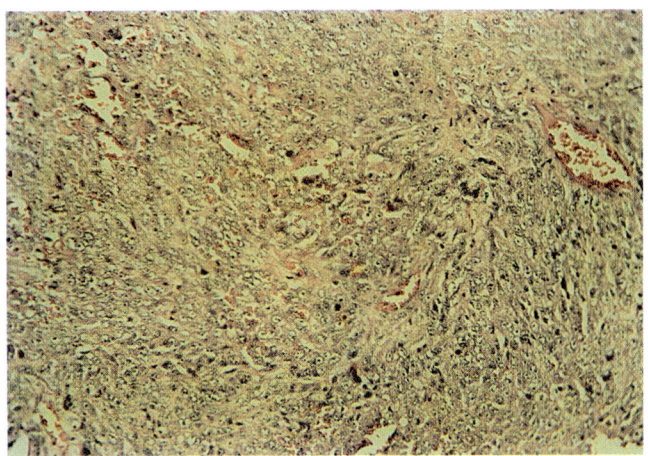

Fig. 11.22a: Malignant mesenchymal tumor in the pericardium. Tumor cells are arranged in flowing bundles. They have ovoid vesicular nuclei. Several blood spaces are noted

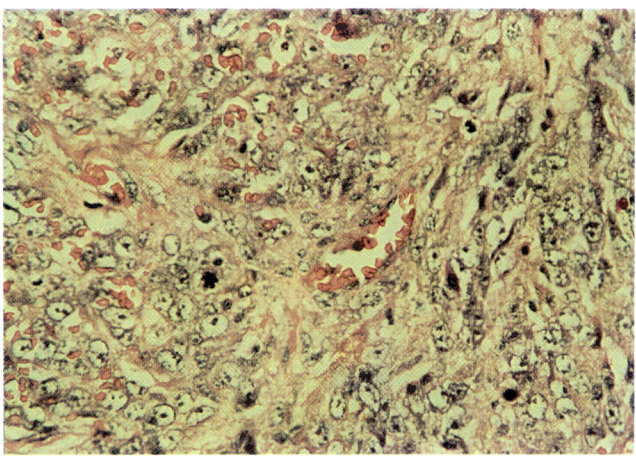

Fig. 11.22b: Malignant mesenchymal tumor in the pericardium. Tumor cells show vesicular nuclei, minimal pleomorphism and mitotic activity. Prominent vascular spaces are present
Note: Patient was a 22 years male who presented with features of constrictive pericarditis. At surgery, hemopericardium (800 ml) was present. The pericardial cavity was filled with a hemorrhagic tumor. Histologically, the tumor was undifferentiated. Tumor markers were noncontributory

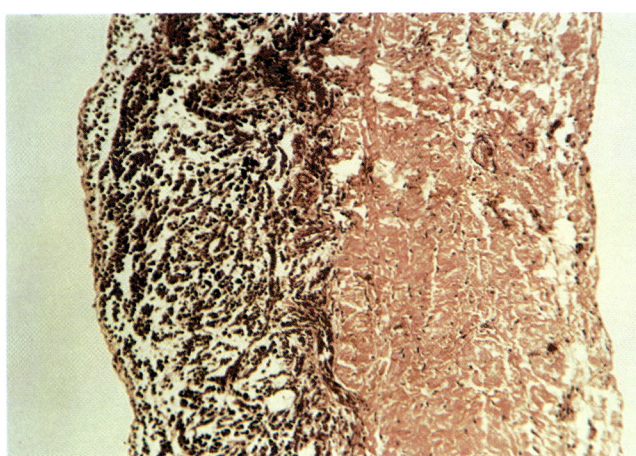

Fig. 11.23: Infiltration of the pericardium by malignant melanoma. Abundant melanin pigment was also recognised

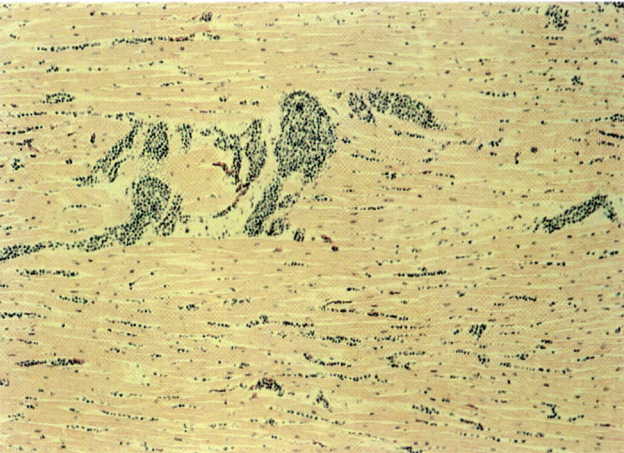

Fig. 11.24: Leukemic infiltrate within the myocardium. The tumor cells are seen in clusters and diffusely within the interstitium of the myocardium

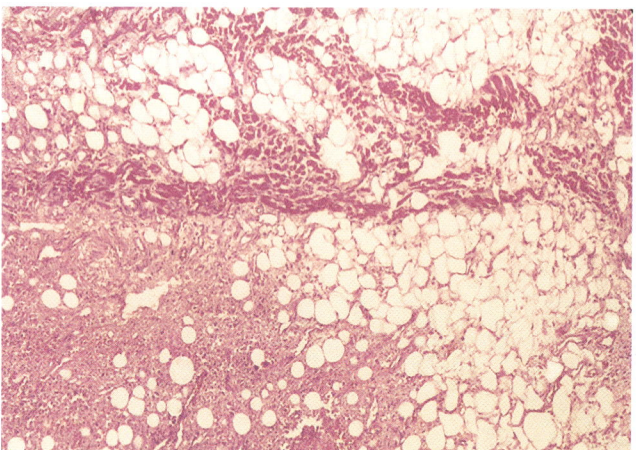

Fig. 11.25a: Photomicrograph showing infiltration of pericardial fat by Hodgkin's lymphoma

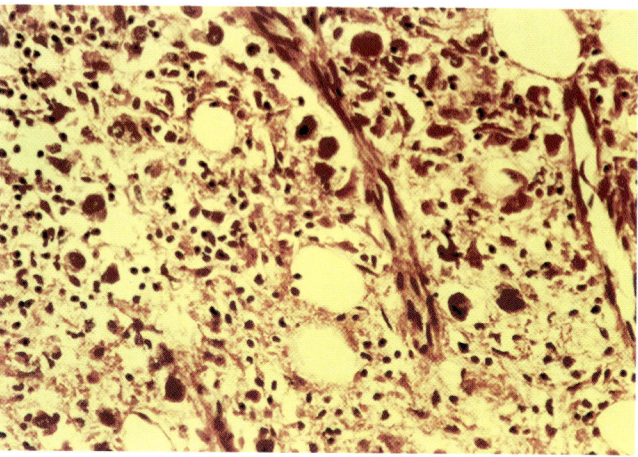

Fig. 11.25b: Higher magnification of Figure 11.25a to show the nature of polymorphic infiltrate which is comprised of lymphocytes, plasma cells and atypical histiocytes. Reed-Sternberg cells are also seen

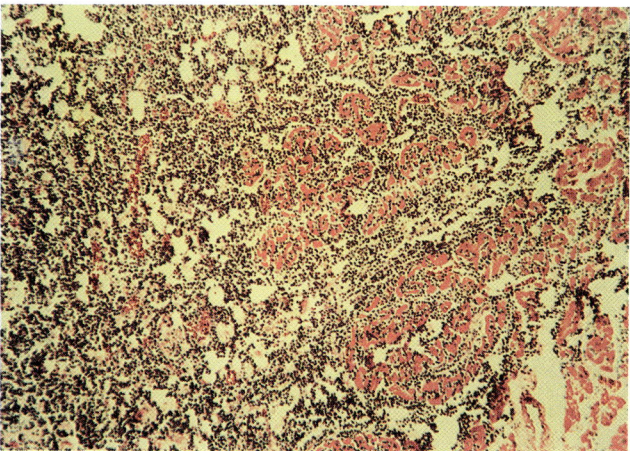

Fig. 11.26: Infiltration by non-Hodgkin's lymphoma of the pericardial fat and myocardium. Sheets of lymphoid cells are observed

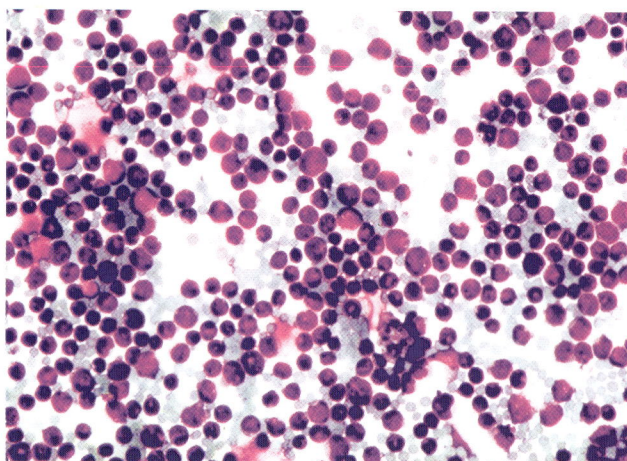

Fig. 11.27a: Non-Hodgkin's lymphoma of the pericardium. Cells are lying singly. They show variation in size, have increased nuclear cytoplasmic ratio large irregular nuclear membrane and coarse chromatin. Minimal cytoplasm is present

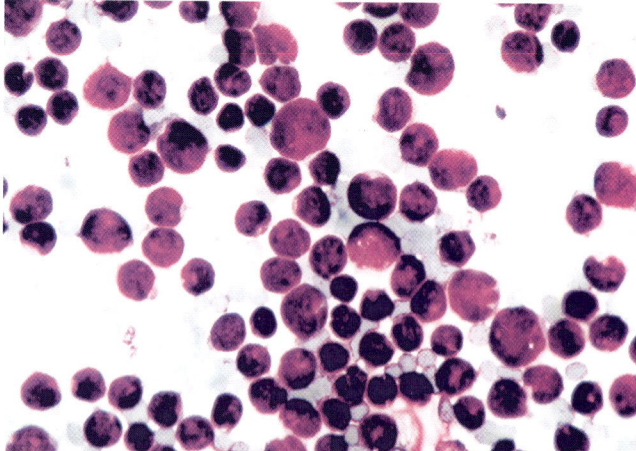

Fig. 11.27b: Non-Hodgkin's lymphoma of the pericardium. Pericardial aspirate is hypercellular and shows sheets of darkly staining monomorphic lymphoid cells

Metastasis to the pericardium has been observed from both carcinomas (Fig. 11.28) and sarcomas.

Mesothelioma Mesothelioma of the pericardium is rare. While pleural and peritoneal mesotheliomas represent over 98% of the total, pericardial mesotheliomas constitute only about 0.7% of malignant mesotheliomas.

Malignant mesotheliomas of the pericardium generally present as nodules that fill the pericardial cavity. The heart and great vessels are usually enveloped by the disease process. The tumor is grey white firm. Areas of hemorrhage, cystic degeneration and necrosis may be present. Microscopically, mesotheliomas may be epithelial, sarcomatoid, biphasic or undifferentiated type. Etiologically, mesothelioma has a link with asbestos exposure. This association is weaker for pericardial than for pleural mesotheliomas. Immunohistochemically most mesotheliomas express cytokeratin both in epithelial and sarcomatoid areas in majority of the cases. Epithelial membrane antigen (EMA) is present in the epithelial areas while vimentin is expressed in the spindle cell areas.

Mesothelioma can often be difficult to distinguish from mesothelial hyperplasia and adenocarcinoma (Table 11.1). This is an exercise which has to be conducted and systematic evaluation needs to be done for a definitive diagnosis. Microscopic features such as cytologic atypia, high nuclear cytoplasmic ratio, pleomorphism, mitotic figures, large cytoplasmic vacuoles, necrosis of cells and infiltration favor a diagnosis of mesothelioma rather than hyperplasia (Figs 11.3, 11.21). Immunohistochemistry is helpful in that membrane staining is obtained with antibody to EMA and HMFG-2 in mesothelioma cells. Differentiation of mesothelioma from adenocarcinoma can also be extremely challenging. Mesothelioma cells generally have

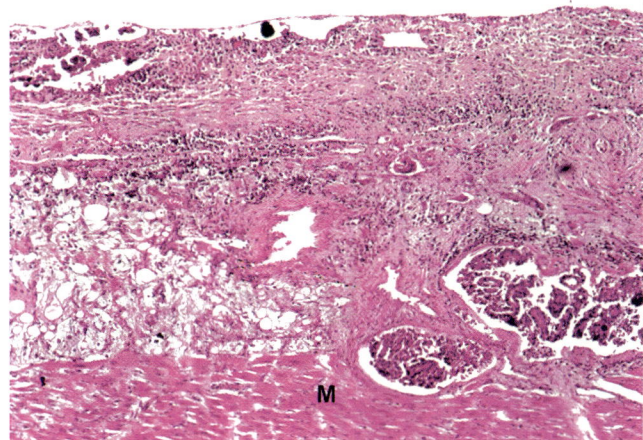

Fig. 11.28a: Metastatic adenocarcinoma pericardium. The pericardium is widened and is infiltrated by groups of epithelial cells. Tiny tumor emboli are also observed. Pericardium shows infiltration by inflammatory cells. Note the epicardial fat and the myocardium (M) in the picture

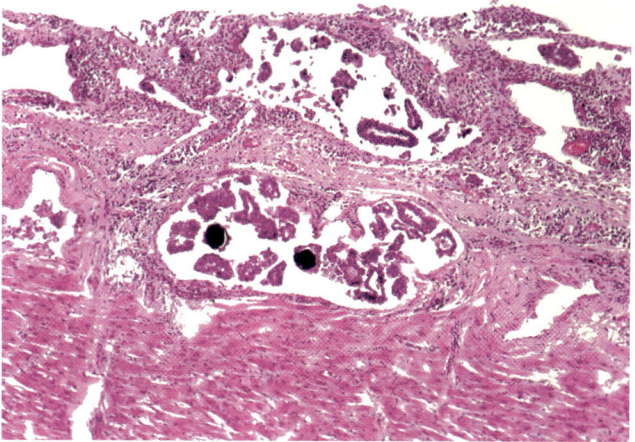

Fig. 11.28b: Metastatic adenocarcinoma pericardium. Islands of tumor cells with psammoma bodies are seen. Myocardium is unremarkable

Note: Patient was a 30 years male who had carcinoma head of pancreas. At autopsy he had disseminated disease

prominent intracytoplasmic vacuoles. There is strong reactivity with colloidal iron and alcian blue which is sensitive to hyaluronidase. This reaction is seen in both reactive mesothelial cells and mesotheliomas. Positive reaction with neutral mucins like hyaluronidase resistant mucicarmine and PAS after diastase digestion suggest adenocarcinoma. This test is relatively insensitive. The histochemical stains suffer several artefacts of interpretation and are less often performed. Immunohistochemistry when judiciously performed aids in the differential diagnosis of mesothelioma. Membrane staining with EMA is observed in mesothelioma cells while carcinoma cells exhibit strong cytoplasmic staining. Adenocarcinoma cells also show strong reaction with CEA.

SUGGESTED READING

1. Agarwal S, Chopra P: Constrictive pericarditis. A histopathologic study of 91 cases. *Ind Heart J* **29**: 278-82, 1977.
2. Chen KY, Liaw YS, Kao HL, Yang PC, Luh KT: Constrictive pericarditis in patients with tuberculous pericarditis. *J Formos Med Assoc* **98(9)**: 599-605, 1999.
3. Darwish Y, Mushannen B, Hussain KM, Nitiham K, *et al:* Pancardiac tuberculosis—A case report. *Angiology* **49**: 151-56, 1998.
4. Ercan Tutar H, Imamoglu A, Atalay S: Recurrent pericarditis as a manifestation of familial Mediterranean fever (letter). *Circulation* **101(5)**: E71-72, 2000.
5. Iizuka B, Yamagishi N, Honma N, Hayashi N: Cardiovascular disease associated with ulcerative colitis. *Nippon Rinsho* **57(11)**: 2540-45, 1999.
6. Janion M, Bakowski D: Diagnosis of pericarditis. *Przegl-Lek* **56(4)**: 286-91, 1999.
7. Myers RB, Spodick DH: Constrictive pericarditis Clinical and pathophysiologic characteristics. *Am Heart J* **138**: 219-32, 1999.
8. Snyder RW, Braun TI: Purulent pericarditis with tamponade in a postpartum patient due to group F streptococcus. *Chest* **115(6)**: 1746-47, 1999.
9. Weber S: Tuberculosis and pericarditis in children. *Trop Doct* **29(3)**: 135-38, 1999.

Tumors of Heart

Tumors of the heart are uncommon. Both primary and metastatic tumors occur in the heart. Metastatic tumors are much more frequent than primary ones and occur in the ratio of 20:1 to 40:1. Of the primary tumors of the heart 75% to 80% are benign and the remaining are malignant tumors. The vast majority of benign tumors of the heart are myxomas. Classification of cardiac tumors is provided in Table 12.1.

BENIGN TUMORS/TUMOR LIKE CONDITIONS OF HEART

Cardiac myxoma This is the most common tumor of the heart. Typically cardiac myxomas are sporadic, benign, non recurring left atrial masses. "A familial" form and a "syndrome" form of cardiac myxoma is well-documented. Majority of the cases are

Table 12.1: Classification of tumors of heart and pericardium

Benign cardiac tumors	Malignant cardiac tumors
Myxoma	Metastatic tumors to heart
Papillary fibroelastoma	Angiosarcoma
Rhabdomyoma	Rhabdomyosarcoma
Fibroma	Unclassified sarcoma
Solitary fibrous tumor of pericardium	Myxosarcoma
Benign fibrous histiocytoma	Fibrosarcoma
Inflammatory pseudotumor	Synovial sarcoma
Hemangioma	Osteosarcoma
Hemangioendothelioma	Malignant schwannoma
Hemangiopericytoma	Kaposi's sarcoma
Lipoma	Malignant germ cell tumors
Lipomatous hypertrophy of atrial septum	Malignant mesothelioma
Mesothelial cysts	
Neurofibroma	
Paraganglioma	
Leiomyoma	
Teratoma	

in the third to sixth decade of life. A female preponderance has been noted in most series. They are most commonly located in the left atrium in the region of the fossa ovalis. Other sites include right atrium (18%) right and left ventricle (4% each) and multiple chambers. In a series of 85 surgically excised cardiac myxomas at the All India Institute of Medical Sciences 71 were located in left atrium, 11 in the right atrium and 3 cases were biatrial.

Cardiac myxomas are oval, round or polypoidal in shape having a smooth, gelatinous and/or hemorrhagic surface (Fig. 12.1). On echocardiography, clot in the left atrium may simulate cardiac myxoma (Fig. 12.2). Cut surface shows a variable appearance namely myxoid, gelatinous, yellow, hemorrhagic, cystic and in some instances firm and calcified foci may also be encountered. **Microscopically,** continuity of the endocardium with the base of the

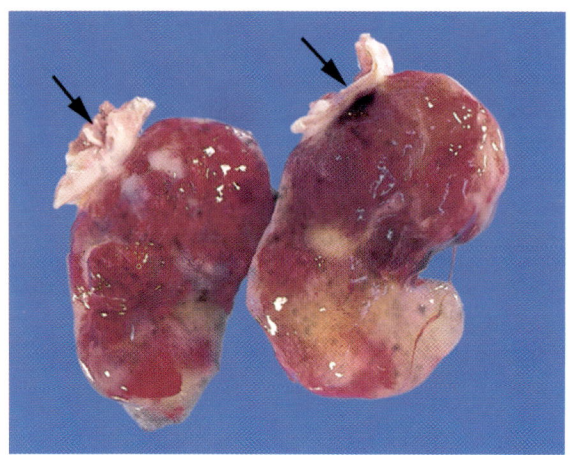

Fig. 12.1a: Cardiac myxoma. This was a mass in the left atrium. It is pedunculated and attached to the septum. The site of attachment is seen as a whitish elevation on the surface (arrows). The mass is lobulated, congested and shows myxoid areas

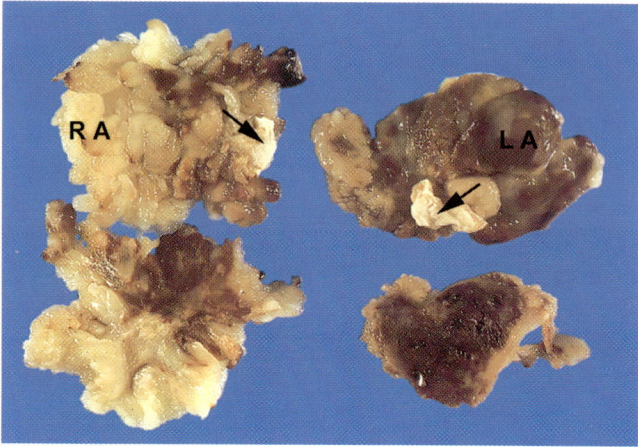

Fig. 12.1b: Bilateral atrial myxoma. The tumor is lobulated, gelatinous/myxoid and congested. Pedicle of the tumor (arrows) is seen. LA—Left atrium; RA—Right atrium

Note: This (Fig. 12.1b) was a case of familial recurrent biatrial cardiac myxoma. The case that is illustrated is from the mother who suffered a recurrence two years later. The son had a left atrial myxoma which recurred 20 years later. The other sibling also had biatrial cardiac myxoma

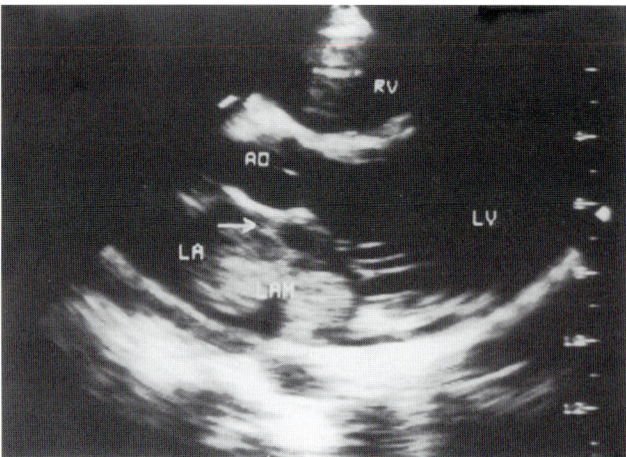

Fig. 12.2a: Echocardiograph in parasternal long axis view showing left atrial myxoma (LAM). Arrow points to the stalk of the tumor

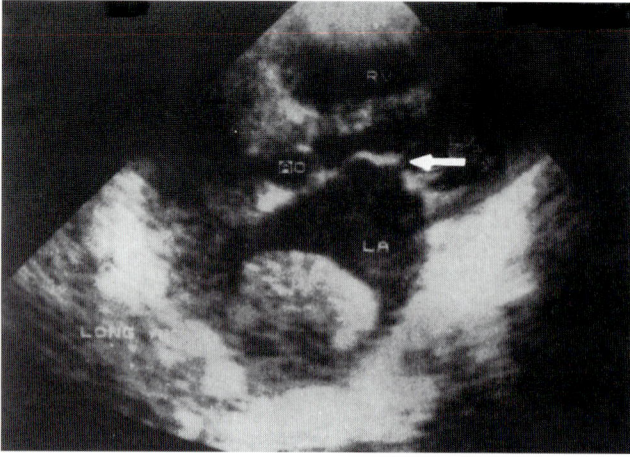

Fig. 12.2b: Echocardiograph in parasternal long axis view in a patient with mitral valve stenosis showing a large thrombus in the left atrial cavity. Mitral valve is thickened (arrow) (Rheumatic heart disease). Left atrial clot is more likely

myxoma can be demonstrated in most cases (Fig. 12.3). Myxomas show a variable cellularity. The cells are dispersed in an abundant eosinophilic and/or myxoid matrix. Surface of the myxoma is lined by cuboidal cells which may be either single or in clusters (Fig. 12.4). In the substance of myxoma, the cells may be either single or multinucleate, round, polyhedral or stellate shaped often arranged in small cords (Figs 12.4 to 12.8). Cells arranged loosely in multilayers around vascular channels are seen in most of the cases (Figs 12.6 to 12.8). These cells are also termed myxoma cells or more commonly as "lepidic" cells. They have an oval nucleus with an open chromatin. In the stroma there is variable degree of inflammatory cells namely lymphocytes (Fig. 12.9), histiocytes (Figs 12.8b and 12.10) and plasma cells. Latter is the predominant cell in some cases.

Other changes in the stroma include foci of hemopoiesis, hemorrhage, necrosis (Fig. 12.11), fibrosis, calcification, and ossification (Fig. 12.11) in some cases. Hemosiderin laden macrophages (Fig. 12.12) are commonly detected. Gamna-Gandy bodies (Fig. 12.13) the like seen in chronic venous congestion of the spleen may be seen occasionally.

Rarely, glandular structures lined by tall columnar cells with or without goblet cells are encountered

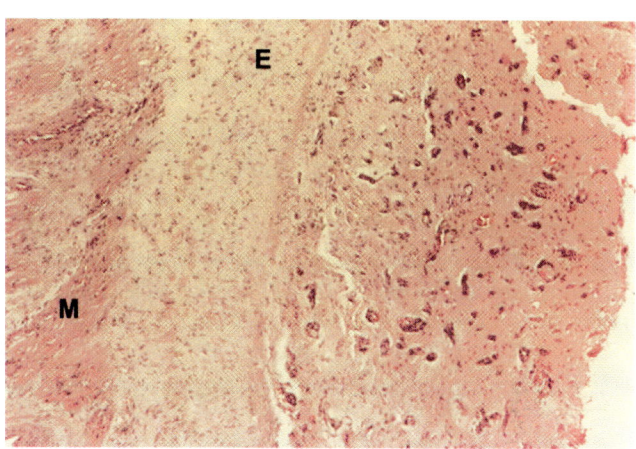

Fig. 12.3: Cardiac myxoma showing its base in continuity with the left atrial endocardium (E). Part of left atrial muscle (M) is also seen in the extreme left of the picture

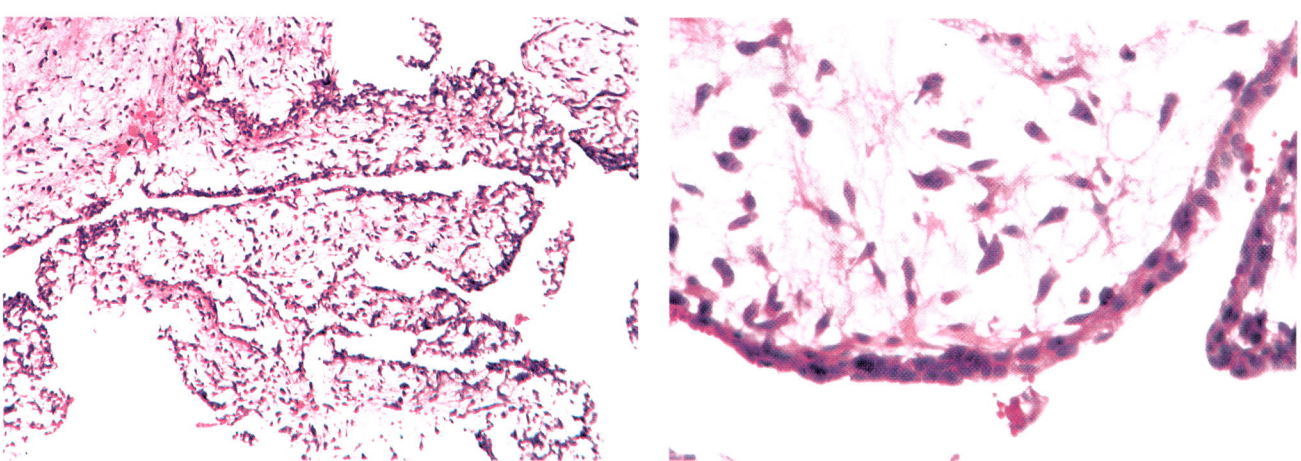

Figs 12.4a and b: Cardiac myxoma (a) the surface lining cells are seen as two rows of flattened attenuated cells. Substance of the myxoma shows stellate cells dispersed in a loose myxoid stroma, (b) higher magnification shows details of surface cells and cells within the myxoid stroma. Cells are ovoid, elongated and stellate shaped and are dispersed within abundant stroma

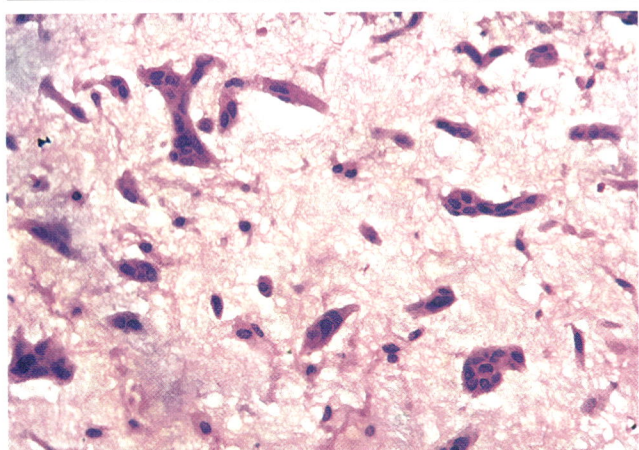

Fig. 12.5: Photomicrograph of cardiac myxoma. Substance of myxoma shows stellate to polyhedral, myxoma cells embedded in abundant loose myxoid stroma

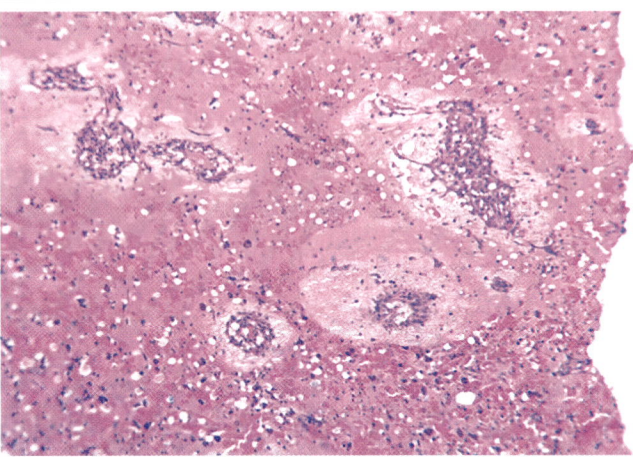

Fig. 12.6: Photomicrograph of cardiac myxoma. Groups of oval to spindle shaped cells are oriented around a vascular space. Stroma surrounding these clusters is relatively acellular and myxoid. Single myxoma (lepidic) cells and sprinkling by inflammatory cells is seen in other areas

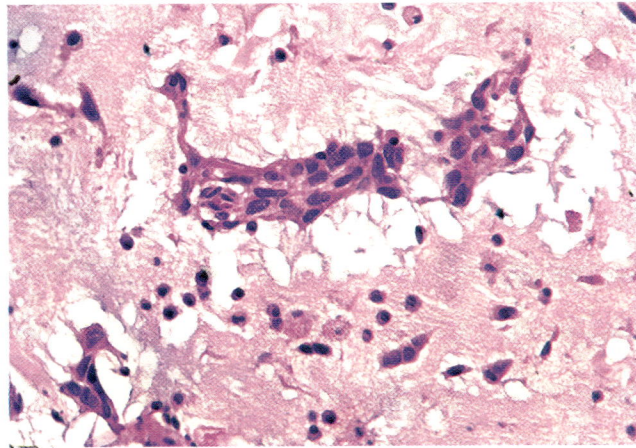

Fig. 12.7: Photomicrograph of cardiac myxoma to show groups of myxoma cells around which the stroma appears vacuolated. The surrounding stroma is loose and myxoid within which stellate to spindle shaped myxoma cells are observed. A few inflammatory cells are also seen

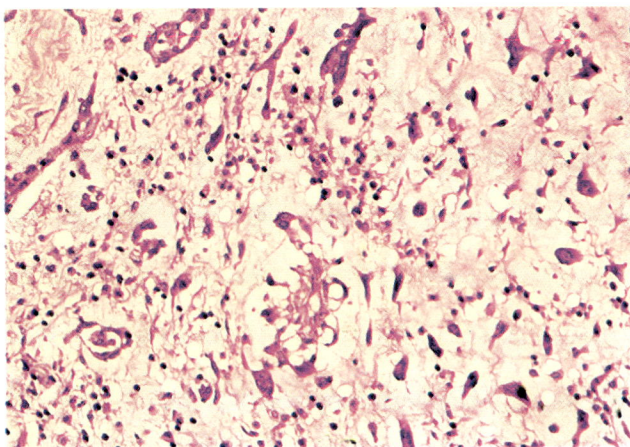

Fig. 12.8a: Cardiac myxoma. Groups as well as single myxoma cells dispersed in myxoid stroma are observed

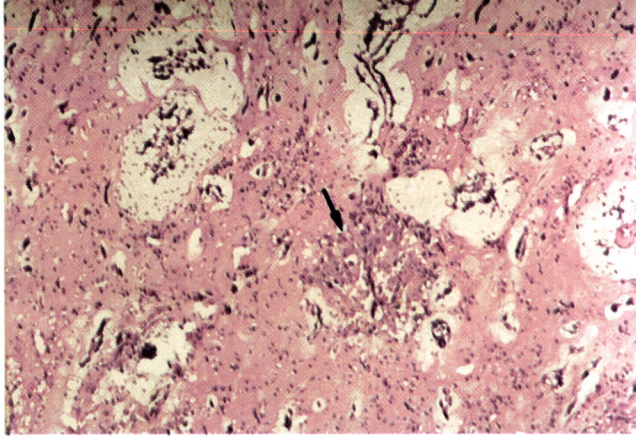

Fig. 12.8b: Cardiac myxoma. Prominent myxoid change is seen around groups of cells. The stroma is loose with interspersed stellate shaped cells. Focal histiocytic aggregate is also seen in the picture (arrow)

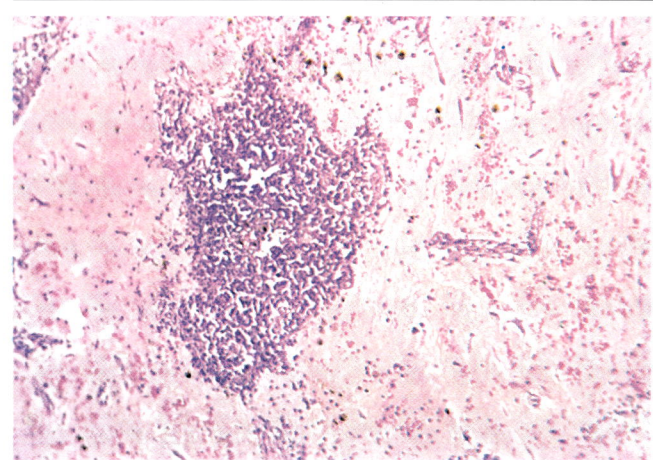

Fig. 12.9: Cardiac myxoma. A large aggregate of lymphocytes is seen in the stroma

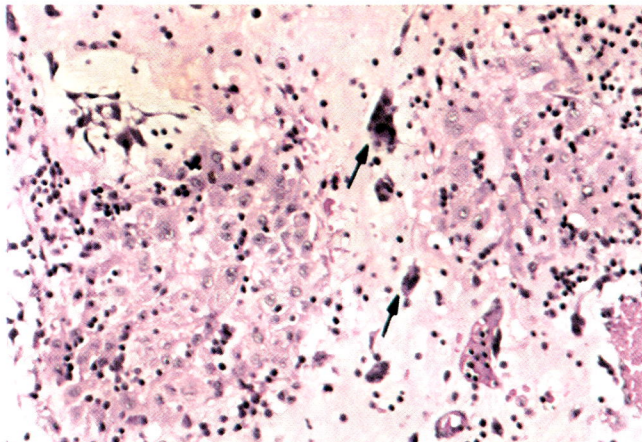

Fig. 12.10a: Cardiac myxoma. Several well-circumscribed aggregates of epithelioid type of cell collections (histiocytes) are seen in the stroma. Lymphocytic infiltration is also noted within these foci. Myxoma cells are present in between these collections (arrows)

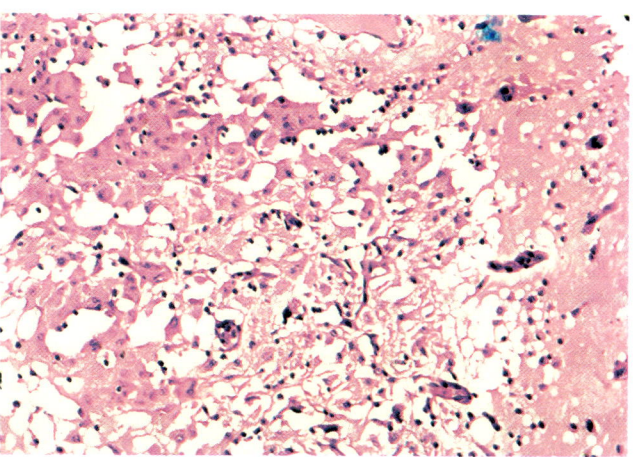

Fig. 12.10b: Cardiac myxoma. Collections of histiocytes are observed within the myxoid stroma. Stellate myxoma cells are noted at the periphery of these foci

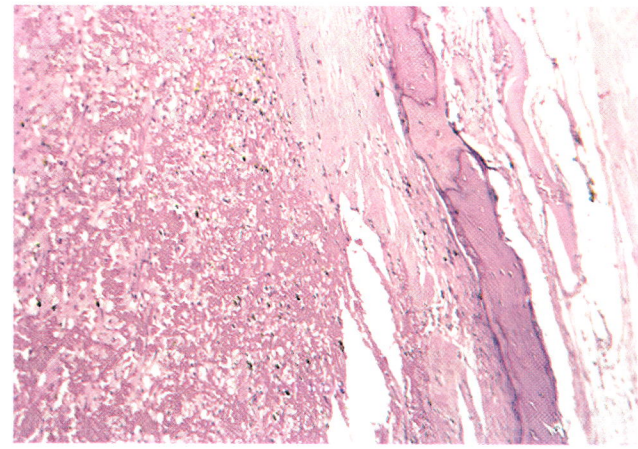

Fig. 12.11: Cardiac myxoma. Large areas of fibrin deposition and necrosis (in other areas) were observed. A focus of ossification is also seen on the right side of picture

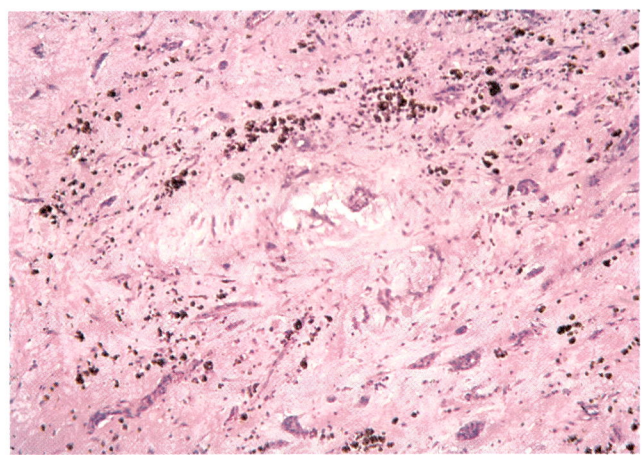

Fig. 12.12a: Cardiac myxoma. Numerous hemosiderin laden macrophages are seen in the myxoid stroma. Myxoma cells are also seen

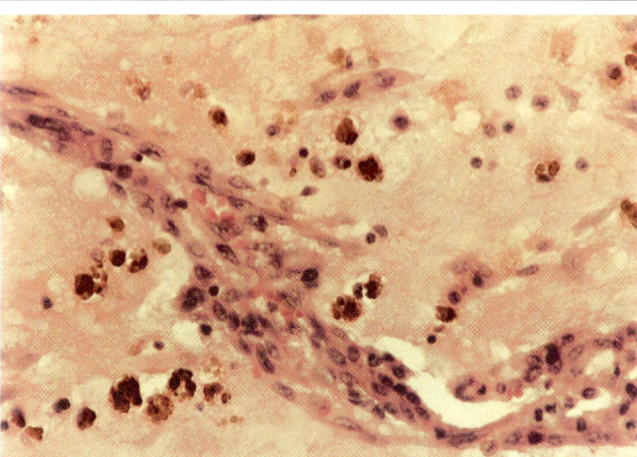

Fig. 12.12b: Cardiac myxoma to show ovoid to spindle shaped cells oriented around a vascular space. Large number of siderophages are noted in the stroma

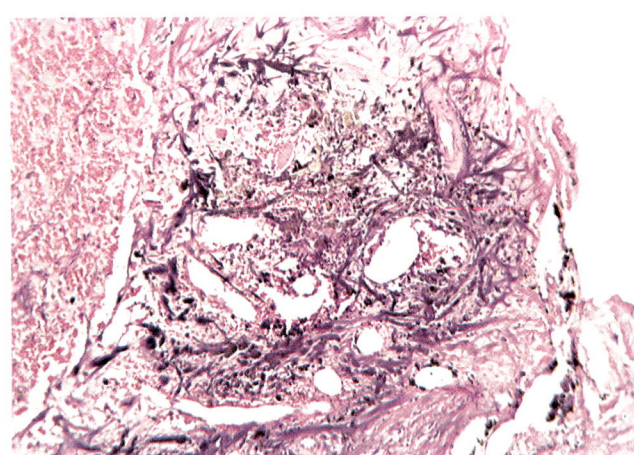

Fig. 12.13a: Cardiac myxoma. A large focal aggregate—Gamna-Gandy body is observed

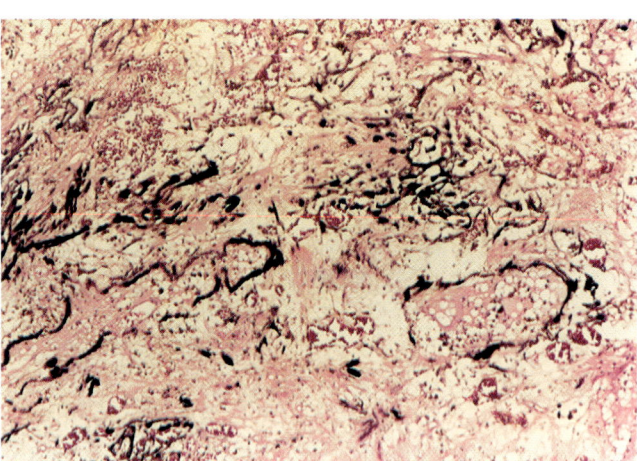

Fig. 12.13b: A focus of degenerative change in a cardiac myxoma showing Gamna-Gandy bodies. These comprise of elongated blackish structures which showed a positive staining reaction for iron and elastic tissue

(Fig. 12.14). We observed this change in 3 of the 85 cases. One was a case of familial cardiac myxoma while the other two were sporadic in nature. Within the glandular component the cells are tall columnar and many of them contain mucin filled vacuoles resembling goblet cells of the gastrointestinal tract. Luminal mucin is also seen within the glandular element. Histochemistry reveal the cells to be mucicarminophilic (Fig. 12.15). The cells showed positive reaction with periodic acid-Schiff's (PAS) reagent which was diastase resistant (Fig. 12.16) and alcian blue PAS (Fig. 12.17). The high iron diamine-alcian blue (HID-AB) stain revealed positivity for both alcian blue (sialomucin) and HIDA (sulphomucin) (Fig. 12.18). Immunohistochemical stains for cytokeratin (CK) (Fig. 12.19) and carcinoembryonic antigen (CEA) (Fig. 12.20) was positive in all the cases (Table 12.2).

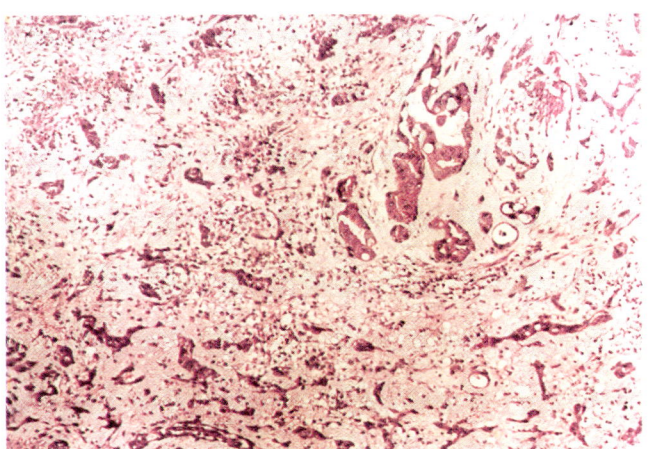

Fig. 12.14a: Cardiac myxoma. Glandular elements are noted in the right upper corner. Notice the myxoma cells arranged singly as well as in groups within a myxoid stroma

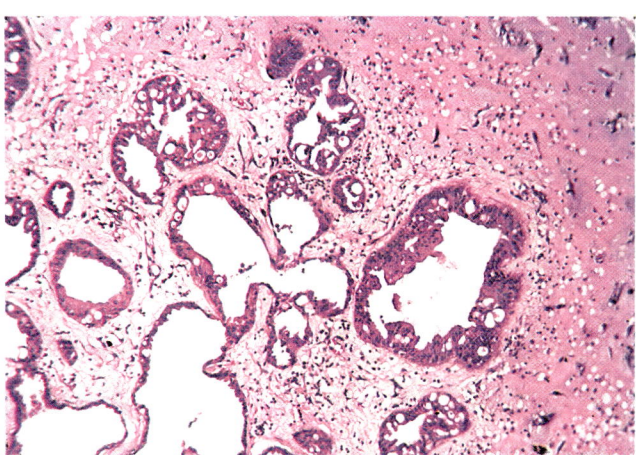

Fig. 12.14b: Recurrent, familial cardiac myxoma showing glandular structures amidst the myxoid stroma. Myxoma cells are also observed in the picture

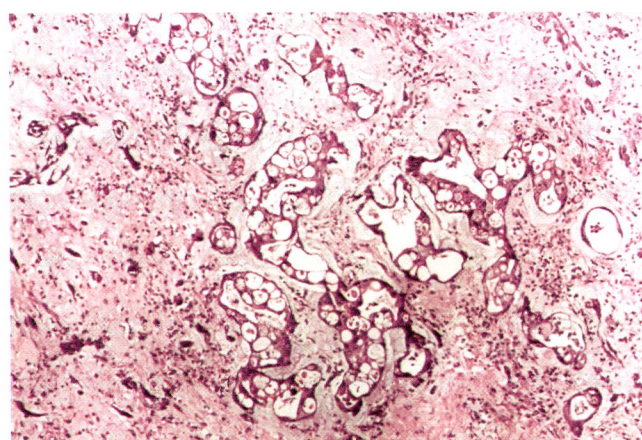

Fig. 12.14c: Left atrial cardiac myxoma excised from a 40-year old female. Prominent glandular structures amidst typical myxoid stroma with myxoma cells arranged singly as well as in groups are recognised

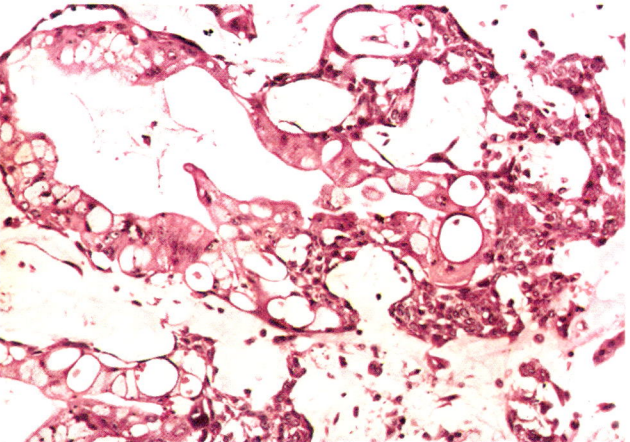

Fig. 12.14d: Cardiac myxoma. Higher magnification of Figure 12.14c to show tall columnar lining cells having vacuolated cytoplasm. Myxoid stroma with myxoma cells is also seen in the photograph

Table 12.2: Histochemical and immunohistochemical reactions in glandular component of cardiac myxoma[3]

Stain	Intensity of reaction	Interpretation
1. Mucicarmine	++	Epithelial mucin
2. Periodic acid-Schiff (PAS)	++	Neutral mucin
3. PAS with Digest	++	Neutral mucin
4. Alcian blue PAS (2.4 ph)	++	Acid mucin
5. High iron diamine-alcian blue (HIDA)		
Blue/Grey	++	– Sialomucin (small intestine)
Dark brown/Black	++	– Sulphomucin (large intestine)
6. Cytokeratin (CK)	++	Epithelial
7. Carcinoembryonic antigen (CEA)	++	Epithelial

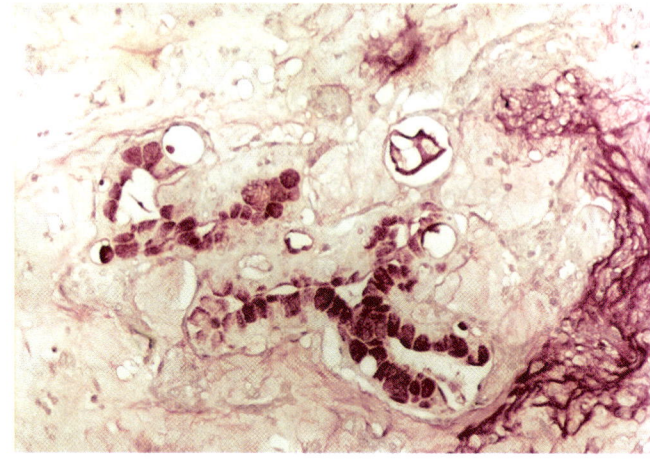

Fig. 12.15: Cardiac myxoma. Mucicarmine stain shows prominent staining reaction of mucin in the cytoplasm of glandular foci within the typical cardiac myxoma

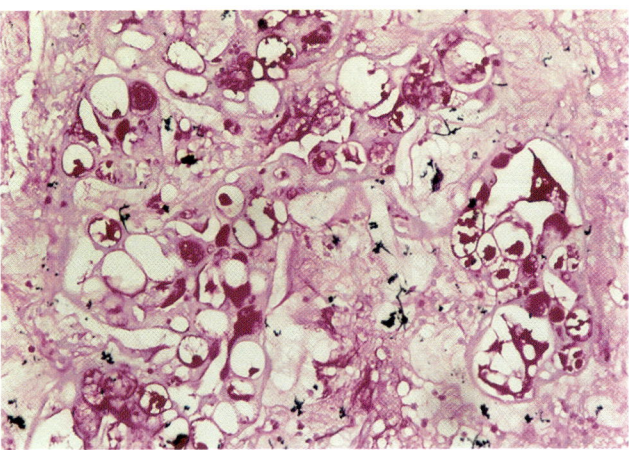

Fig. 12.16a: Cardiac myxoma. Periodic acid-Schiff reaction. The tall columnar lining cells of the glandular component show intense positive reaction of the cytoplasm

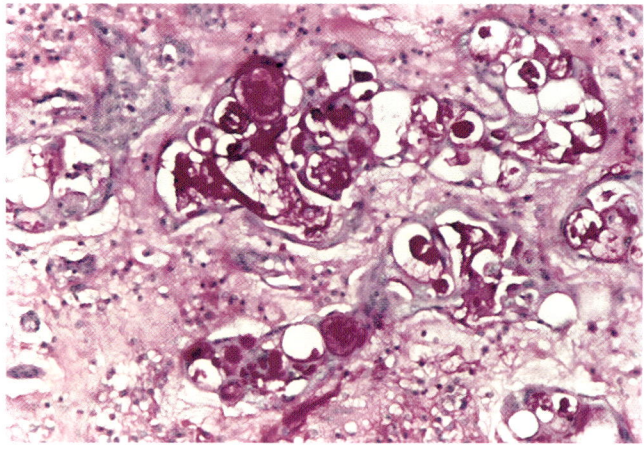

Fig. 12.16b: Cardiac myxoma. Periodic acid-Schiff reaction with diastase. The PAS material in the lining cells is resistant to diastase digestion

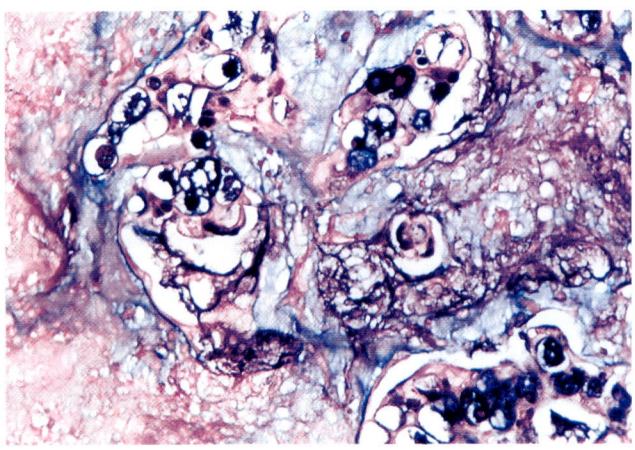

Fig. 12.17: Cardiac myxoma. Alcian blue PAS stain. The lining cells of the glandular component show positive reaction. The stroma also shows staining for acid mucin

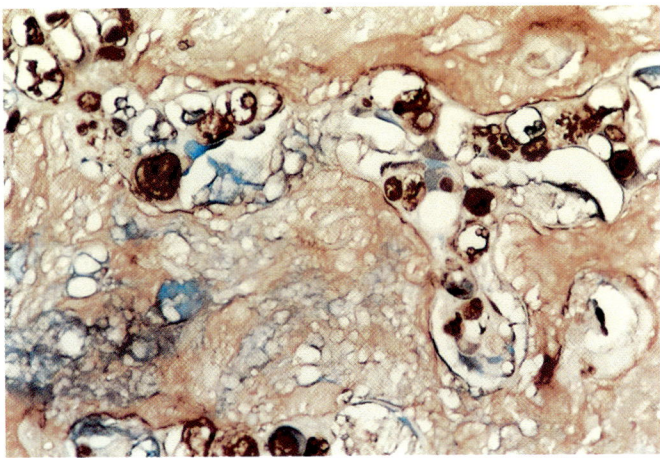

Fig. 12.18: Cardiac myxoma. High iron diamine (HIDA) stain shows 2 types of staining pattern. The light grey blue color represent sialomucin (small intestine) whereas the brown black color suggests sulphomucin (large intestine)

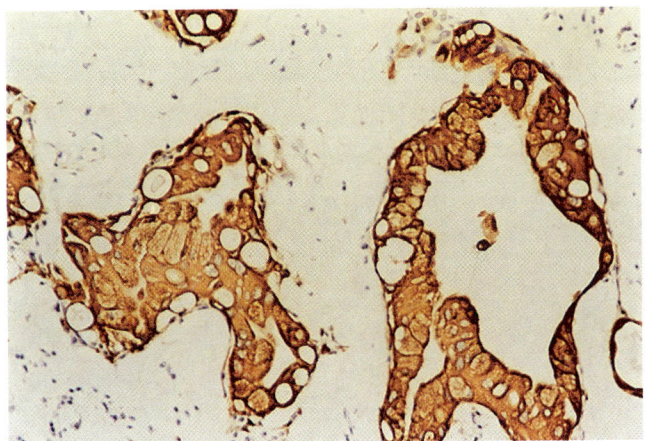

Fig. 12.19: Cardiac myxoma. The glandular component shows strong immunoperoxidase reaction for cytokeratin

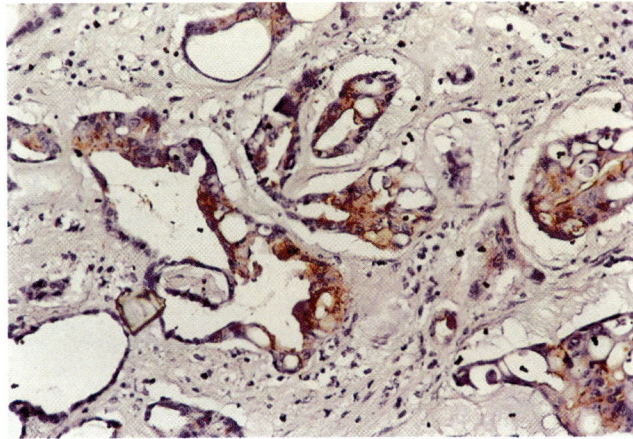

Fig. 12.20: Cardiac myxoma. The lining cells of the glandular component show focal positive immunoperoxidase staining reaction for carcinoembryonic antigen

Ultrastructure

The myxoma cell has ultrastructural features resembling smooth muscle cells, fibroblasts, endothelial cells and myofibroblasts. The cell membrane of most of the myxoma cells is thrown into prominent folds. Variable numbers of cellular organelles are encountered. Some cells show numerous microfilaments present in parallel bundles which crisscross in various directions enclosing and encircling the other organelles. These lack periodicity and resemble myofilaments. Other cells show varying amounts of rough endoplasmic reticulum, pinocytotic vesicles, smooth endoplasmic reticulum and Golgi apparatus (Figs 12.21 to 12.26).

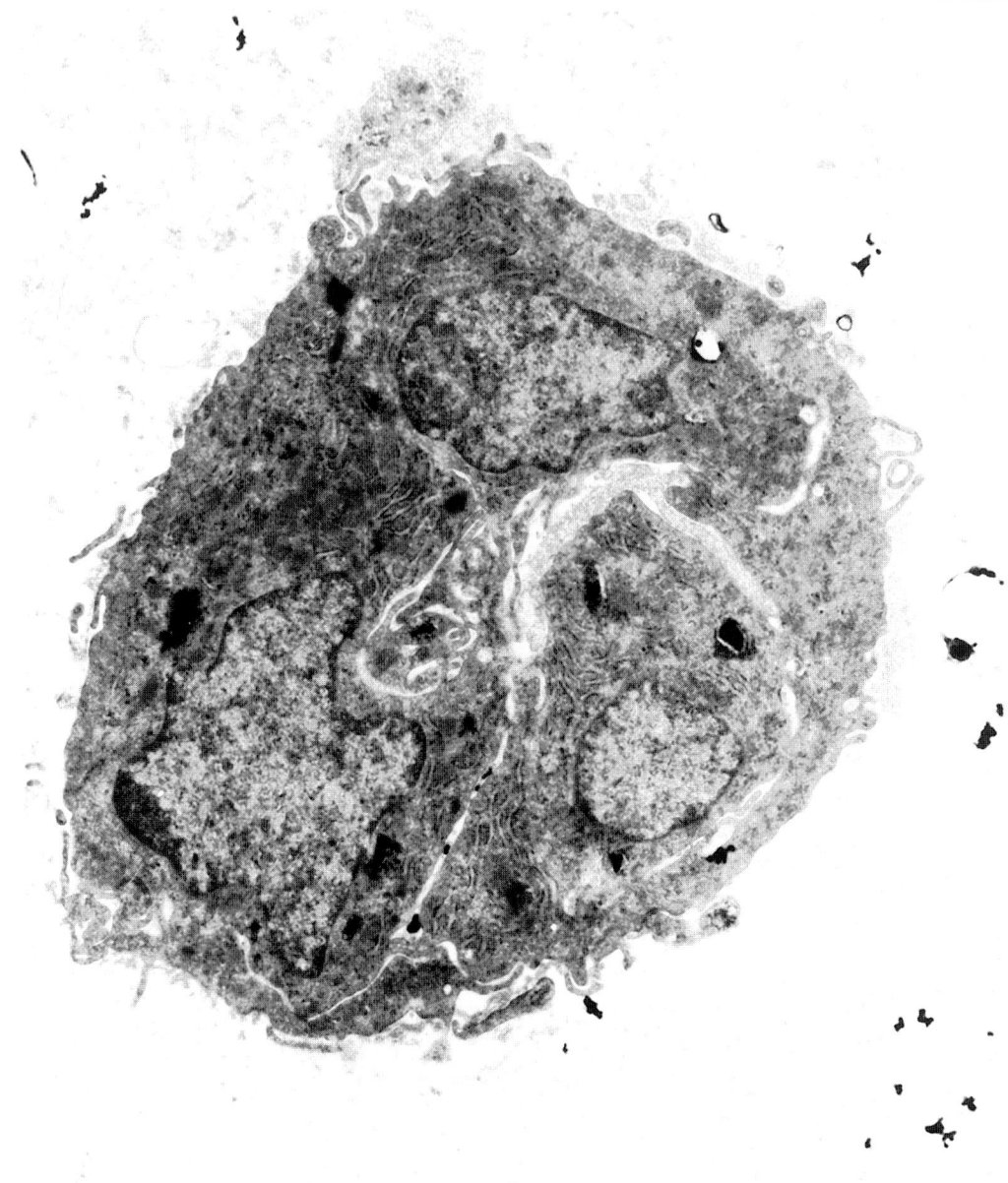

Fig. 12.21: Cardiac myxoma. A group of three cells which show prominent folds of the cell membrane are observed. Cell junctions are ill-defined. The nuclei are variable in shape with prominent indentations of the nuclear membranes. Cytoplasmic organelles are few to moderate in number

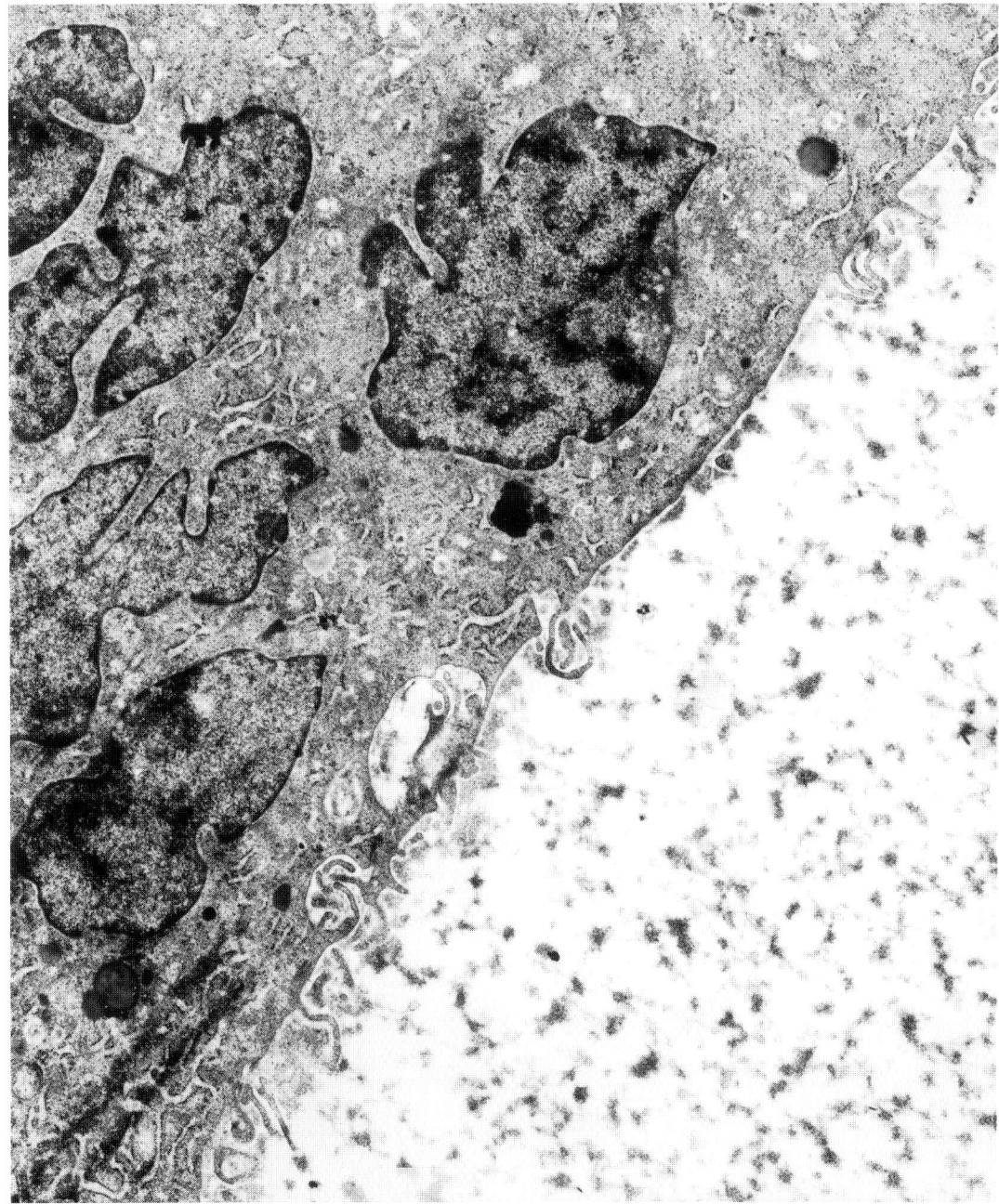

Fig. 12.22: Cardiac myxoma. A group myxoma cells are seen. Notice the prominent infoldings of the cell membrane giving a villous appearance. Ill defined cell junctions are present. Nuclear membrane shows deep indentations. Cytoplasmic organelles are few in number

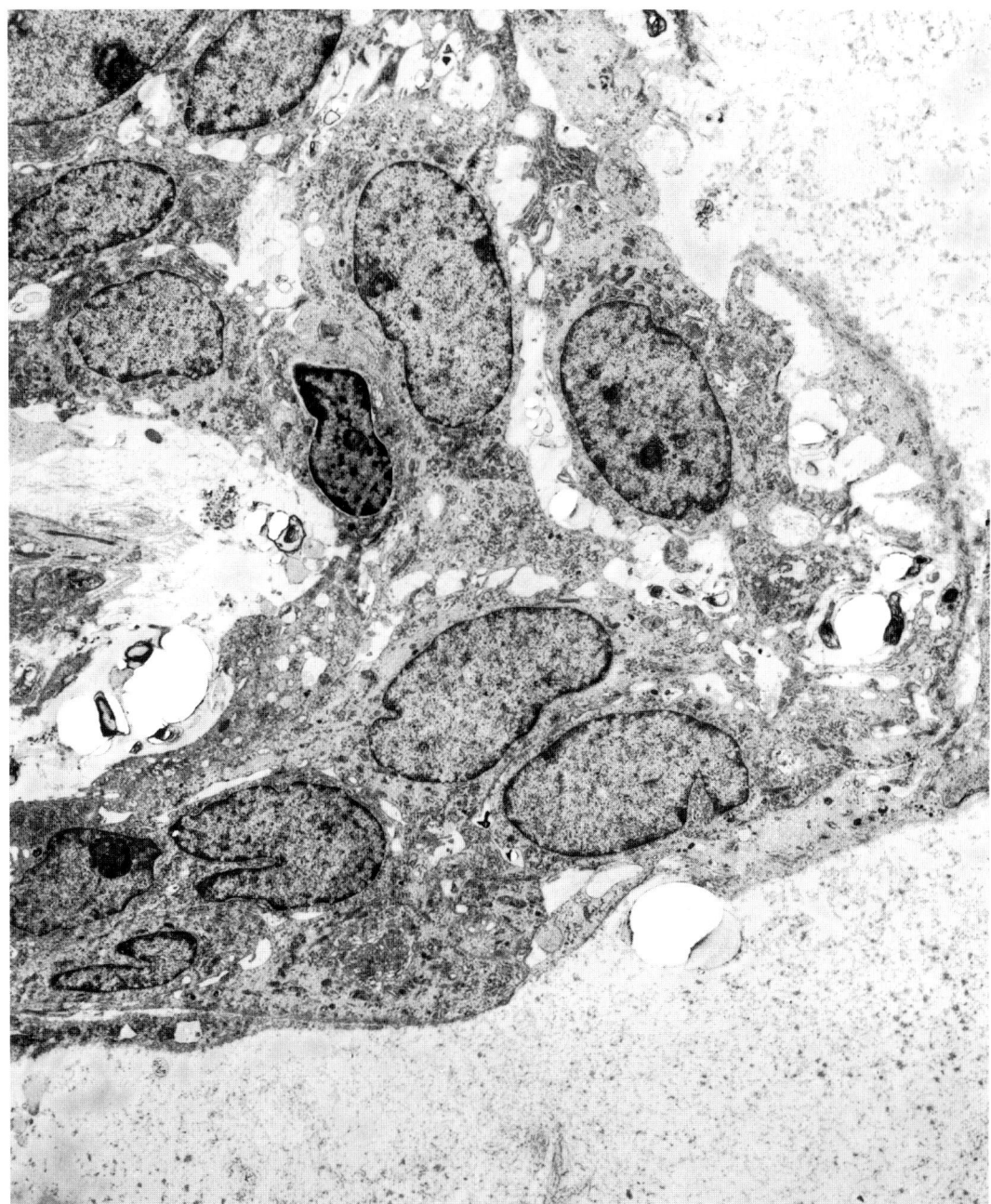

Fig. 12.23: Cardiac myxoma. A group of myxoma cells which are oriented around a blood vessel are seen. Cytoplasmic organelles are moderate in number. Notice the intercellular junctions

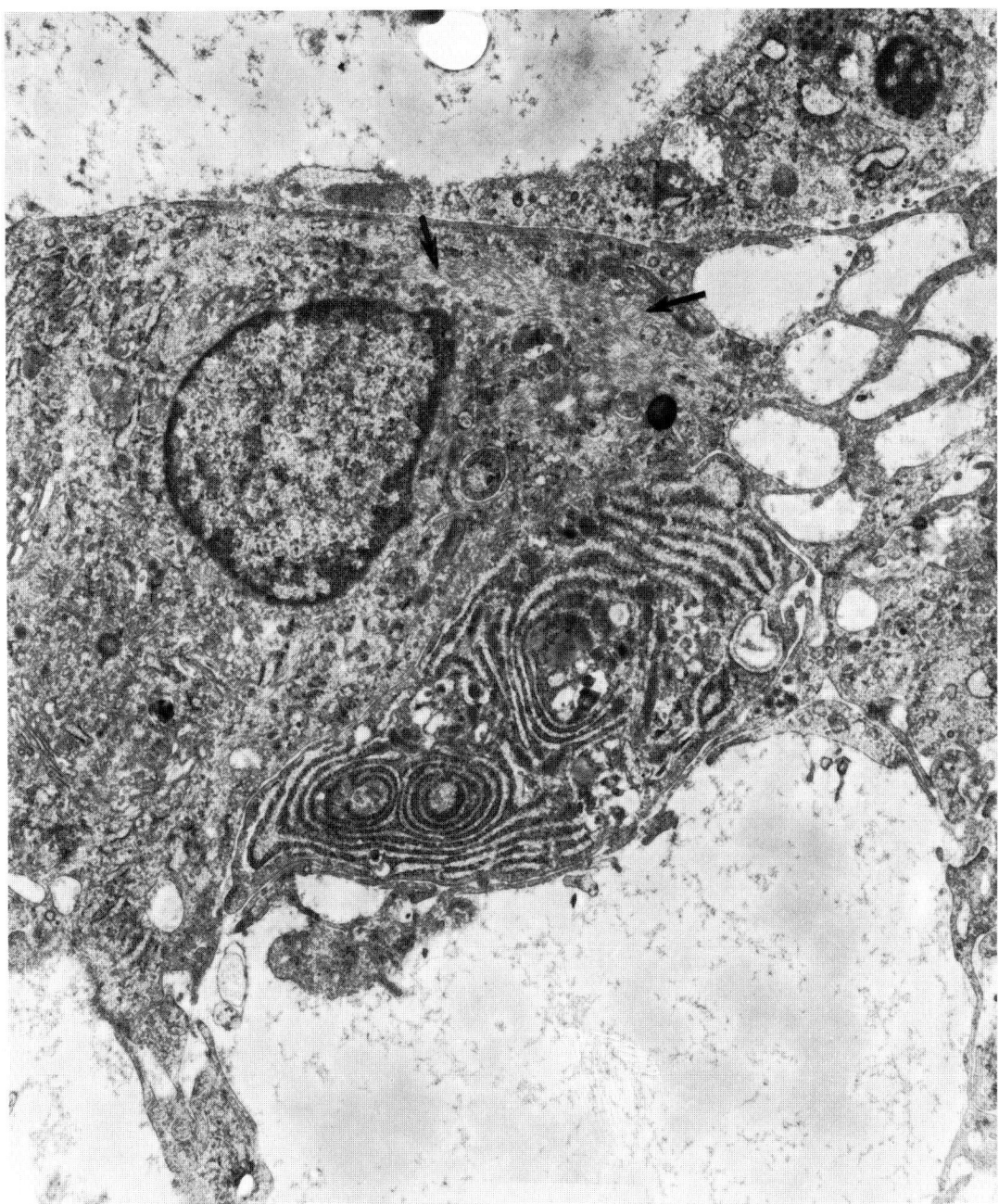

Fig. 12.24: Cardiac myxoma. Higher magnification shows numerous RER profiles arranged in a concentric fashion. Compactly arranged microfilaments are seen arranged in flowing bundles (arrows)

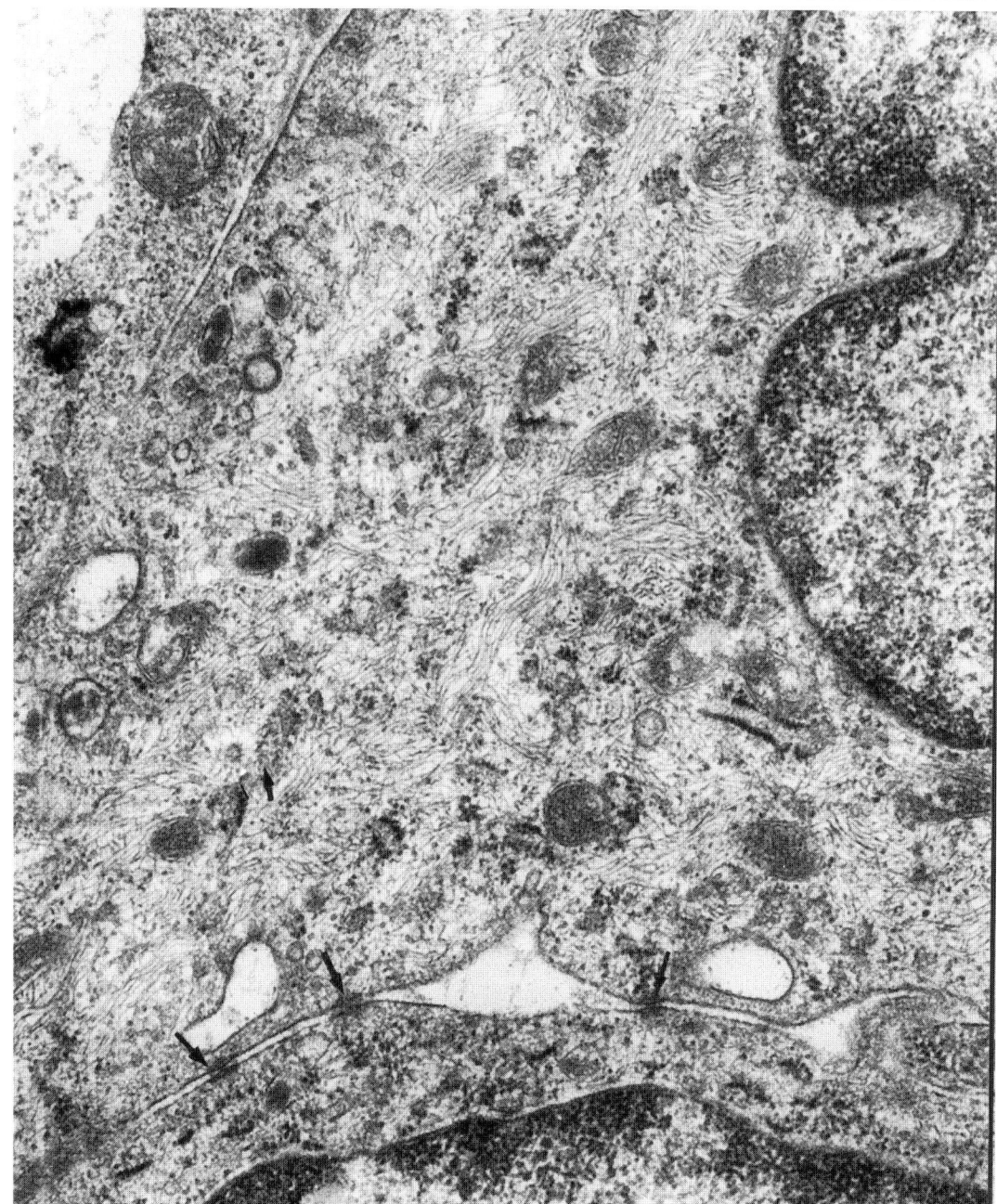

Fig. 12.25: Cardiac myxoma. Parts of two myxoma cells are seen. Numerous microfilaments are seen crisscrossing around the mitochondria and RER (Rough Endoplasmic Reticulum) profiles in the cytoplasm. Notice the intercellular junctions closely resembling the desmosomes (arrows)

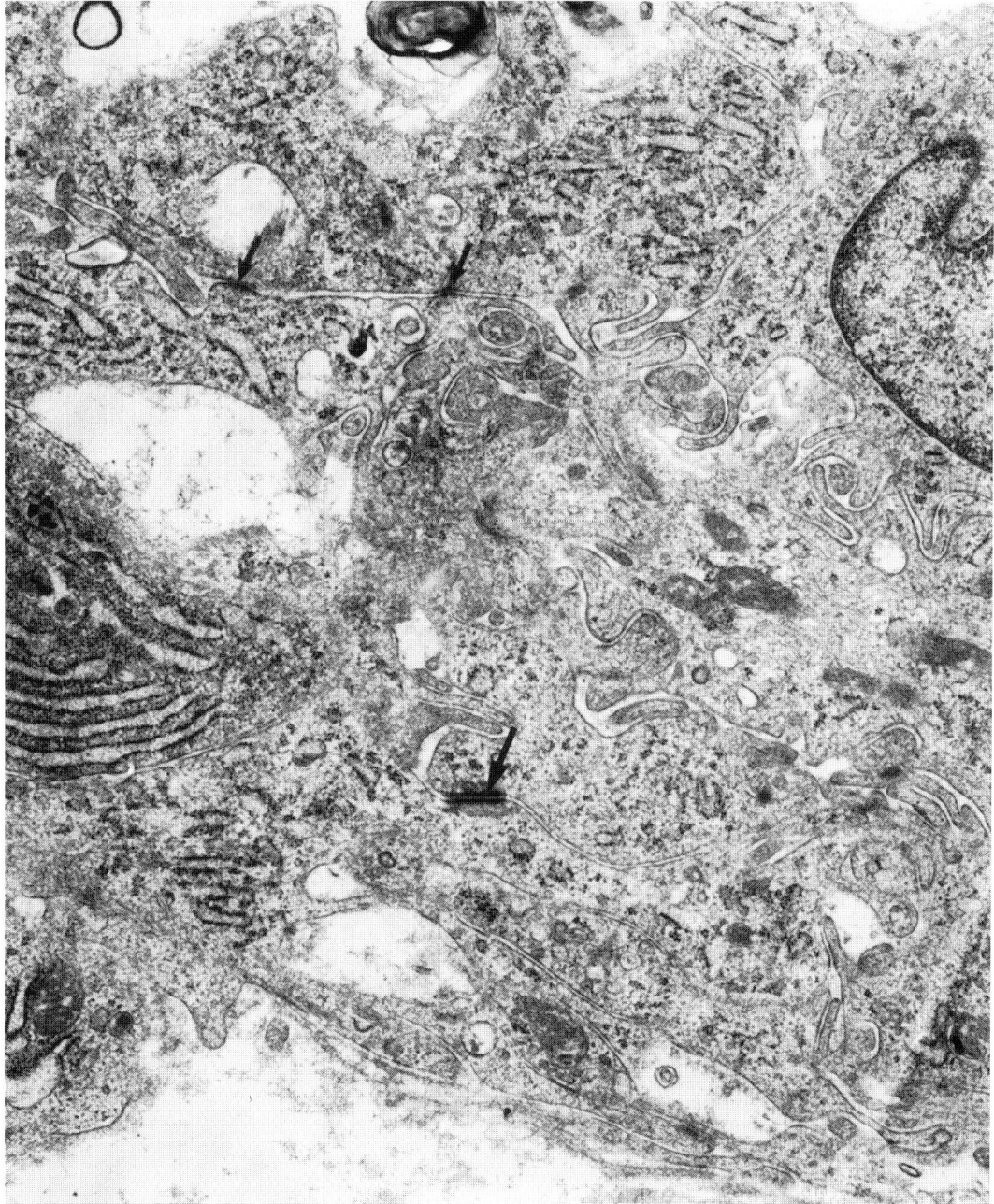

Fig. 12.26: Cardiac myxoma cell. Cytoplasm shows a variety of organelles namely, profiles of RER, microfilaments, glycogen, lysosomal bodies and mitochondria. Prominent cell membrane invaginations are also present. Notice the cell junctions (arrows)

Familial cardiac myxomas Most cases of cardiac myxoma are sporadic. However, in approximately 5% of patients these may be familial and may be associated with extracardiac lesions. The latter group has been categorised as **Myxoma syndrome**. Familial cardiac myxoma has an autosomal dominant inheritance pattern. A combination of features namely nevi, atrial myxoma, myxoid neurofibroma, ephelides-**NAME** has been recognised. Similarly another syndrome named **LAMB** (lentigines, atrial myxoma, mucocutaneous myxomas, blue nevi) has also been described. A complex comprising atrial myxoma, skin pigmentation, sertoli cell tumors of testis, cutaneous myxoma, myxoid fibroadenoma of the breast, adrenal cortical hyperplasia and pituitary hyperactivity has also been documented. To date 22 familial cardiac myxomas have been reported worldwide. We have encountered one family comprised of mother, daughter and son with recurrent biatrial (mother) cardiac myxoma.

Clinical presentation of cardiac myxoma includes constitutional features, obstructive effects and embolic phenomenon. The presenting features in over 90 percent cases are dyspnea on exertion, fever, malaise, arthralgia, rash, clubbing of fingers, etc. Features of mitral valve stenosis, pulmonary hypertension and systemic embolisation may be encountered. Laboratory findings of anemia, increased sedimentation rate, hypergammaglobulinemia, thrombocytosis, polycythemia have been documented in cardiac myxoma. Elevated levels of interleukin-6 (IL-6) have also been reported. Detection and precise anatomical location of cardiac myxomas has been facilitated by several diagnostic techniques namely 2D-echocardiography (Fig. 12.2a), computerised tomography and magnetic resonance imaging. A high degree of clinical suspicion coupled with various investigative modalities have increased the yield of these tumors which are then surgically excised successfully.

Histogenesis The two major controversies regarding the nature of cardiac myxoma have been that, is cardiac myxoma a neoplasm or a thrombus? Several observations/investigations almost certainly are in favor of it being a neoplasm. Studies which support neoplastic nature of cardiac myxoma include recurrence with local invasion, multiplicity, embolisation with intimal and vessel wall invasion, chromosomal abnormalities, tissue culture and DNA ploidy status. Tissue culture of cardiac myxomas yield an overgrowth of cells of the kind seen within the myxoma whereas tissue culture of thrombus show overgrowth of fibroblasts. DNA analysis of cardiac myxoma has revealed some cases to be aneuploid and/or tetraploid. Immunohistochemistry to a panel of antibodies suggest that cardiac myxoma arises from multipotent cells that have the potential to differentiate along several mesenchymal cells and epithelial cells as concurrent reactivity for both mesenchymal and epithelial markers has been reported in some cases. An interesting facet of histogenesis is provided by the epithelial/glandular component of cardiac myxoma which we observed in 3 cases. The epithelial cells showed evidence of neutral mucin, sialomucin and sulphomicin (Figs 12.15 to 12.18). The cells also showed reaction to CK and CEA (Figs 12.19 and 12.20). These observations suggest that the epithelial islands exhibit gastrointestinal phenotype which possibly represent intracardiac endodermal heterotopia.

Papillary fibroelastoma is a papilloma of the endocardium over valves. This has several synonyms namely giant Lambl's excrescences, myxofibroma, myxoma of valves, fibroma of valves, fibroelastic papilloma, etc. There is a great deal of similarity between Lambl's excrescences and papillary fibroelastomas, however, latter are larger and more gelatinous than Lambl's excrescences and are present on valves away from the line of closure. This is generally an incidental finding and may assume clinical significance when they embolise. Grossly, it has papillary or finger like appearance and is often gelatinous to feel. Microscopically the papillae are lined by endothelial cells. The supporting matrix is loose and myxoid with elastic fibers and occasional smooth muscle cells and fibroblasts. Both papillary fibroelastoma and Lambl's excrescences are believed to be organising thrombi.

Rhabdomyoma This is exclusive to the heart and is believed to be a hamartoma. Rhabdomyoma is the most common mass lesion in infancy and childhood. It may occur by itself or more commonly associated either with tuberous sclerosis or congenital heart disease. About 50 percent of patients with cardiac rhabdomyoma have features of tuberous sclerosis syndrome namely intracranial hamartomas, subungual fibromas, epidermal nevi, angiomyolipoma of kidney, etc.

Rhabdomyomas may exist either as a single large mass, multiple lobulated nodules or numerous minute lesions distributed on the entire surface of heart. Size of the lesion varies from 1 mm to 10 cm. Microscopically the lesion is well-circumscribed and produces compression of the adjacent myocardium.

The cells of rhabdomyoma are quite characteristic. They are large with abundant clear cytoplasm in which slender cytoplasmic strands extend from the nucleus to the cell wall. Latter have the appearance of "spider" cells. These cells possess abundant glycogen which is well brought out with periodic acid-Schiff stain. They also show positive reaction with antisera to myoglobin, desmin and actin (Fig. 12.27c). Ultrastructural features include abundant glycogen, irregular myofilaments with Z bands and other organelles. Large and single rhabdomyomas can be subject to surgery with good long-term results.

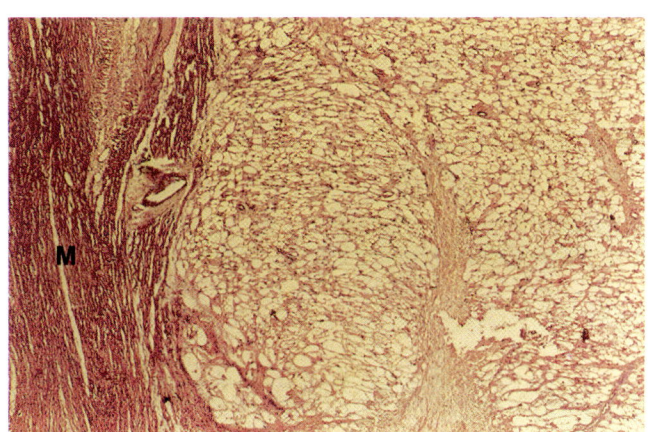

Fig. 12.27a: Cardiac rhabdomyoma. The lesion consists of a fairly well circumscribed mass comprised of sheets of vacuolated cells. Compression of the adjacent myocardium (M) is observed

Note: Patient was a 2 months old infant who presented with features of congestive cardiac failure. Multiple small whitish nodules in the wall of the right atrium and right ventricle were present. Surgical excision was done

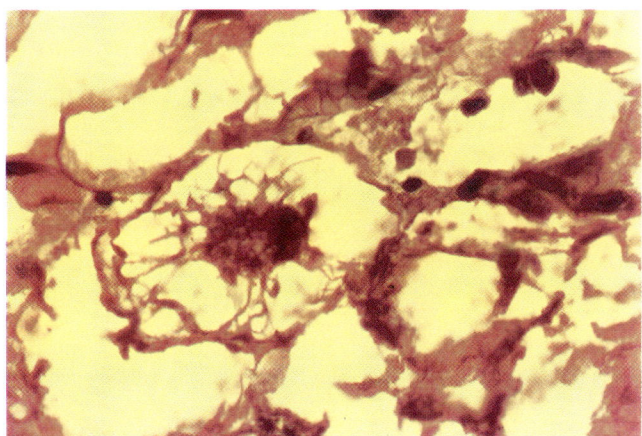

Fig. 12.27b: Cardiac rhabdomyoma. Photomicrograph shows typical cells having vacuolation of the cytoplasm, large nucleus and delicate cytoplasmic strands between the nucleus and cell wall (spider cell)

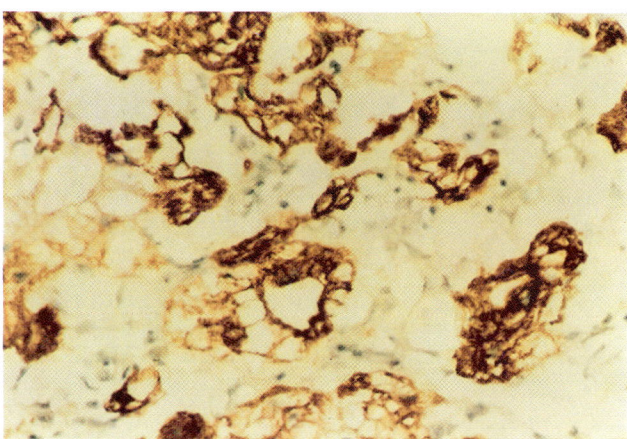

Fig. 12.27c: Cardiac rhabdomyoma. The tumor cells show strong immunoreactivity with antiserum to myoglobin

Benign tumors of fibrous tissue included in this group are cardiac fibroma, solitary fibrous tumor of the pericardium, benign fibrous histiocytoma and inflammatory pseudotumor. Amongst these rare tumors cardiac fibroma is the most common tumor of childhood after rhabdomyoma. *Cardiac fibroma* is a benign congenital tumor occurring as a discrete mass in the ventricular septum, left ventricular free wall, right ventricle and atria in that order. Microscopically, spindle shaped proliferating fibroblasts with variable amount of collagen is seen. Inflammatory cell infiltration consisting of lymphocytes and histiocytes is often encountered. The treatment is surgical excision (Figs 12.28 and 12.29).

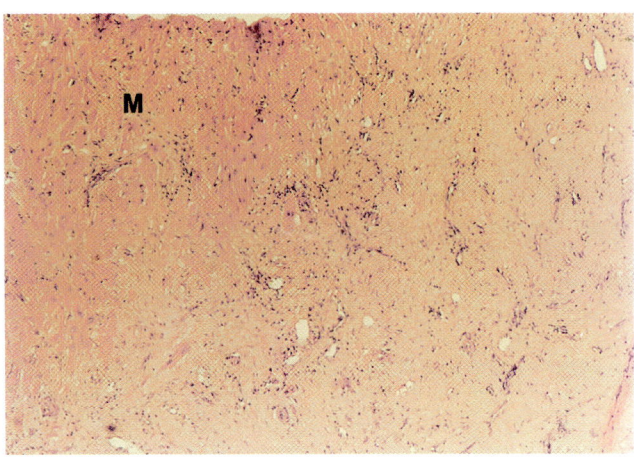

Fig. 12.28a: Cardiac fibroma right ventricle. Large areas of vascular collagen are seen in the right half of the picture. A few lymphocytes are also sprinkled. This process is seen to extend into the myocardium (M)

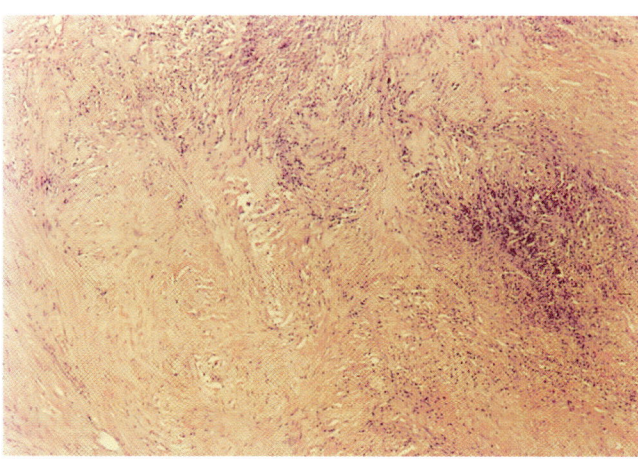

Fig. 12.28b: Cardiac fibroma. Sections from other areas of the lesion show variable numbers of chronic inflammatory cell infiltration mostly lymphocytes within dense fibrocollagen tissue. Inflammatory cells were present both diffusely and in aggregates

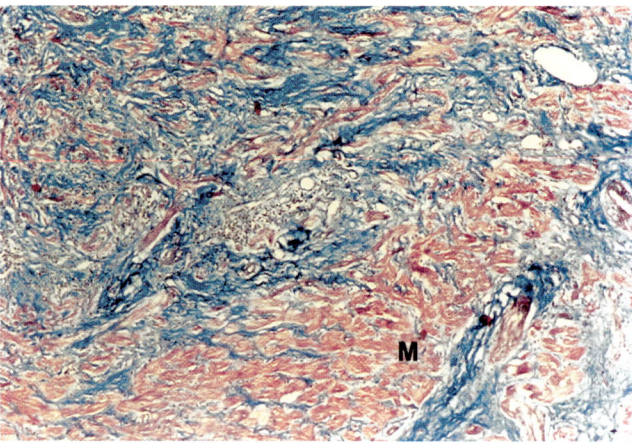

Fig. 12.28d: Cardiac fibroma. Masson trichrome stain to highlight the fibroconnective tissue and inflammatory cells with extension into the adjacent myocardium (M)

Note: The patient was a 26 years old male who presented with dyspnea and abdominal distension for 5 months. ECHO/MRI revealed a mass in the right ventricular outflow tract which showed fibrosis. The tricuspid valve also appeared fibrotic. It was excised piece meal (3 × 2 × 1 cm)

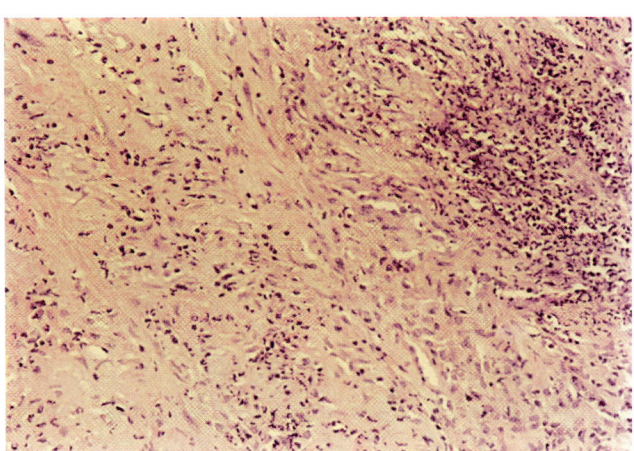

Fig. 12.28c: Cardiac fibroma. Higher magnification of Figure 12.28b to show a large numer of inflammatory cells including polymorphs in this focus. Plump fibroblasts are also noted

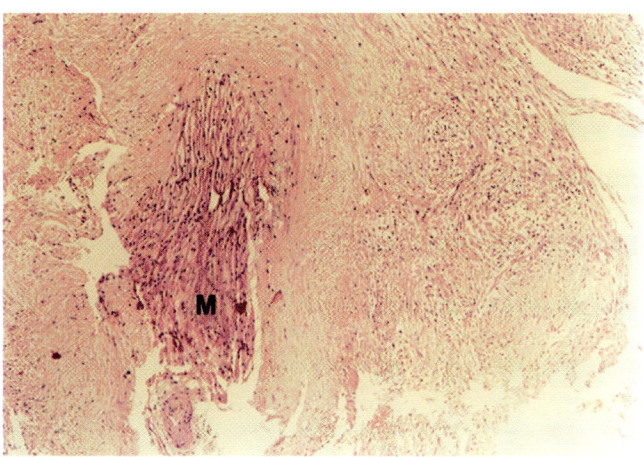

Fig. 12.29a: Cardiac fibroma, right atrium. The tumor is sparsely cellular with large areas of hyalinisation. Tumor cells are arranged in short fascicles. Inflammatory cells are admixed with the tumor cells. The stroma has a myxomatous appearance. Myocardium (M) is trapped within the fibrous tissue. Compare with fibroma of right ventricle illustrated in Figure 12.28

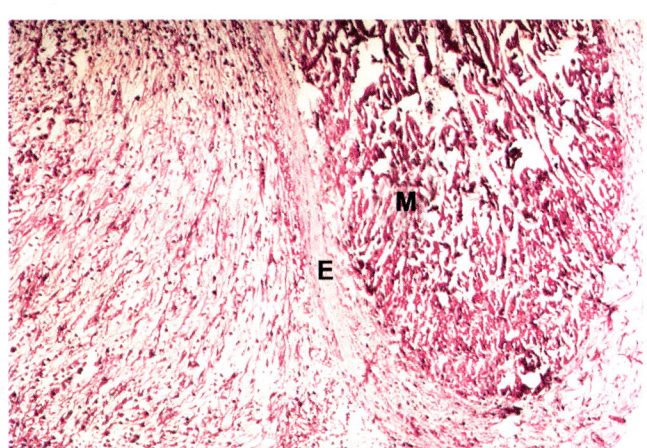

Fig. 12.29b: Cardiac fibroma. The lesion is seen to be continuous with left atrial endocardium (E). Myocardiuim (M) is entrapped within the tumor

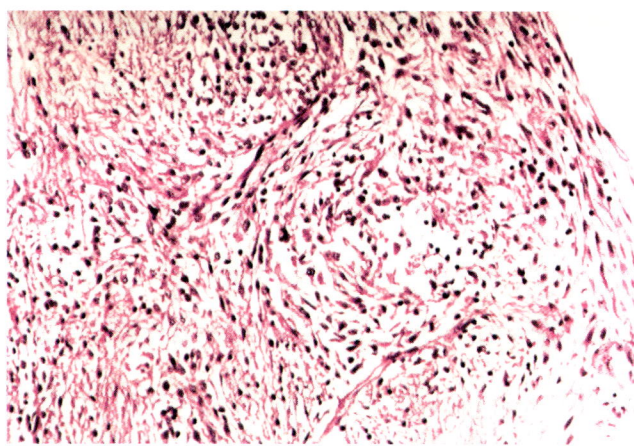

Fig. 12.29c: Cardiac fibroma. Tumor cells are spindle shaped and arranged in small fascicles that have a faint whorling arrangement. A few inflammatory cells are interspersed. No nuclear pleomorphism or mitotic activity is observed

Note: Patient was a 3 years old male child. Pedunculated mass having papillary appearance in foci was found attached to right atrium at the level of atrioventricular groove. Base of mass was extending into full thickness of right atrial wall. Tiny papillary nodules were also seen to be attached to chordae tendinea and papillary muscle

Benign tumors of fatty tissue The lesions of interest in this group are lipomatous hypertrophy of the interatrial septum and lipoma. Lipomatous hypertrophy of the atrial septum is a rare lesion and comprises accumulation of fat within it. This is possibly a hamartomatous lesion. On naked eye examination the atrial septum is thickened and may assume large proportions. Microscopically, adipose tissue, variable amounts of brown fat admixed with myocytes which may have bizarre shapes and sizes is seen.

Lipomas of heart are generally encountered on the epicardial surface of the atria or ventricles. Other fatty tissue lesions include lipomatous hamartoma of cardiac valves and diffuse fatty infiltration of the heart (fatty heart).

Vascular tumors Benign vascular tumors of the heart are rare. They may present as **blood cysts** over the endocardium. **Hemangiomas** of the heart and pericardium are uncommon. The morphological features are identical to those in the soft tissues. Other vascular tumors documented in the heart and pericardium are hemangioendothelioma, hemangiopericytoma and lymphangioma.

MALIGNANT TUMORS OF HEART

Malignant mesenchymal tumors of heart These are either primary or secondary. All soft tissue sarcomas have been described in the heart (Figs 12.30 and 12.31). The most common primary sarcomas of the heart are angiosarcoma (Fig. 12.32) and unclassified undifferentiated sarcoma (Fig. 12.33). Latter is a term applied when mesenchymal tumors lack any specific recognisable morphologic pattern or differentiation and the immunohistochemical findings and ultrastructural features are also noncontributory. Other sarcomas reported in the heart and pericardium are malignant fibrous histiocytoma, osteosarcoma, leiomyosarcoma, myxosarcoma, liposarcoma, synovial sarcoma, etc. The morphology and behavior of these tumors is as encountered in the soft tissues.

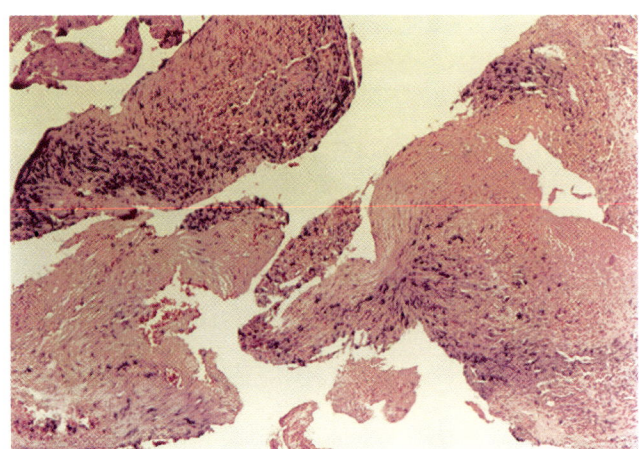

Fig. 12.30a: Malignant mesenchymal tumor, right atrium. Cellular foci are seen admixed with fibrous ones. Areas of congestion are also observed

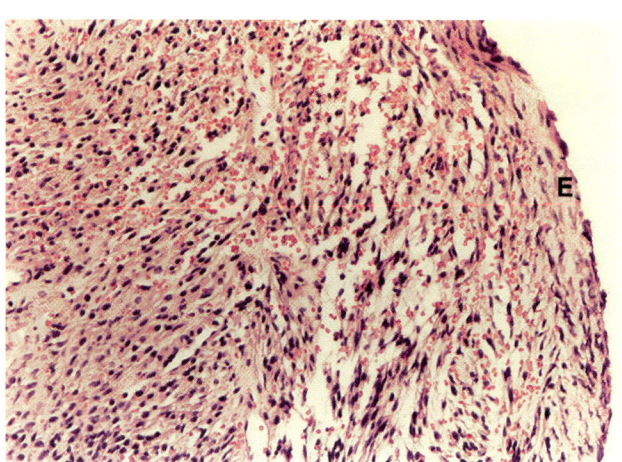

Fig. 12.30b: Malignant mesenchymal tumor right atrium. Tumor cells are arranged in flowing bundles. The tumor extends beneath the endocardium (E). Mild nuclear pleomorphism is noted. Few mitotic figures were also recognised. Extravasation of red blood cells is seen

Note: The patient was a 22 years male who presented with rapidly accumulating recurrent, pericardial and pleural effusion. ECHO revealed a large mass in right atrium, interatrial septum and left atrium. Bilateral pulmonary metastases were detected

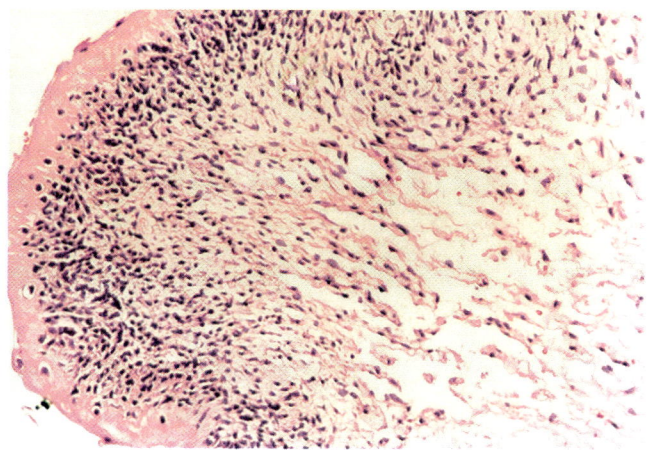

Fig. 12.31a: Photomicrograph of a mass in the right ventricle. Spindle shaped cells are seen in the subendocardial region. The deeper portion is sparsely cellular with loose myxoid stroma. Markers for myogenic differentiation were negative. Histological changes are those of a fibrosarcoma

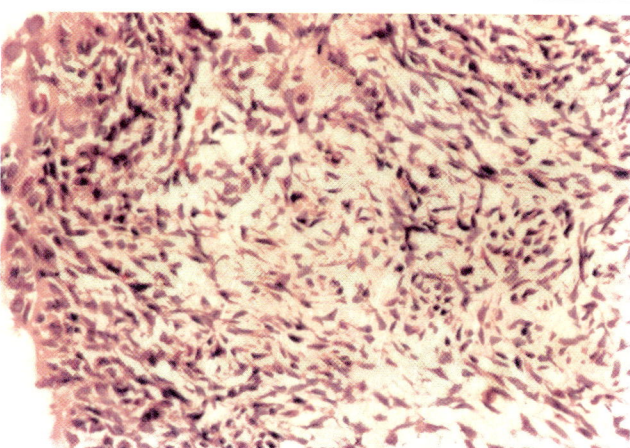

Fig. 12.31b: Higher magnification of the Figure 12.31a to demonstrate pattern of the tumor. The tumor cells are spindle shaped and have elongated nuclei showing moderate pleomorphism. Stroma is loose and myxoid

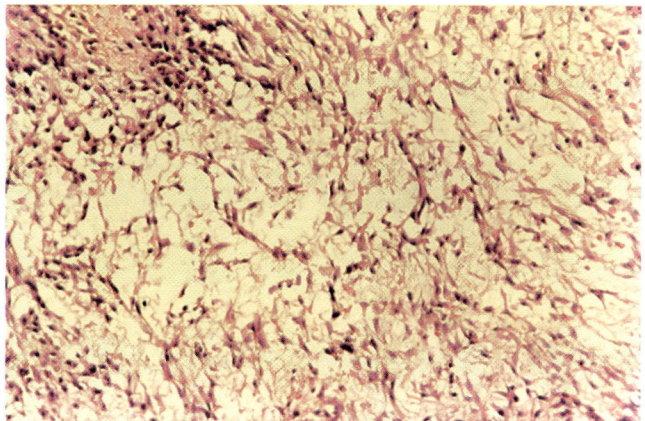

Fig. 12.31c: Fibrosarcoma heart. Another area of the tumor illustrated in Figures 12.31a and b showing loose myxomatous stroma in which ovoid to spindle shaped tumor cells are dispersed

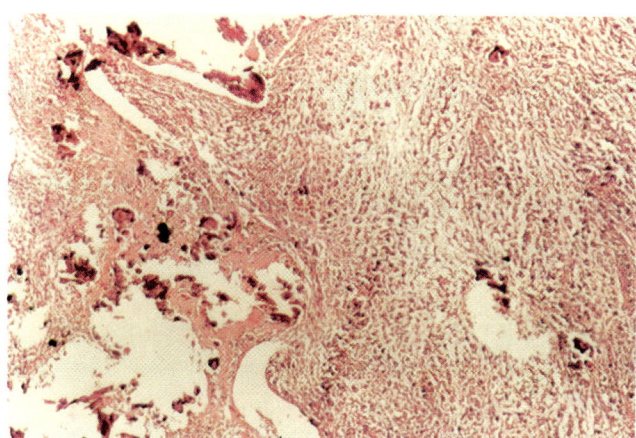

Fig. 12.31d: Fibrosarcoma heart. Several foci of calcification were detected within the tumor

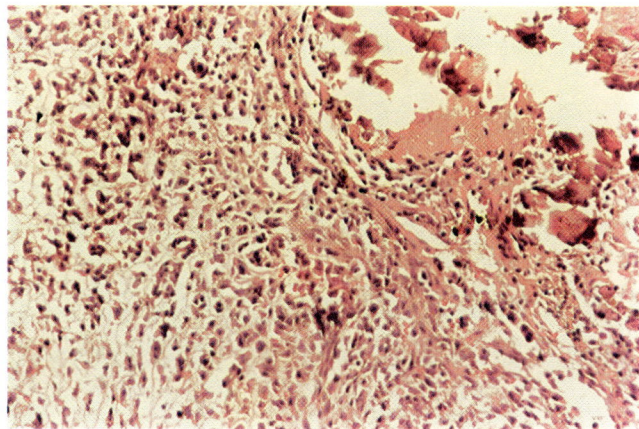

Fig. 12.31e: Fibrosarcoma heart. Higher magnification to demonstrate focus of calcification along with round to ovoid tumor cells. The cells in this focus are arranged in a compact manner

Note: The patient was a 25 years old young man who presented with shortness of breath for 3 months. A lobulated grey white mass measuring 8 × 3 × 1.6 cm and weighing 60 gm was removed from the right ventricular cavity. The mass was also attached to anterior leaflet of tricuspid valve

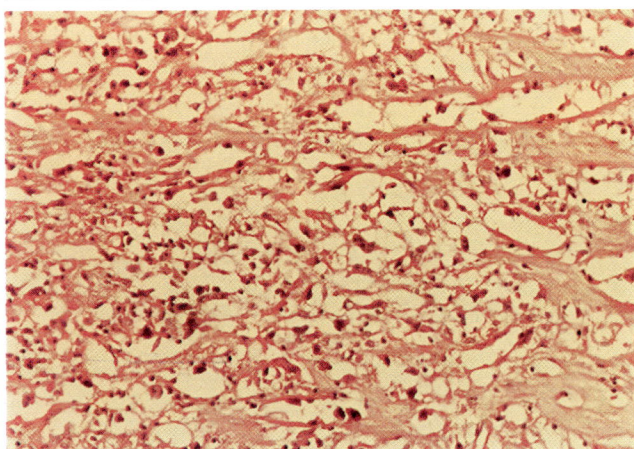

Fig. 12.32a: Angiosarcoma heart. Several well-defined vascular spaces are seen to be lined by pleomorphic cells

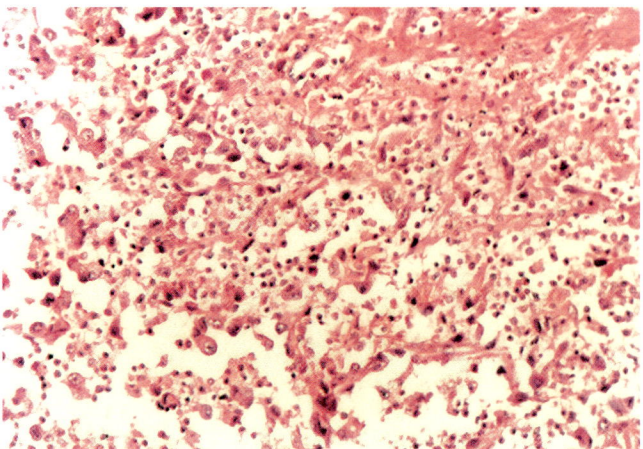

Fig. 12.32b: Angiosarcoma heart. Round to polyhedral tumor cells showing pleomorphism line anastomosing vascular channels

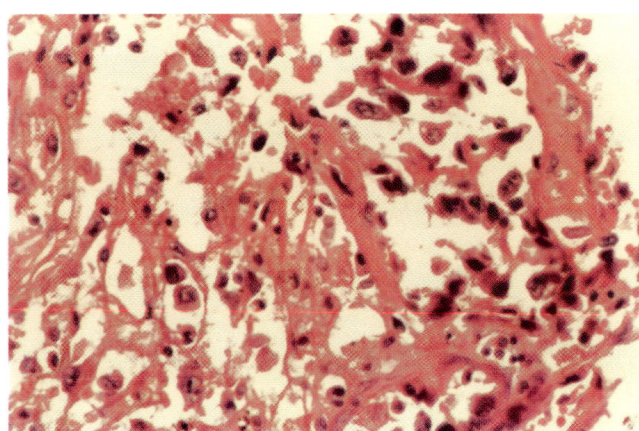

Fig. 12.32c: Angiosarcoma heart. Higher magnification of Figure 12.32b to demonstrate morphologic features of tumor cells which are round to polyhedral, have pink cytoplasm and show pleomorphism. Cells seem to be projecting into the lumen

Note: The patient was a known case of rheumatic heart disease with aortic and mitral valvulitis. Mitral stenosis was present. A large soft friable mass was seen in the left atrium that was encroaching on the stenosed mitral valve. Cut surface was dark brown in color. Tumor involved the entire thickness of the left atrial endocardium but did not extend into the myocardium. Cerebral metastasis (3 cm diameter) was also detected.

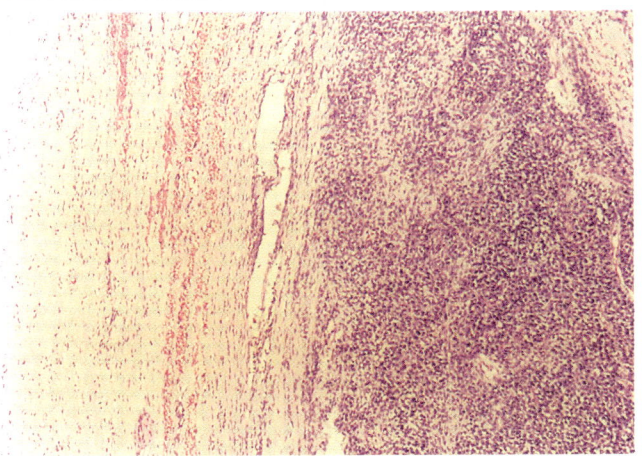 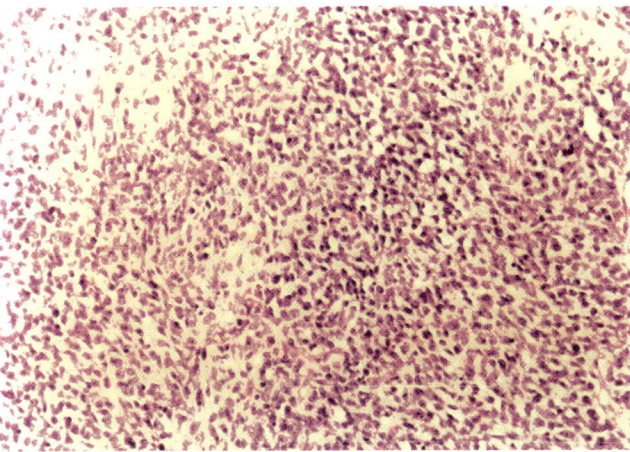

Fig. 12.33a: Undifferentiated sarcoma right ventricle. Tumor cells are arranged in fascicles/sheets and comprise of plump to spindle shaped cells. Tumor was attached to the septal leaflet of the tricuspid valve which is seen in left of the picture

Fig. 12.33b: Undifferentiated sarcoma right ventricle. Tumor cells are round to polyhedral to spindle shaped. Mild nuclear pleomorphism is noted. Mitosis was variable being 3-4/HPF in most active areas

Note: Patient was a 26 years male who presented with congestive heart failure. Echocardiography revealed a large right ventricular mass attached to the interventricular septum which was prolapsing into right atrium in systole. At surgery a mass was seen in the right ventricle (5 × 4 × 1.5 cm) which was attached to septal leaflet of tricuspid valve. It was extending into the pulmonary artery (2 × 2 × 0.5 cm) and right atrium (4 × 4 × 1.5 cm)

Hematologic tumors Malignant lymphoma may be primary when the bulk of the tumor is present within the heart and pericardium or they may be involved secondarily to lymphoma elsewhere in the body. Primary cardiac lymphoma is extremely uncommon whereas secondary cardiac involvement occurs in about 10% to 25% of patients having disseminated lymphoma. The heart and pericardium may also be involved in leukemia. Autopsy series have reported infiltrates in both heart and pericardium in 20% to 40% of patients with acute leukemia.

Malignant mesothelioma of pericardium Primary mesothelioma of the pericardium is rare. The rarity is appreciated by documented reports of its incidence being 0.7% as compared with pleural and peritoneal mesotheliomas which are 98% or more of the total. As in other sites, pericardial mesothelioma also is related to asbestos exposure and other mineral fibers. In a sizeable number of cases, however, there is either no history of exposure to asbestos or at best only a weak association is documented.

Malignant mesotheliomas of the pericardium present as large, nodular masses filling the pericardial cavity often encircling the heart and great vessels. Like in the soft tissues, epithelial, sarcomatoid or biphasic pattern of tumor cells is seen microscopically. Both intracellular and extracellular glycosaminoglycans can be demonstrated in most cases. Since pericardial mesothelioma is rare it needs to be differentiated from metastatic adenocarcinoma, reactive mesothelial hyperplasia, angiosarcoma and other mesenchymal tumors using appropriate stains, immunohistochemistry and electron microscopy (Figs 11.2, 11.3, 11.21 and Table 11.1) Surgical treatment at best is palliative. Radiation and combination chemotherapy has also been applied. The prognosis is poor.

Tumors metastatic to heart and pericardium

Metastatic tumors to the heart and pericardium are much more common than primary neoplasms (Figs 11.28 and 12.34). In majority of the cases the primary tumor is within the thoracic cage which reaches the heart usually by direct contiguous spread. Other routes of spread are hematogenous, via lymphatics and extension from the inferior vena cava into the cavity of the heart. Tumors that have propensity to spread to the heart include malignant melanoma, carcinoma of kidney, lung, breast, choriocarcinoma, rhabdomyosarcoma, other sarcomas, lymphoma, etc.

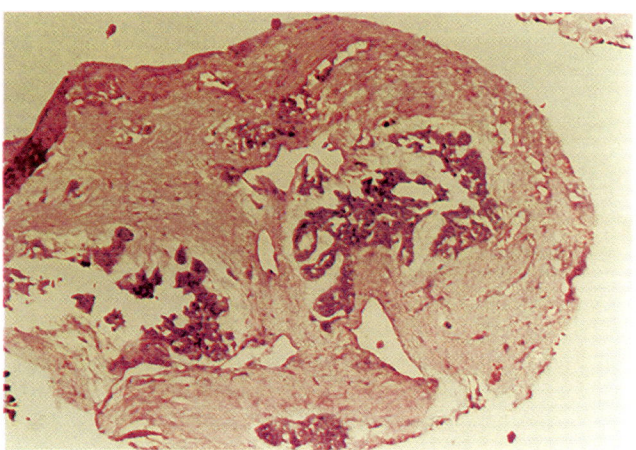

Fig. 12.34a: Endomyocardial biopsy from a mass in right ventricle in a 52-year-old female. The mass was extending into the pulmonary trunk. Groups of cells are present amidst vascular fibroconnective tissue

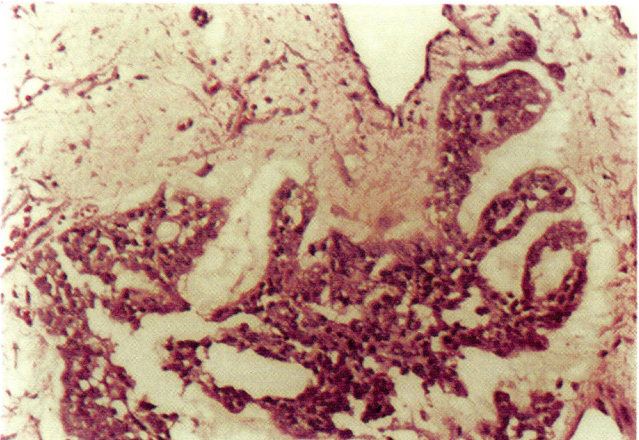

Fig. 12.34b: Higher magnification of tumor cells illustrated in Figure 12.34a. Tumor cells are arranged in groups and gland formation is noted. Mucicarmine stain was negative. A metastatic epithelial tumor was suggested. However, no primary tumor was detected elsewhere in the body

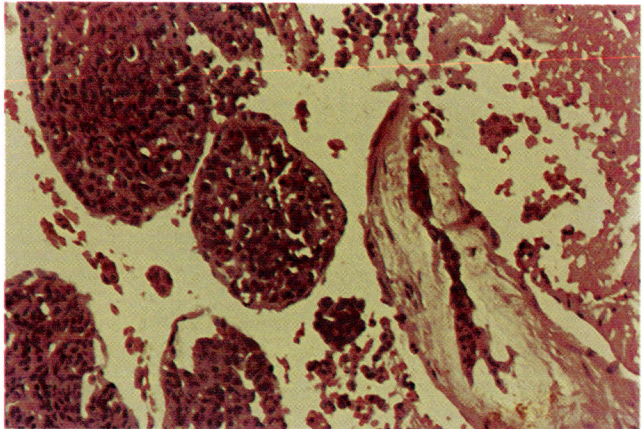

Fig. 12.34c: Excised tumor in the heart that was subjected to endomyocardial biopsy (Figs 12.34a and b). It shows identical histology to that seen in the endomyocardial biopsy (Fig. 12.34b). Groups of tumor cells are present. Infiltration of fibroconnective tissue by tumor is also seen. The tumor cells showed a strong reactivity with antiserum to cytokeratin

Presenting features of metastatic cardiac tumors include dyspnea, cough, chest pain, palpitations, symptoms and signs of superior vena cava syndrome, right ventricular outflow tract obstruction, hemorrhagic pericardial effusion and others. Causes of death may be cardiac tamponade, congestive heart failure, rhythm disorders of the heart, coronary artery embolism, etc.

Metastatic cardiac tumors can be localised using two dimensional echocardiography, computerised tomography, magnetic resonance imaging and gallium scans. Diagnosis of heart and pericardial tumors may be made by endomyocardial biopsy and pericardial biopsy respectively. These procedures are worthwhile and if applied judiciously they may provide a definitive clue to the nature of the lesion and thereby appropriate management of the case. Metastatic lesions may be treated by surgical resection, radiation and/or chemotherapy depending upon the extent and the type of the tumor.

SUGGESTED READING

1. Angrish K, Shankar SK, Manchanda SC, Chopra P: Primary angiosarcoma of the hearts. *Jap Heart J* **20**: 375-80, 1979.
2. Bire F, Roudaut R, Chevalier JM, Quiniou G, Dubecq S, Marazanoff M, Choussat A: Cardiac myxoma in patients over 75 years of age. Report of 19 cases. *Arch Mal Coeur Vaiss* **92(3)**: 323-28, 1999.
3. Butany J, Yu W: Cardiac angiosarcoma: two cases and a review of the literature. *Can J Cardiol* **16(2)**: 197-205, 2000.
4. Chopra P: Intracardiac myxoma an evaluation by scanning electron microscopy. *Jap Heart J* **26/3**: 457-62, 1985.
5. Chopra P, Ray R, Airan B, Talwar KK, Venugopal P: Appraisal of histogenesis of cardiac myxoma: Our experience of 78 cases with review of literature. *Ind Heart J* **51/1**: 69-74, 1999.
6. Chopra P, Sharma V: Left atrial myxoma: A morphologic and histogenetic study. *Jap Heart J* **22**: 353-61, 1981.
7. Deshpande A, Venugopal P, Sampath Kumar A, Chopra P: Phenotypic characterisation of cellular components of cardiac myxoma. A light microscopy and immunohistochemistry study. *Human Pathol* **27(10)**: 1056-59, 1996.
8. Lindner V, Edah Tally S, Chakfe N, Onody T, Eisenmann B, Walter P: Cardiac myxoma with glandular component: case report and review of the literature. *Pathol Res Pract* **195(4)**: 267-72, 1999.
9. Majumdar N, Ray R, Venugopal, Chopra P: DNA ploidy and proliferative index of cardiac myxoma. *Ind Heart J* **50/5**: 535-38, 1998.
10. Roskell DE, Biddolph SC: Proliferating cell nuclear antigen expression grossly over-estimates cellular proliferation in cardiac myxomas. *Eur J Med Res:* **26/4(3)**: 105-06, 1999.
11. Srivastava S, Chopra P, Sampath Kumar A: Fibrosarcoma of the right ventricle. *Int J Cardiol* **9**: 234-37, 1985.
12. Suzuki J, Takayama K, Mitsui F, Kono T, Yazaki Y, Takei M, Amano J, Isobe M: *In situ* interleukin-6 transcription in embryonic nonmuscle myosin heavy chain expressing immature mesenchyme cells of cardiac myxoma. *Cardiovasc Pathol* **9(1)**: 33-37, 2000.
13. Vander Salm TJ: Unusual primary tumors of the heart. *Semin Thorac Cardiovasc Surg* **12/25**: 89-100, 2000.

13. Diseases of Blood Vessels

Vasculitis is inflammation of the vessel wall that is often accompanied by necrosis. It comprises a heterogeneous group and may be either focal or more commonly it is generalised with multisystem and/or multiorgan involvement. In fact it is a clinicopathological entity to the extent that several pathologic findings are common to different types of vasculitides. Thus morphologic findings need to be correlated with the clinical presentation and/or laboratory data to reach a diagnosis. Classification and nomenclature of vasculitis has been a subject of much discussion and no single satisfactory classification which encompasses the clinical, pathologic and laboratory spectrum exists. However, for practical purposes it may be useful to classify vasculitides on the basis of the size of vessel involved (Table 13.1).

Table 13.1: Classification/nomenclature of systemic vasculitides

Large vessel vasculitis	: Takayasu arteritis
	: Giant cell (Temporal) arteritis
Medium sized vessel vasculitis	: Polyarteritis nodosa (classic)
	: Kawasaki disease
	: Wegener granulomatosis
	: Churg-Strauss syndrome
Small vessel vasculitis	: Wegener granulomatosis
	: Churg-Strauss syndrome
	: Microscopic polyangiitis (Microscopic polyarteritis)
	: Cutaneous leukocytoclastic vasculitis
	: Henoch-Schönlein purpura
	: Essential cryoglobulinemic vasculitis
In some vasculitis, association with other disorders is described. Thus the vasculitis is secondary to these conditions.	
Vasculitis associated with connective tissue diseases (generally affects the small vessels)	: Systemic lupus erythematosus
	: Dermatomyositis
	: Scleroderma
	: Rheumatoid arthritis
	: Mixed connective tissue disease
Vasculitis associated with infections (affects both the small and medium sized vessels)	: Hepatitis B and C viruses
	: HIV
	: Infective endocarditis
Vasculitis associated with paraproteins (affects the small vessels)	: Cryoglobulinemia
	: Macroglobulinemia
Hypersensitivity vasculitis (involves small vessels)	: Drug related
Malignancy related vasculitis	

Diseases of Blood Vessels

Takayasu arteritis Commonly designated as nonspecific aortoarteritis is a panarteritis affecting the large and medium sized vessels of predominantly women of 20 to 30 years of age. The typical manifestation is one of "pulseless disease" due to obliterative arteritis of the arch vessels (aortic arch syndrome) (Fig. 13.1). However, the disease process may affect any segment of the aorta and medium sized arteries, pulmonary arteries, etc. (Figs 13.1 to 13.12). Involvement of the thoraco-abdominal segment of the aorta including the renal arteries is frequently seen (Figs 13.5 to 13.8). Renal artery narrowing/stenosis is a common cause of hypertension of the young in this country (Figs 13.6a, 13.7 to 13.9b). Extent, severity and type of vascular involvement can be clearly delineated by intra-arterial digital subtraction angiography/angiography. Percutaneous transrenal angioplasty is routinely carried out to restore the lumen (Fig. 13.9b).

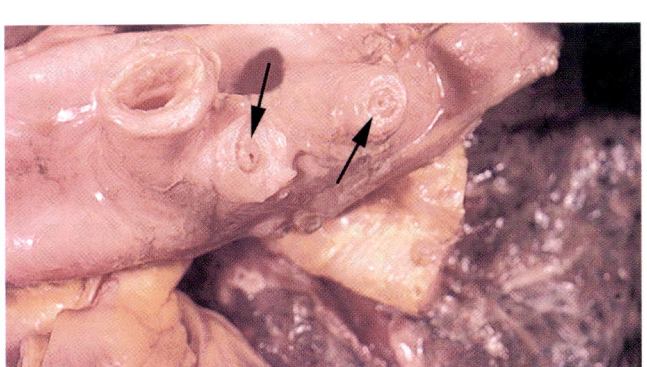

Fig. 13.1a: Non-specific aortoarteritis (Takayasu disease). Thickening of wall of all the branches of the arch of aorta leading to obliteration of the arterial lumina (arrows) is observed

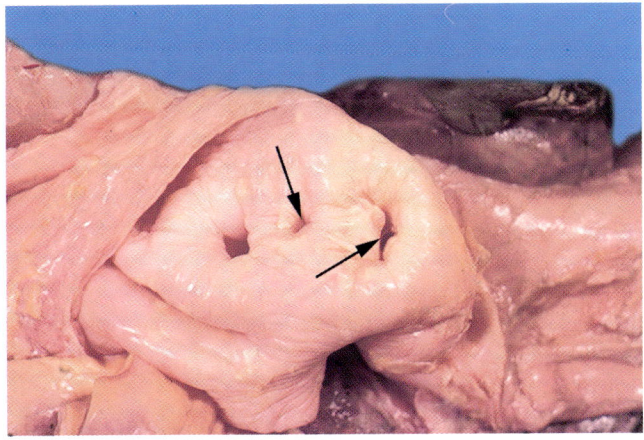

Fig. 13.1b: Non-specific aortoarteritis (Takayasu disease). Photograph shows the intimal aspect of the aortic arch vessels. The intima is puckered leading to narrowing at the origin (arrows)

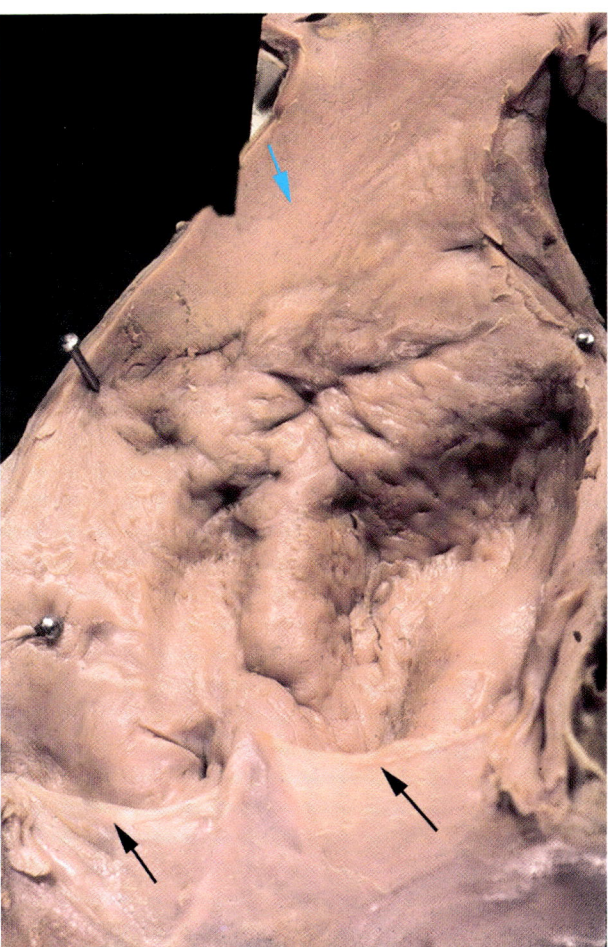

Fig. 13.2: Non-specific aortoarteritis (Takayasu arteritis). The root and part of the ascending aorta is diseased. The wall of aorta is thickened. Intima is wrinkled, roughened and resembles the bark of a tree. The lesion ends abruptly beyond which the intima of the ascending aorta is relatively normal (Blue arrow). The origin of all arch vessels were involved in the disease process. Aortic valve cusps are unremarkable (Black arrows).

Note: The appearance of the lesion and the location in the ascending aorta is much like syphilitic aortitis. With this kind of lesion one must consider and exclude this possibility. In this case the renal artery ostia were also affected by the disease process. Serology for syphilis was negative

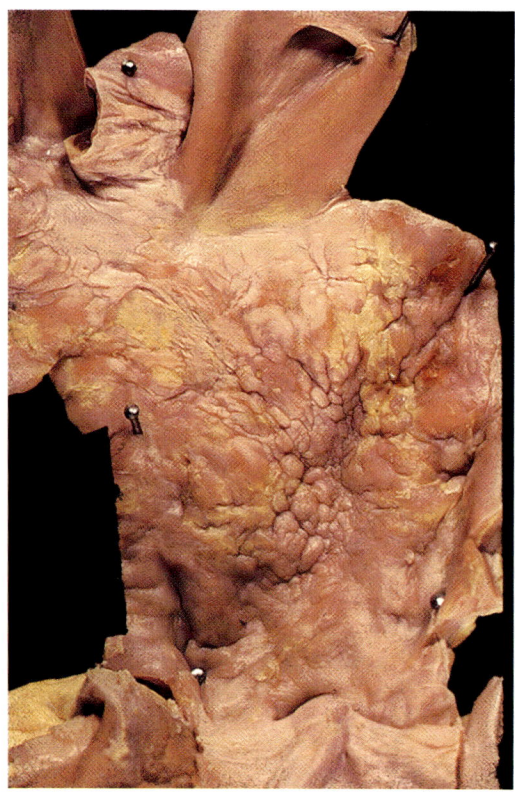

Fig. 13.3: Non-specific aortoarteritis (Takayasu arteritis). The root of the aorta and ascending aorta is affected by the disease process. The intima is puckered, wrinkled and irregular in contrast with the intima of the arch vessels

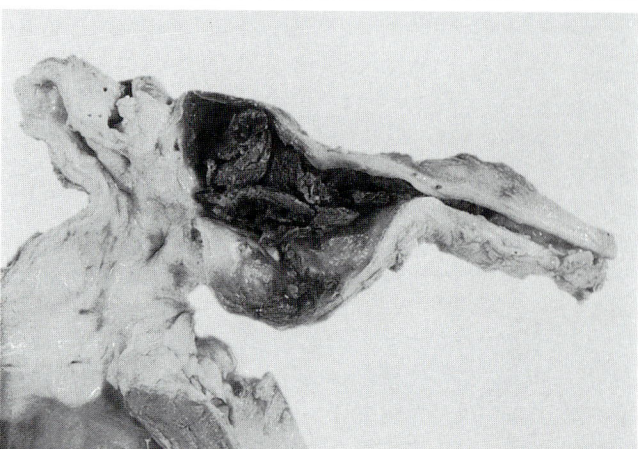

Fig. 13.4: Non-specific aortoarteritis (Takayasu arteritis). The entire aorta, right from its root till below the renal arteries was involved. The ascending aorta and its branches show severe thickening of the vessel wall resulting in tubular narrowing of the aorta in foci. There is segmental dilatation of the thoracic aorta which is filled with an organised thrombus. Abdominal aorta distal to the renal arteries also showed a thrombus (not in picture)

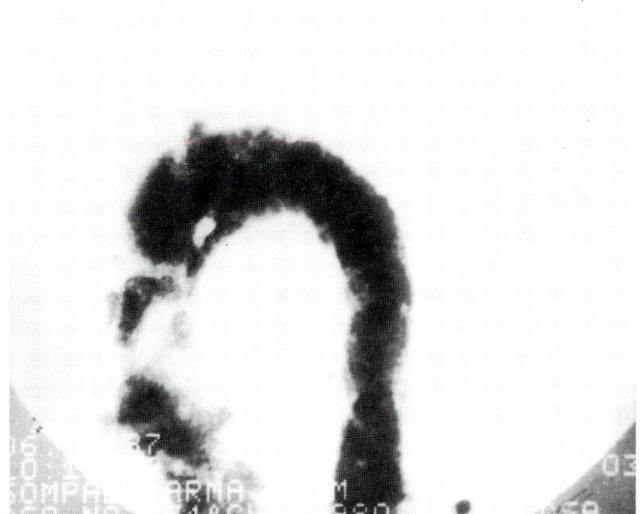

Fig. 13.5a: Intra-arterial digital subtraction angiography of aortic arch (IA-DSA) in left anterior oblique (LAO) view shows occlusion of all neck branches-innominate, left carotid and left subclavian arteries

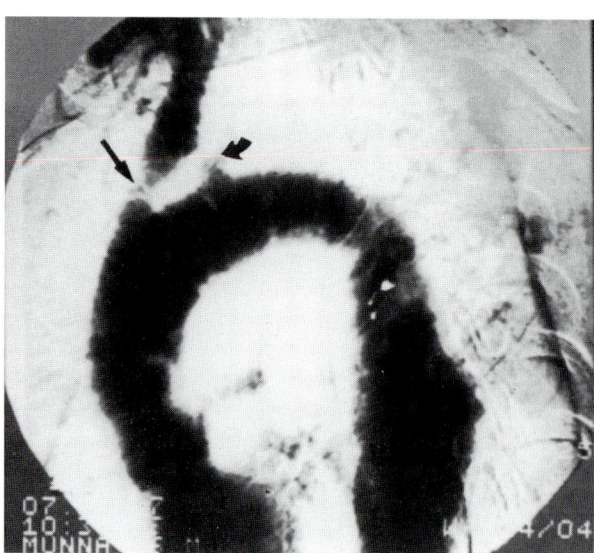

Fig. 13.5b: Aortic arch DSA in LAO view shows a focal stenosis of the innominate (arrow), and occlusion of left common carotid artery (thick arrow)

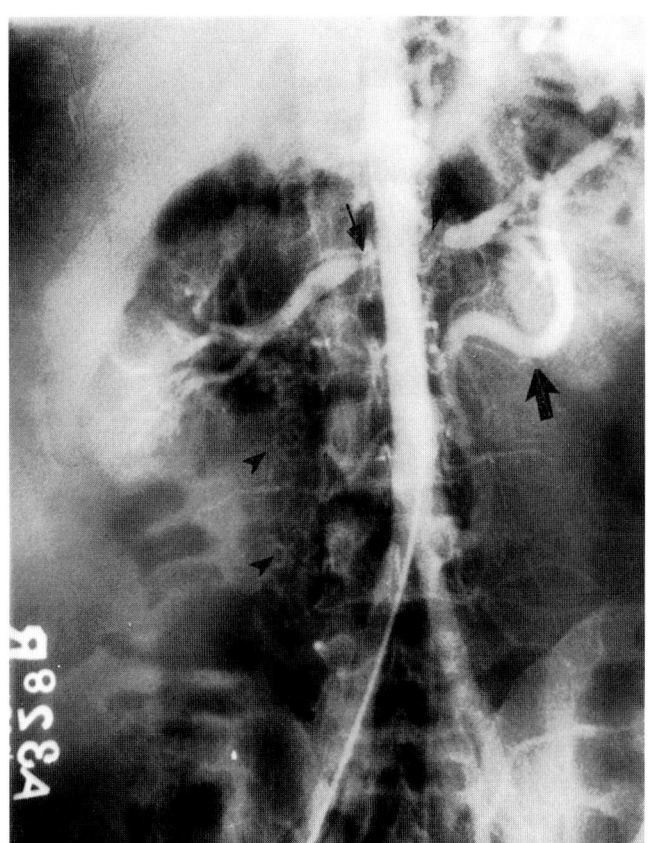 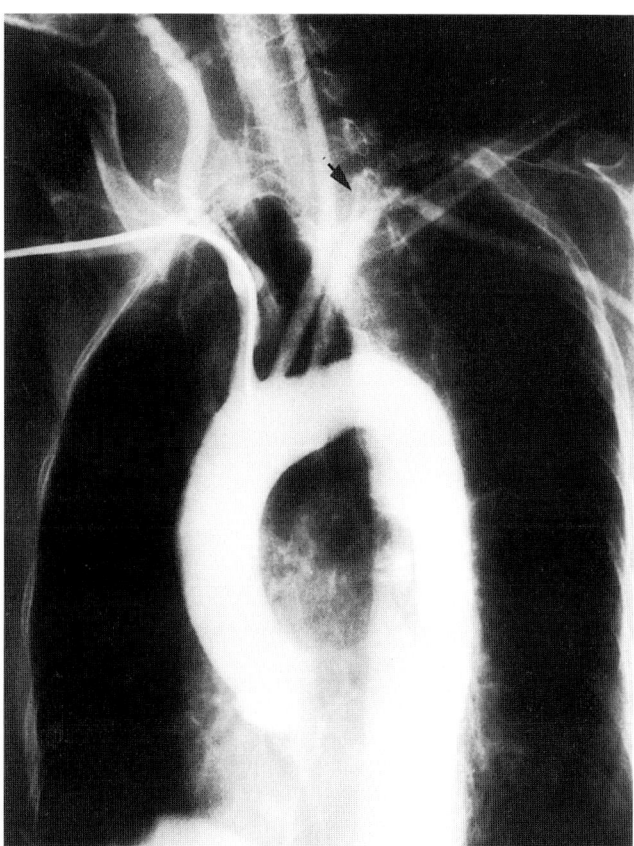

Figs 13.6a and b: Non-specific aortoarteritis (Takayasu arteritis) in a young hypertensive female (a) bilateral renal artery stenosis (arrow) and multiple renal hilar and periureteric collaterals (arrowheads) are seen in this flush abdominal aortogram. The superior mesenteric artery is not visualised (occluded) and a large meandering collateral arising from the inferior mesenteric artery (large arrow) is seen to supply its territory, (b) thoracic aortogram shows a blocked left vertebral artery (arrow) soon after its origin from left subclavian artery

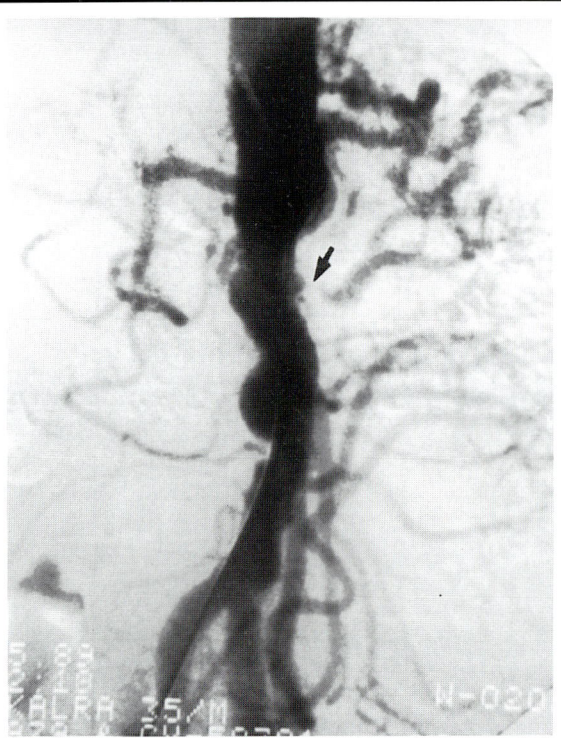

Fig. 13.7: Intra-arterial (IA) digital subtraction angiography (DSA) of abdominal aorta in AP view. Multiple saccular aneurysms with long mild stenosis of perirenal segment is observed. There is a tight post-ostial stenosis of left renal artery (arrow). Right renal artery and superior mesenteric artery are blocked. There is a large meandering collateral

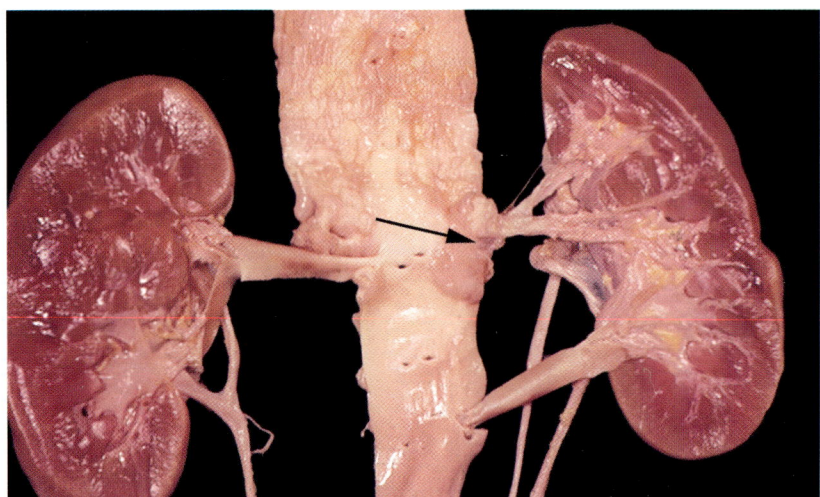

Fig. 13.8: Non-specific aortoarteritis (Takayasu disease). The suprarenal segment of the abdominal aorta is diseased (compare with the normal infrarenal segment of aorta). Intimal surface appears fleshy, irregular and bears resemblance to a tree bark

Note: The origin of intercostal arteries is narrowed. The disease process extends to ostia of renal arteries resulting in narrowing (arrow) (Same case as illustrated in Figure 13.1)

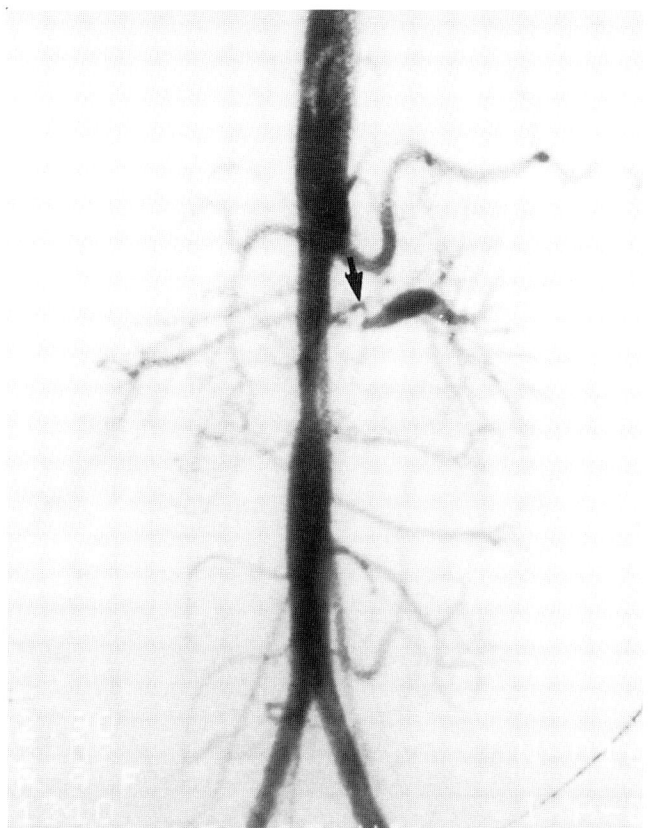
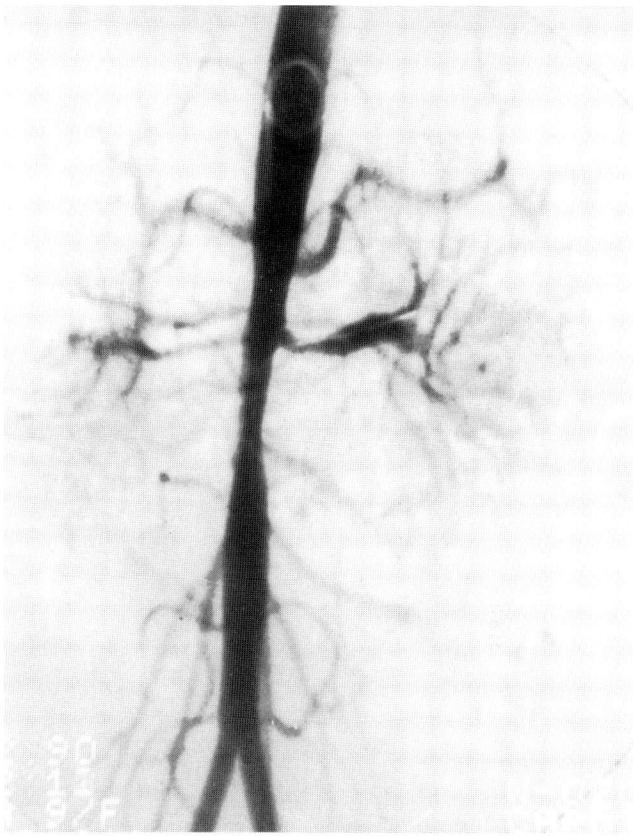

Fig. 13.9a: IA-DSA of the abdominal aorta in AP view shows a focal stenosis of juxta renal segment of the aorta, tight left renal artery segment (arrow) and diffuse disease of right renal artery

Fig. 13.9b: The same case as in Figure 13.9a after left percutaneous transrenal angioplasty (PTRA). Notice the restored lumen

Gross examination reveals thickening of all layers of the vessel wall leading to narrowing/obliteration of the lumen. The intimal surface is pale white, irregular and wrinkled (Figs 13.1 to 13.4 and 13.8). Though thickening and narrowing of the affected vessel is most commonly observed, diffuse dilative type of involvement of aorta with or without aneurysm formation has also been observed in Takayasu arteritis (Figs 13.7, 13.10 and 13.11). Microscopically all the layers are affected. The adventitia shows thickening by fibrocollagen tissue. Perivascular cuffing by lymphocytes predominantly is seen (Figs 13.13 to 13.15). Media reveals variable degrees of destruction of the elastic tissue and replacement fibrosis (Fig. 13.15). Chronic inflammation may be seen. In the early stages marked chronic inflammation with or without granulomatous inflammation is observed (Fig. 13.14). In our limited experience granulomatous inflammation is present only infrequently the granulomas are few and ill-defined. At autopsy features of end stage disease are evident by varying degrees of fibrosis with only mild focal or no inflammation. Intima shows thickening by myofibroblast proliferation, and myxoid fibroconnective tissue in varying proportions. Healing leads to fibrosis and morphological expressions such as arterial stenosis and/or narrowing, occlusion, dilatation of segments and aneurysm formation in some cases. **Etiology** of Takayasu arteritis is ill understood. Immunological abnormalities like, circulating immune complexes and circulating antibodies to some unidentified antigen in the arterial wall have been reported. Tuberculosis, *Chlamydia pneumoniae*, and viral infections have also been suggested in the causation of Takayasu arteritis. Some workers have demonstrated the role of cellular immune mechanisms in the pathogenesis of this disease. Genetic factors have also been documented.

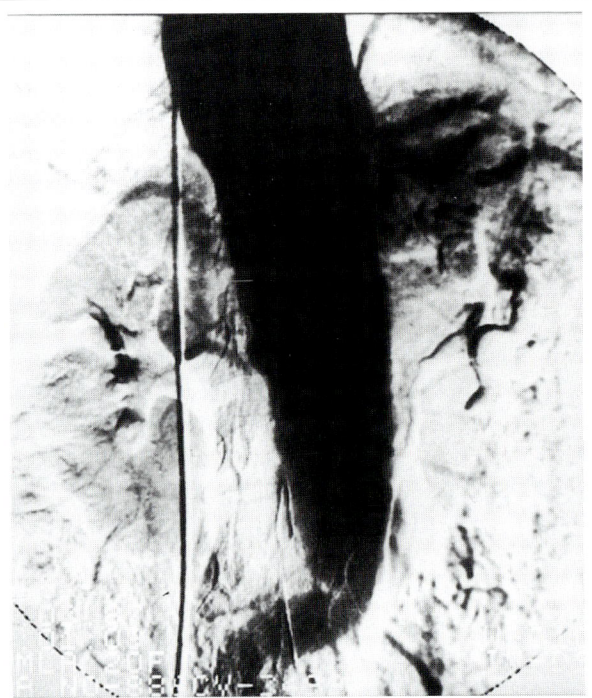

Fig. 13.10: Non-specific aortoarteritis. Diffuse dilative type of involvement of abdominal aorta

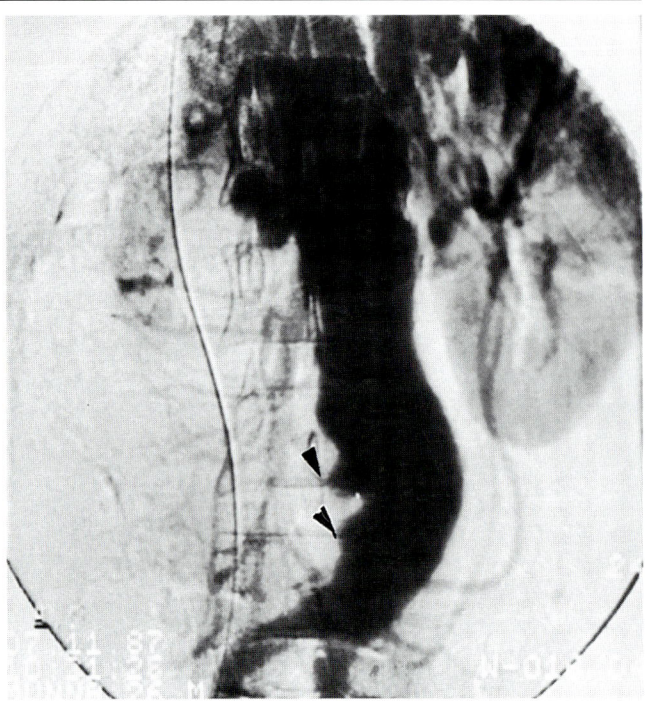

Fig. 13.11: Non-specific aortoarteritis. Diffuse dilative type of involvement of abdominal aorta with localised saccular aneurysms (arrow heads)

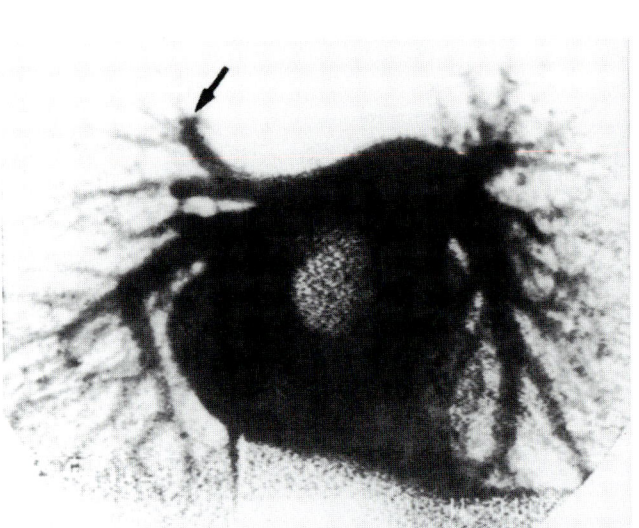

Fig. 13.12: Non-specific aortoarteritis. Digital subtraction pulmonary angiogram in AP view shows occlusion of the right upper lobe branch of right pulmonary artery (arrow)

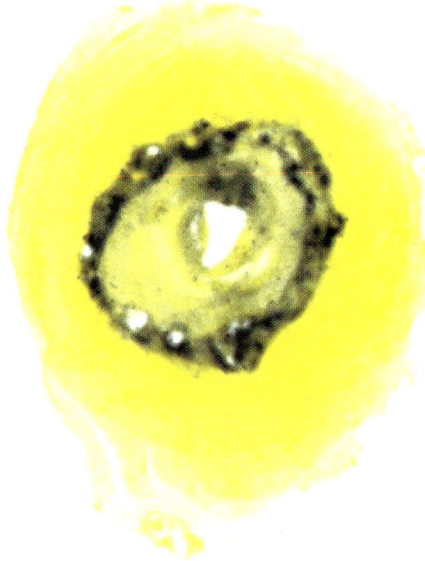

Fig. 13.13: Non-specific aortoarteritis. Whole slide mount of a cross-section of the left subclavian artery. All layers of the artery are thickened. The lumen is severly compromised. Elastic tissue of the media is fragmented and has a moth eaten appearance. Elastic van Gieson's stain

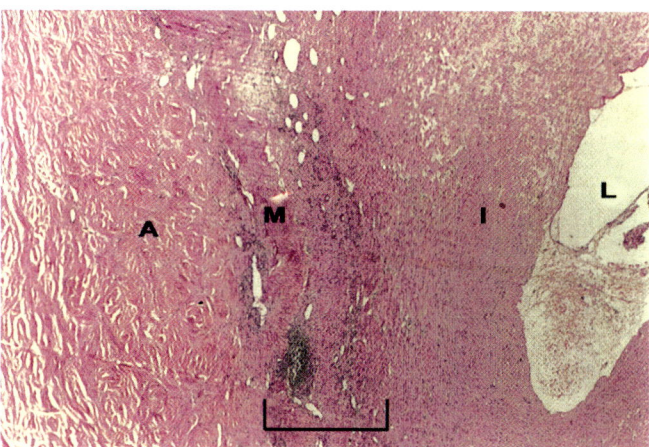

Fig. 13.14a: Non-specific aortorateritis. Photomicrograph of diseased arch of aorta shows marked thickening of all layers. Media (M) is thinned out, distorted and reveals patchy infiltration by lymphocytes and focal fibrosis. The intima (I) and adventitia are markedly thickened, (L=lumen)

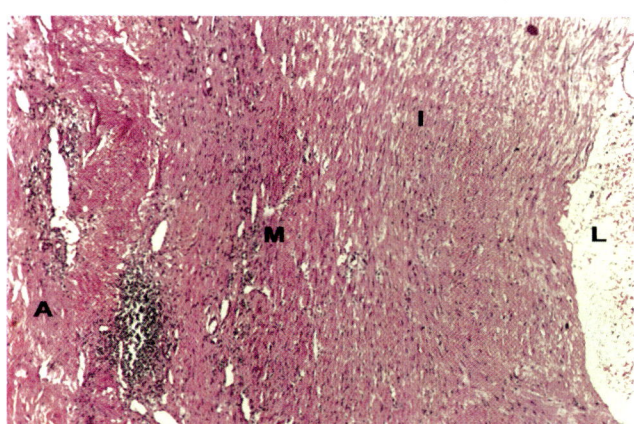

Fig. 13.14b: Non-specific aortoarteritis. Intima is thickened due to prominent myofibroblasts. Media reveals marked fibrosis and focal chronic inflammation. Part of the adventitia (A) included in the picture shows dense collagenisation and focal mononuclear cell infiltration. L=Lumen, M=Media, I=Intima

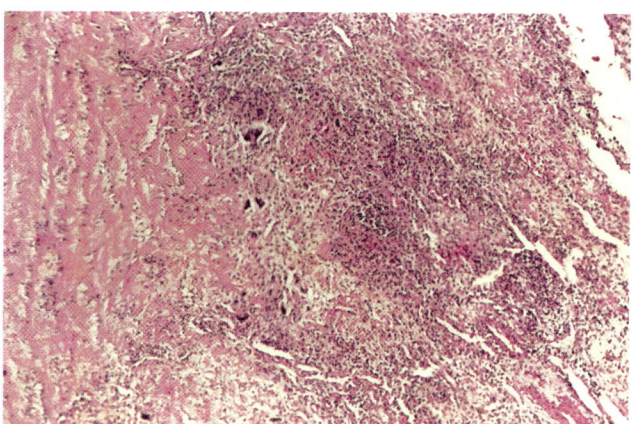

Fig. 13.14c: Non-specific aortoarteritis. Section from the abdominal aorta shows marked inflammatory cell infiltration of the media, increased vascularity and several multinucleated giant cells

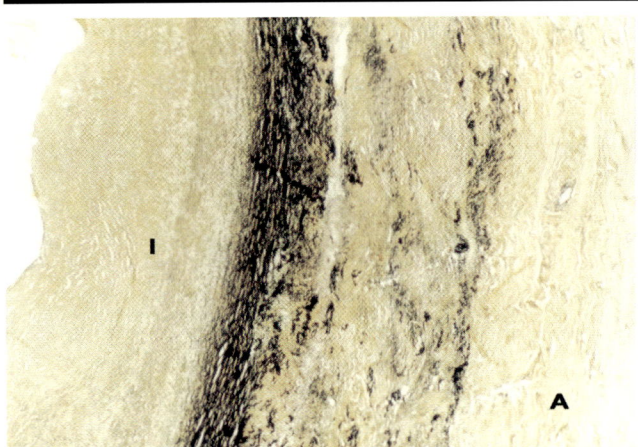

Fig. 13.15a: Non-specific aortoarteritis. Verhoeff-van Gieson stain reveals severe destruction of the elastic tissue within the media and thickening of intima (I) and adventitia (A)

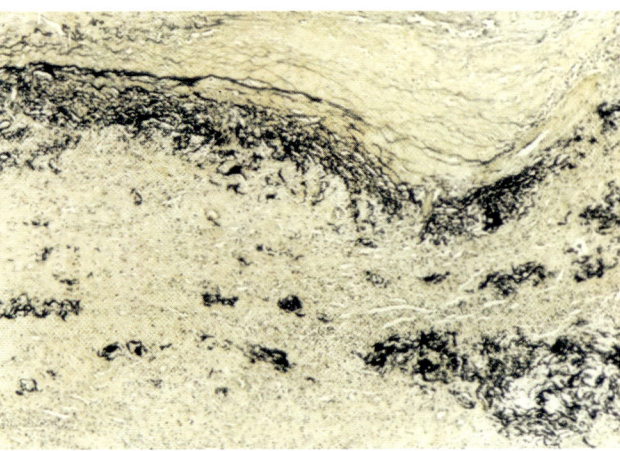

Fig. 13.15b: Non-specific aortoarteritis. Verhoeff-van Gieson stain demonstrates marked destruction of the elastic tissue of media

Note: Patient was a twenty six years female who presented with severe headache. On examination radial, brachial and carotid pulsations were feeble. At autopsy, obliterative arteritis involving the thoracic and abdominal aorta and marked occlusion of left common carotid, left subclavian and left renal arteries was detected

Mucoid vasculopathy is a non-atherosclerotic and non-inflammatory degenerative vascular disease, characterized by premature arteriosclerosis with generalized narrowing (Figs 13.16 and 13.17) and deposition of large quantities of abnormal acid mucopolysaccharides (**AMPS**, also called, glycosaminoglycans or **GAGs**) throughout the vessel wall (Figs 13.18 to 13.19). Affected arteries, especially medium sized muscular arteries, resemble narrow thick walled rubber tubes. They are more prone to dystrophic mineralization (Figs 13.18b and 13.20), thrombosis, and dissection (Fig. 13.16) with rupture. The disorder, seen in young individuals, causes vascular disease syndromes such as coronary, cerebrovascular, aortic, renal and peripheral vascular diseases. The condition is often associated with endomyocardial fibrosis and nutritional endocrinopathies particularly goiter and pancreatic atrophy with or without lithiasis and diabetes mellitus, all of which are common in tropical and developing regions of the world. A bonnet monkey model for mucoid vasculopathy and associated diseases was successfully developed. The model has established that the condition is an acquired metabolic disorder caused by nutritional imbalance owing to consumption of low-protein high-starch diet.

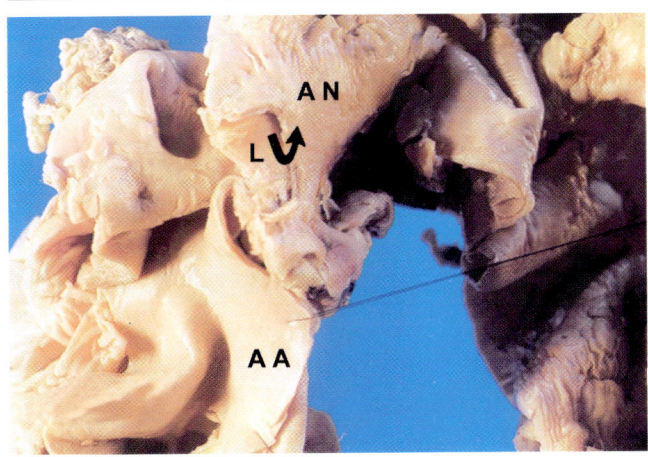

Fig. 13.16: Mucoid vasculopathy. The ascending aorta (AA) has a thick rubbery wall with glistening boggy intima. A few fibromucoid plaques are seen in the arch of the aorta, at the origin of brachiocephalic vessels. There is extensive dissection and aneurysm of the thoracoabdominal aorta. Arrow indicates site of communication between aneurysm (AN) and true lumen of aorta

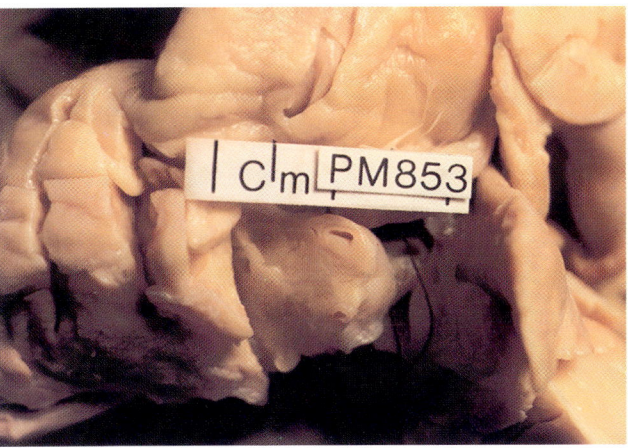

Fig. 13.17: Mucoid vasculopathy. Left anterior descending coronary artery shows concentric thickening of intima and media by gelatinous mucoid intimal plaque and luminal narrowing

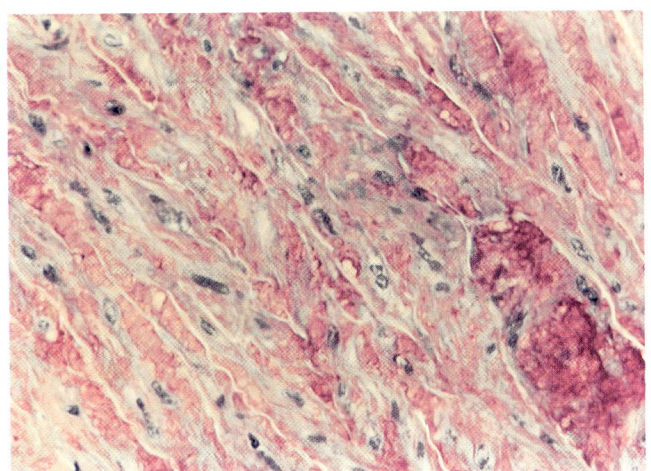

Fig. 13.18a: Mucoid vasculopathy. Toludine blue stain shows metachromasia due to the acid mucopolysaccharides in between the smooth muscle cells of the media

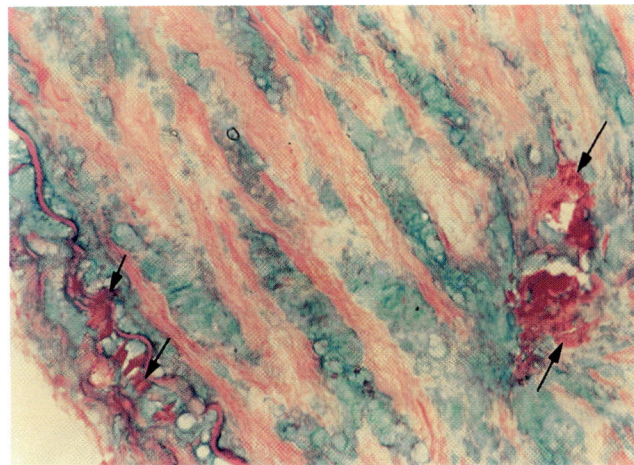

Fig. 13.18b: Mucoid vasculopathy. Alcian blue pH 2.5 shows alcinophilia indicating presence of acid mucopolysaccharides in the vessel wall. Dystrophic mineralisation of fragmented internal and medial elastic laminae is also seen (arrows)

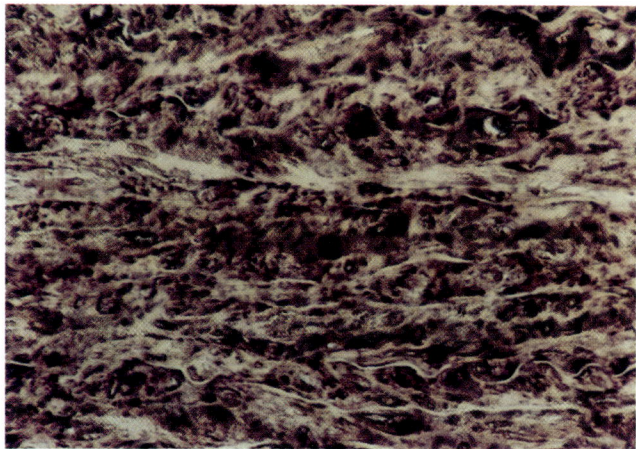

Fig. 13.19a: Mucoid vasculopathy. Immunohistochemistry to demonstrate large quantities of acid mucopolysaccharides in the vessel wall

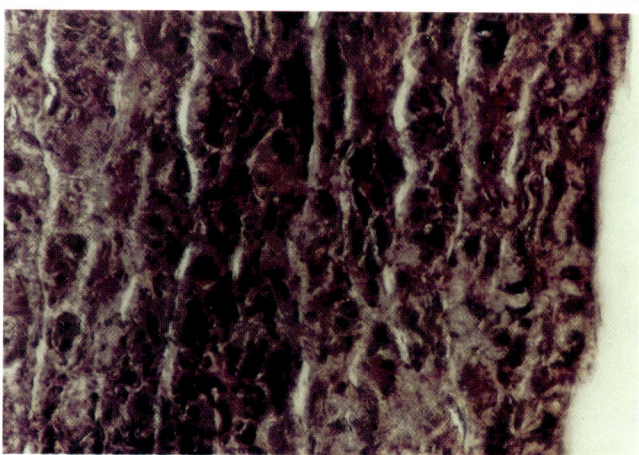

Fig. 13.19b: Mucoid vasculopathy. Immunohistochemistry to demonstrate large quantities of abnormal mucopolysaccharides-heparan sulfate

Note: Immunohistochemistry was done using monoclonal antibodies to detect proteoglycan core proteins after digestion with appropriate enzymes

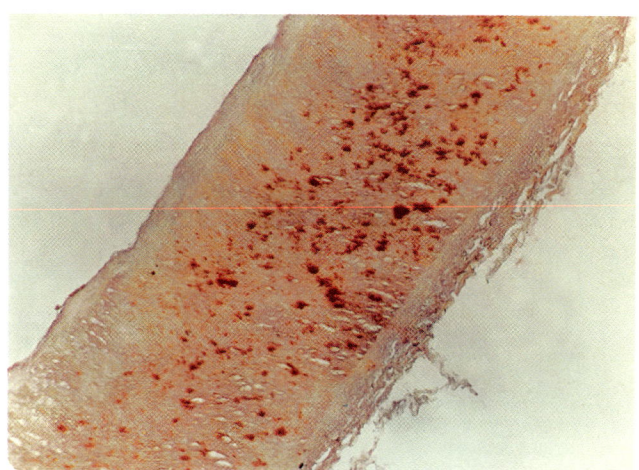

Fig. 13.20: Mucoid vasculopathy. The wall of an artery with mucoid material shows extensive foci of dystrophic mineralisation largely calcium (Alizarin red) *(Figs 13.16 to 13.20 are Courtesy: Dr Sandhya Mani)*

Temporal arteritis occurs in elderly individuals generally over the age of 50 years affecting women more often than men. Amongst the extracranial arteries temporal artery is most commonly involved. Headache and throbbing pain in the temporal region is a common presentation. Other features include scalp tenderness, polymyalgia, fever, malaise and visual symptoms. Anemia and raised erythrocyte sedimentation rate are commonly associated. Microscopically, it is characterized by panarteritis with infiltration by lymphocytes, plasma cells, macrophages, epithelioid cells and occasional eosinophils. Inflammatory cell infiltration is most marked in the media. Internal elastic lamina is fragmented and giant cell reaction in relation to it is frequently observed. Intima is thickened leading to narrowing of the lumen (Figs 13.21 and 13.22). **Etiology** is unclear. Both humoral and cell-mediated immunity have been demonstrated. It is also believed that the elastic tissue may excite a local immunological response. Cytokines namely IL-1, IL-6 and tumor necrosis factor have also been implicated in the pathogenesis.

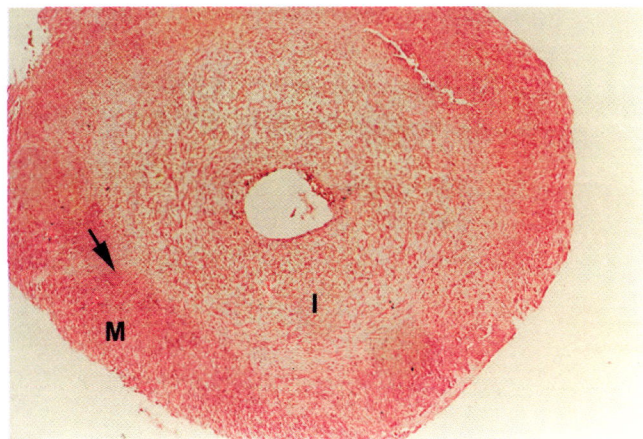

Fig. 13.21a: Giant cell arteritis. Biopsy of the temporal artery shows marked luminal narrowing due to extensive concentric intimal thickening. Giant cells (arrow) are seen at the intima (I) media (M) interphase

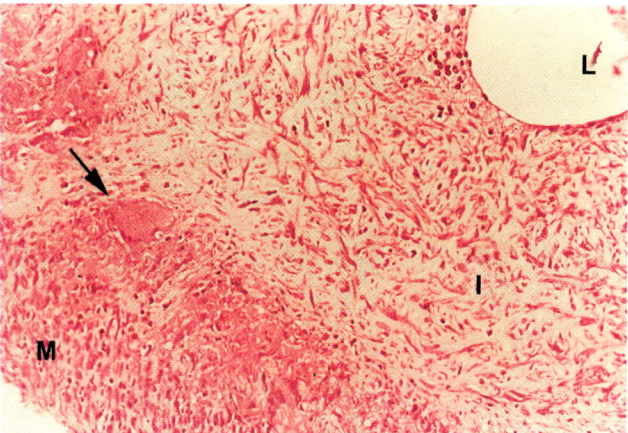

Fig. 13.21b: Marked intimal thickening comprised of plump myofibroblasts in a loose background are seen. Notice the giant cells (arrow) at the intima (I) media (M) interphase. L—Lumen

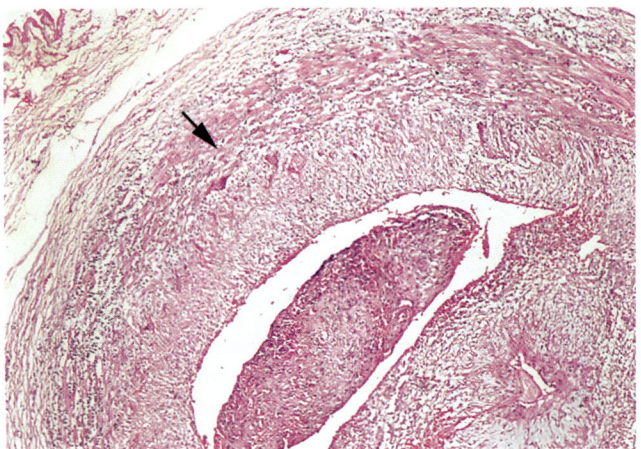

Fig. 13.22a: Giant cell arteritis. Multinucleated giant cells are present in relation to the fragmented internal elastic lamina (arrow). Epithelioid cells in a palisade arrangement are seen in the intimal region

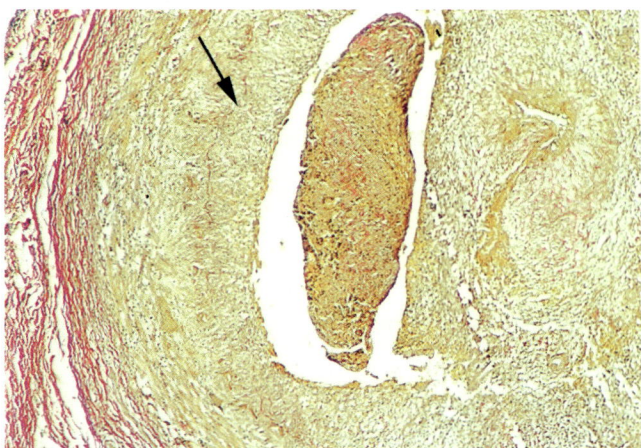

Fig. 13.22b: Elastic van Gieson's stain to highlight the fragmented internal elastic lamina (arrow)

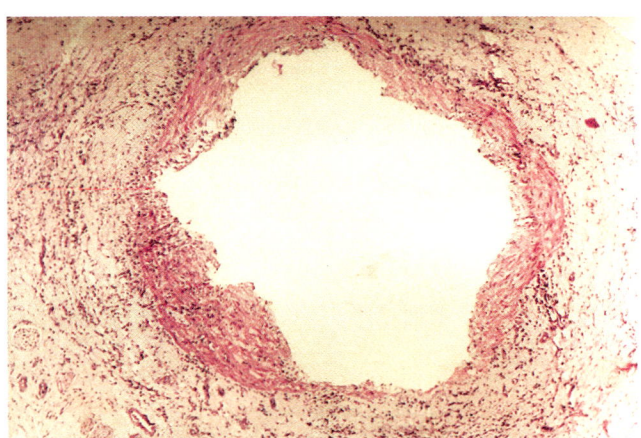

Fig. 13.22c: Giant cell arteritis. A vein was included with the temporal artery biopsy. The wall of vein and the perivenular tissue is infiltrated by lymphocytes

Polyarteritis nodosa (PAN) also known as classic or macroscopic form of PAN, is a multisystem disease characterized by involvement of medium sized arteries which reveal inflammation and necrosis. Aneurysm formation and/or thrombosis may occur (Fig. 13.23). Most frequently affected blood vessels include renal, coronary, mesenteric (Fig. 13.24), hepatic arteries, etc. Classically, a segment of the vessel is necrosed leading to weakness of the vessel wall which has the potential for aneurysm and/or thrombus formation. These lesions can be clearly demonstrated by angiography (Fig. 13.23). Microscopically, PAN is characterised by fibrinoid necrosis of the vessel wall which usually affects part of the circumference of the vessel. In early lesions, infiltration by polymorphs, mononuclear cells and occasional eosinophils is present. Fresh thrombus may be seen (Figs 13.25 to 13.27).

In older lesions fibrosis often along with fibrinoid necrosis is encountered. Inflammatory cells mostly plasma cells, lymphocytes and macrophages are recognised. Organisation of thrombosis occurs at this stage (Figs 13.25 and 13.26a and b). Due to vessel involvement of various organ systems it is not uncommon for a case of PAN to present with symptoms in relation to involvement of the heart, kidney, gastrointestinal tract, brain etc. A limited type of PAN also exists where vasculitis is restricted to the skin, nerves and/or the musculoskeletal system (Fig. 13.26). Differentiation between limited and systemic forms is important from therapy point of view. **Etiology** of PAN is not known. In 25-30% cases of PAN, HBsAg has been detected in the serum. The association between ANCA and classic PAN is insignificant. However, p-ANCA has been reported to be positive in about 20% cases.

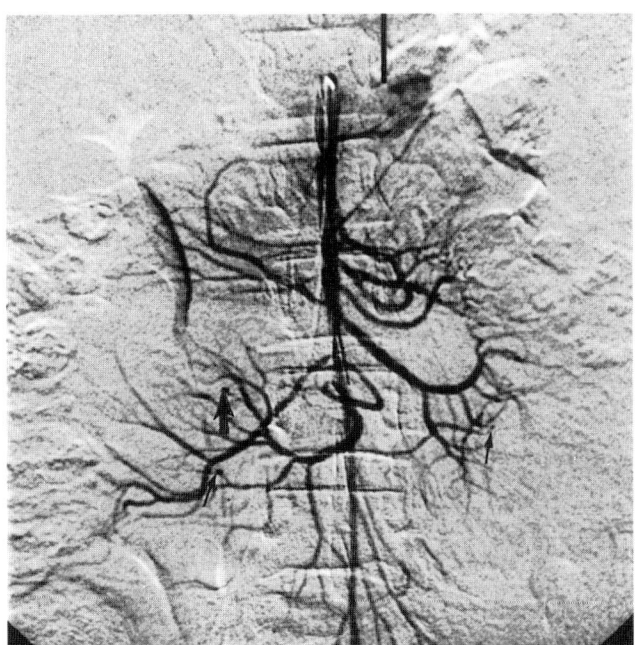

Fig. 13.23a: Polyarteritis nodosa. A selective right renal angiogram showing pruning of the arterial tree and both micro (small arrow) and macro aneurysms (large arrow)

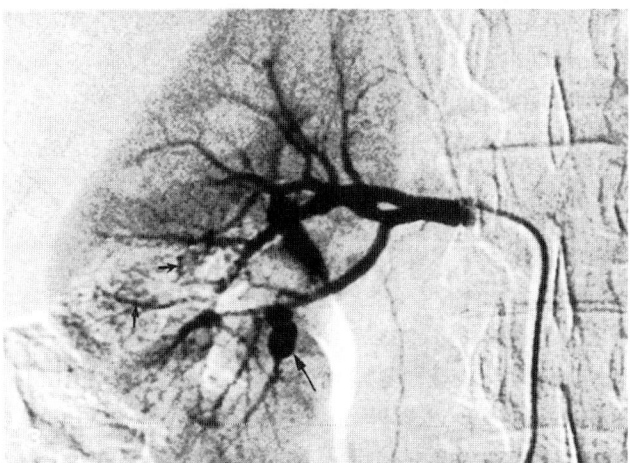

Fig. 13.23b: Polyarteritis nodosa. A selective superior mesenteric angiogram demonstrates multiple micro aneurysms (arrows)

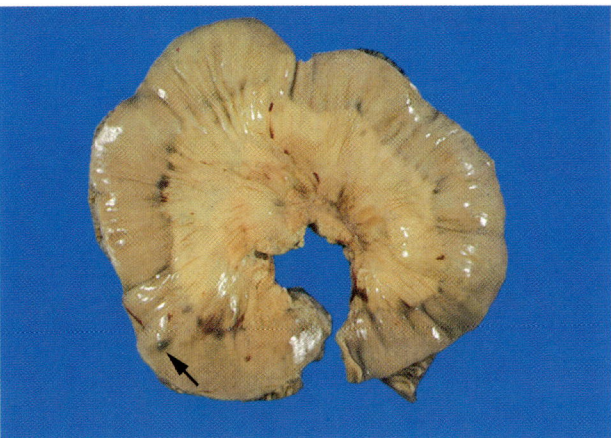

Fig. 13.24: Polyarteritis nodosa. Excised segment of small intestine. An elevated bluish nodule is seen through the serosa (arrow). Microscopic observations of this nodule are illustrated in Figure 13.27

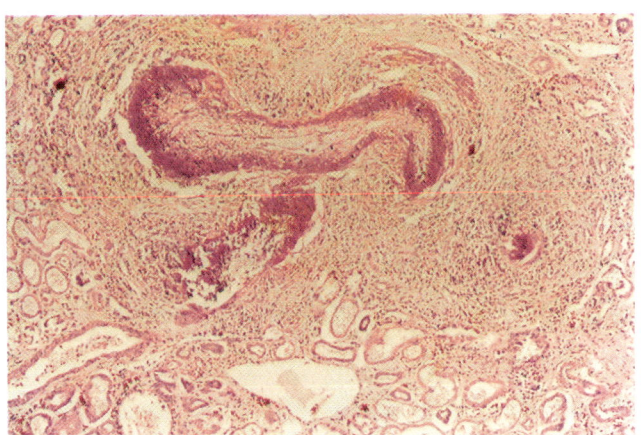

Fig. 13.25a: Polyarteritis nodosa. Medium sized artery in the kidney shows extensive fibrinoid necrosis of vessel wall and obliteration of lumen. The perivascular tissue shows marked inflammation

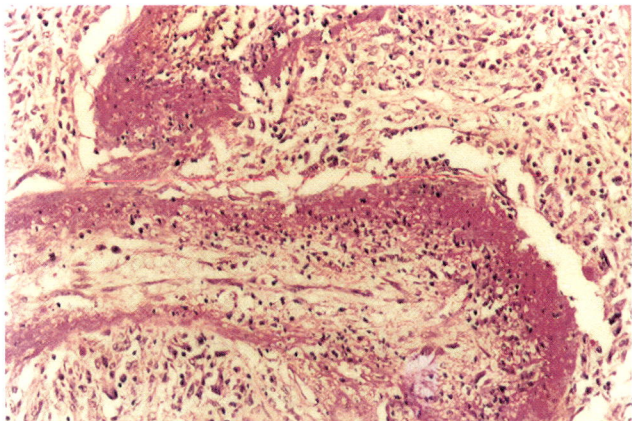

Fig. 13.25b: Polyarteritis nodosa. Higher magnification of Figure 13.25a reveals fibrinoid necrosis and destruction of the vessel wall. Nuclear debris, polymorphs and some histiocytes are present. An organising thrombus is seen in the lumen of the vessel. The perivascular tissue also shows inflammation

Diseases of Blood Vessels

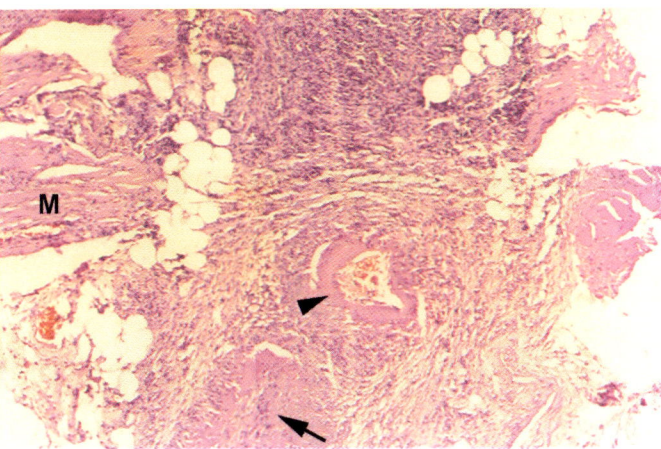

Fig. 13.26a: Polyarteritis nodosa. Calf muscle biopsy was done for diagnostic purposes. Muscle (M) is seen in the left upper hand corner of the picture. Medium sized artery shows fibrinoid necrosis of the blood vessel wall (arrowhead). Part of thrombosed artery is also seen in the picture (thin arrow)

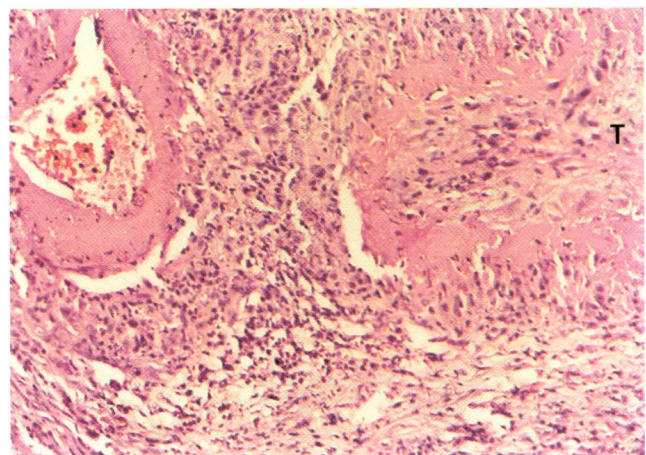

Fig. 13.26b: Higher magnification of Figure 13.26a to highlight fibrinoid necrosis of the vessel wall, thrombus (T) in one blood vessel and marked periarterial inflammation

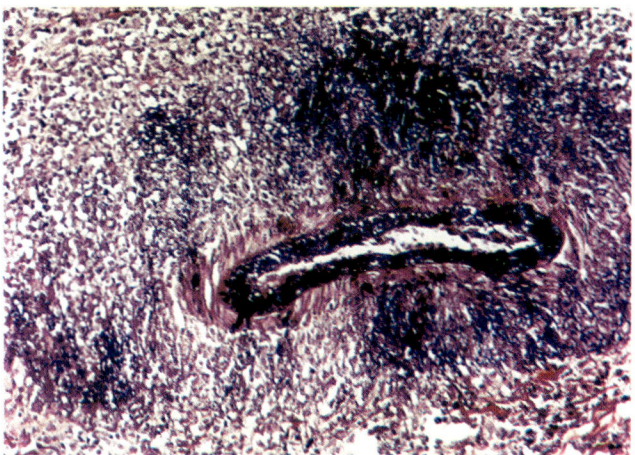

Fig. 13.26c: Polyarteritis nodosa. Fibrinoid necrosis is well appreciated with PTAH stain where the necrosis appears deep blue in color

Note: The patient was a 50 years male who complained of pain on walking as well as difficulty in walking. A clinical diagnosis of polymyositis was made. Calf muscle biopsy was performed to rule out the clinical suspicion. This is a rewarding site to detect vasculitis as exemplified by this case. This case is an example of limited PAN where vasculitis is restricted to the skin, nerves and/or musculoskeletal system

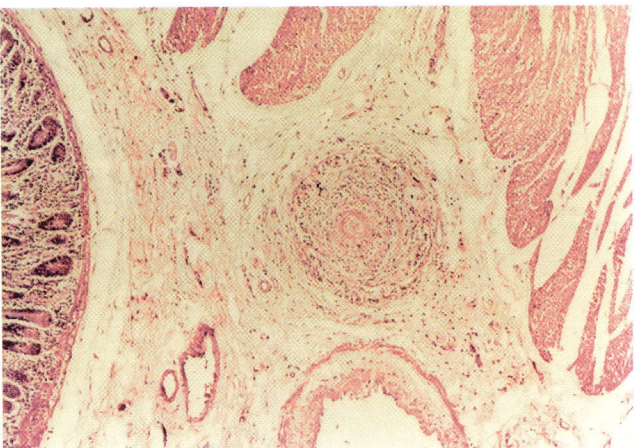

Fig. 13.27a: Polyarteritis nodosa. Vasculitis of small artery is seen in the submucosa. Intestinal mucosa and muscularis are seen in the left and right side of the picture respectively

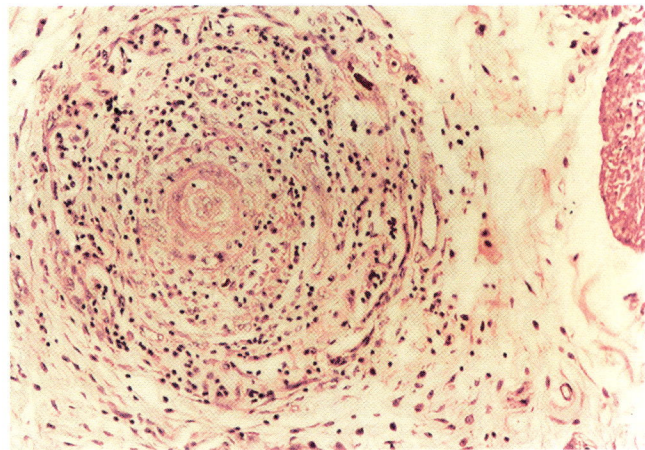

Fig. 13.27b: Polyarteritis nodosa. Higher magnification of Figure 13.27a to demonstrate inflammatory cell infiltration of all layer of blood vessel wall. A large number of eosinophils wave noted amidst the infiltrate

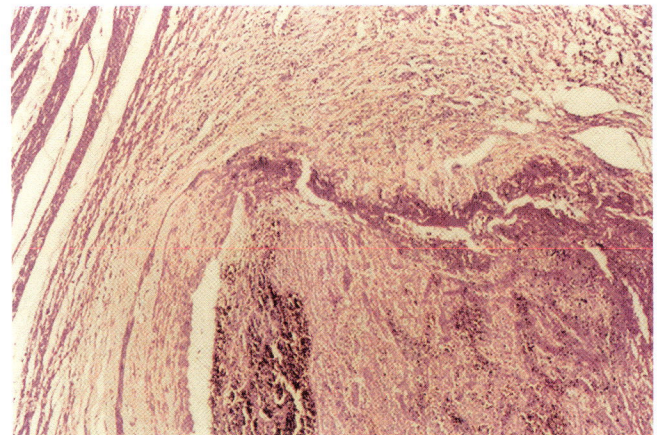

Fig. 13.27c: Polyarteritis nodosa. Medium sized artery in the submucosa contains a fresh thrombus. Part of attenuated muscularis is seen in left upper hand of picture. In other areas an organised thrombus was also detected

Note: This was a thirty years old female patient who had fever for 4 months. She presented with malena for 7 days. She was detected to be hypertensive. Angiography revealed aneurysms in superior mesenteric artery and bleeding point in the jejunum on the mucosal surface (4 mm). The affected segment was excised. Specimen of the excised intestine is illustrated in Figure 13.24

Wegener granulomatosis is characterized by systemic, necrotizing vasculitis of small to medium sized arteries, necrotizing granulomatous inflammation of the lungs, ear, nose, throat and paranasal sinuses with associated necrotizing/crescentic glomerulonephritis. Some cases may present with isolated lung or renal involvement. Cases without renal involvement are termed as limited Wegener granulomatosis. Males are affected more often than females. The peak incidence is the fifth decade of life. High mortality is associated with untreated cases.

Microscopically, necrosis of medium to small sized arteries, arterioles, capillaries and venules is characteristically observed. Necrotizing granulomatous inflammation comprising of large areas of necrosis, epithelioid cell granulomas, multinucleated giant cells and infiltration by polymorphs, lymphocytes and prominent nuclear cell debris is seen (Figs 13.28 and 13.29). The necrotizing process is often invasive resulting in destruction of tissues and nasal septal perforation resulting in saddle nose deformity. When kidneys are involved necrotizing glomerulonephritis and/or crescentic glomerulonephritis

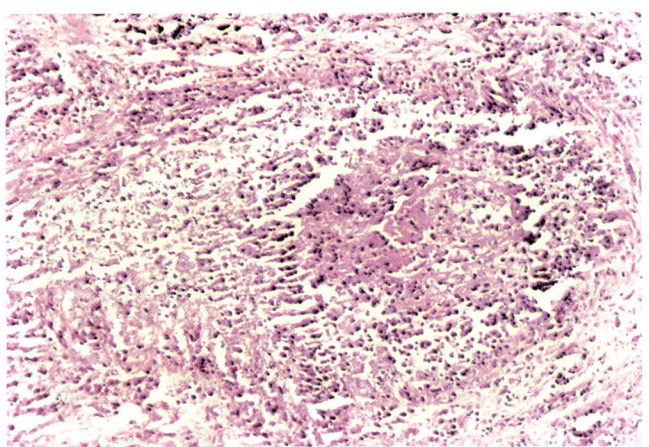

Fig. 13.28a: Wegener granulomatosis lung. Extensive necrotizing inflammation with granulomatous angiitis is observed

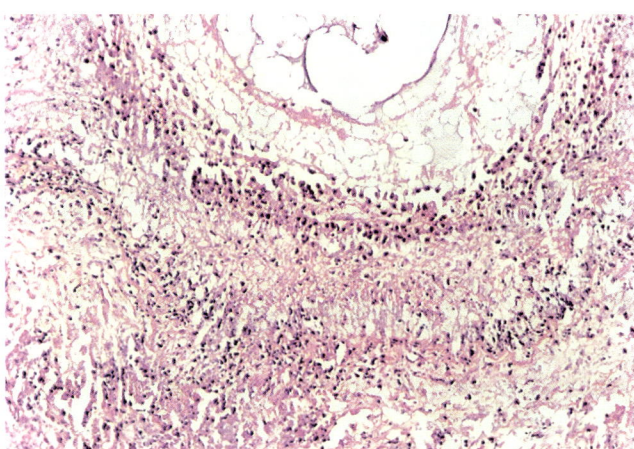

Fig. 13.28b: Wegener granulomatosis lung. Another area to demonstrate extensive necrosis and inflammation of the vessel wall

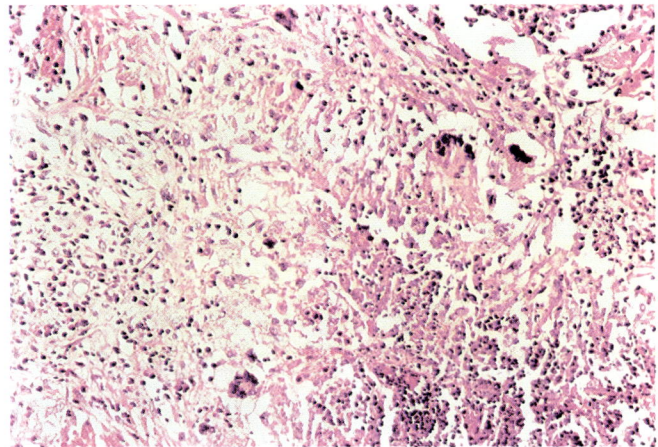

Fig. 13.28c: Wegener granulomatosis lung. Epithelioid cell granulomas with giant cells are seen within the necrotic blood vessels

Note: Other areas showed hemorrhagic infarcts and inflammatory cell infiltration. At autopsy, kidney, spleen and intestinal tract were also involved

is observed (Fig. 13.30). **Etiology** of Wegener granulomatosis is unknown and ill understood. It is believed that in a predisposed individual exposure of the airways to unidentified substances leads to systemic autoimmune disease. Immunoglobulin deposits on the glomerular basement membrane and/or circulating immune complexes have been demonstrated in some patients. Cell mediated immunity has also been implicated. Antinuclear cytoplasmic autoantibodies (c-ANCA) have been demonstrated in about 85-90% patients with active Wegener granulomatosis and about 40% of patients in remission. Serial measurements of c-ANCA have been used to monitor disease activity and effect of therapy.

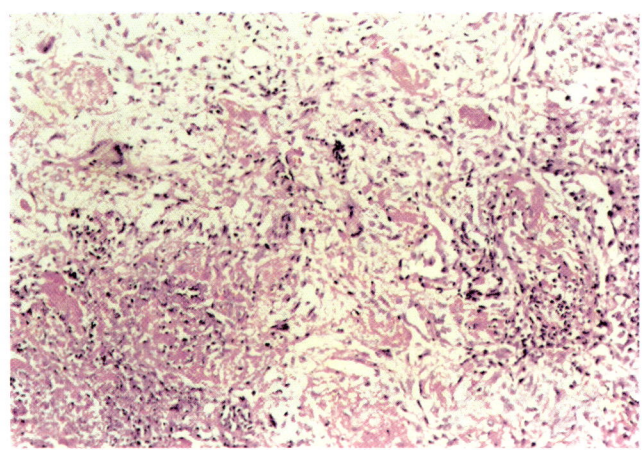

Fig. 13.29a: Wegener granulomatosis, lung. Necrotizing inflammation along with epithelioid giant cells are seen

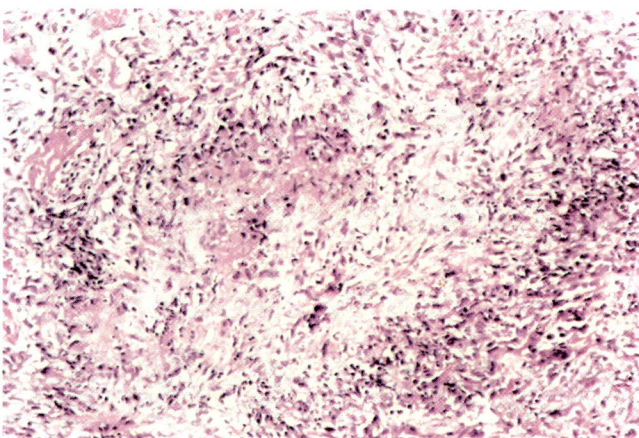

Fig. 13.29b: Wegener granulomatosis, lung. Necrotizing angiitis is observed

Note: Lung biopsy was done for diagnostic purposes

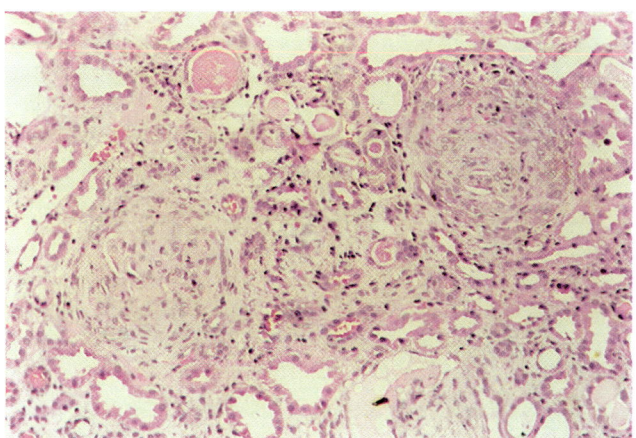

Fig. 13.30a: Wegener granulomatosis, kidney. Fibrocellular crescents are seen. Other glomeruli showed either sclerosis or necrosis

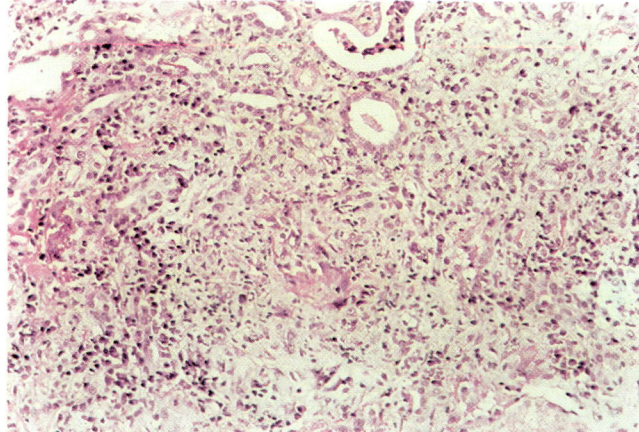

Fig. 13.30b: Wegener granulomatosis, kidney. Necrotizing granulomatous inflammation along with giant cells is seen within the interstitium of the kidney

Note: Kidney biopsy was done for diagnostic purposes

Churg-Strauss syndrome also known as allergic granulomatous angiitis is characterized by systemic vasculitis affecting small to medium sized vessels, asthma and hypereosinophilia. Microscopically, necrotizing vasculitis with a prominent infiltrate by eosinophils is seen (Fig. 13.31). Granulomas including giant cells may also be observed. p-ANCA has been detected in several cases (about 70% cases).

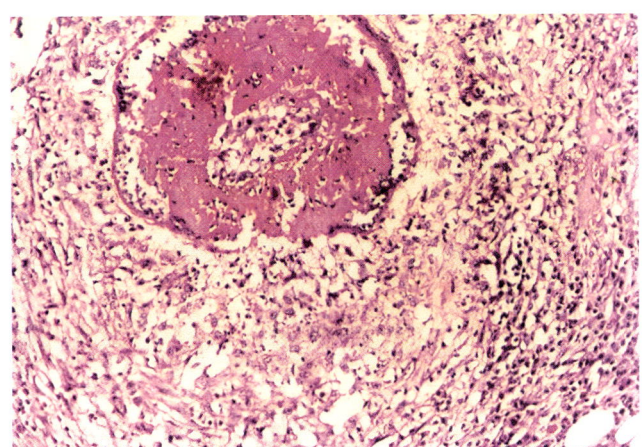

Fig. 13.31a: Churg-Strauss disease. Photomicrograph of blood vessel in the mesentery shows marked fibrinoid necrosis and destruction of the vessel wall. Inflammatory cell infiltration is seen around the blood vessel. Mixed type of infiltrate including eosinophils was present

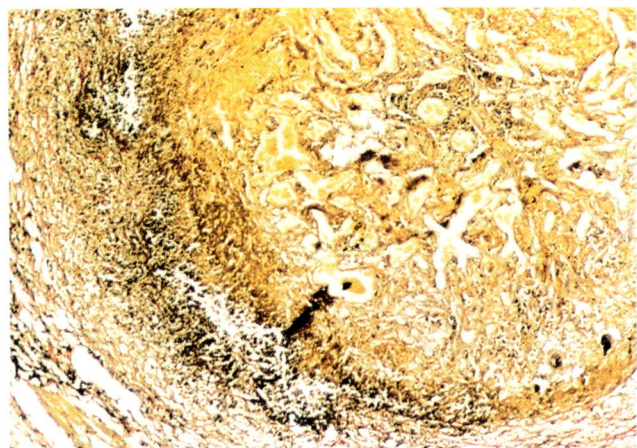

Fig. 13.31b: Churg-Strauss disease. Another area from the case illustrated in Figure 13.31a shows an organised thrombus within the blood vessel. Fresh thrombi were also observed in other arterial branches

Note: Patient a 16 years old male was an asthmatic since 2 years. Peripheral smear showed absolute eosinophilia. He complained of pain in abdomen for two months and had features of peritonitis. At surgery, a segment of ileum showed ulceration and perforation. Microscopically, large areas of mucosal ulceration and necrosis were recognized. Eosinophils dominated the inflammatory infiltrate. Sections from the mesentery revealed vasculitis of small and medium sized arteries with both fresh and organized thrombi

Kawasaki syndrome also known as mucocutaneous lymph node syndrome, is a febrile illness which affects infants and children below five years of age. It is characterized by vasculitis of the medium sized arteries with frequent involvement of the coronary arteries. Latter present as ectasia, aneurysm which may rupture or show thrombosis. Consequently myocardial infarction and sudden death can occur. In addition to arteritis, reddening and desquamation of palms and soles, a maculopapular rash, conjunctival congestion, reddening of lips and tongue and nonpurulent cervical lymphadenopathy are often associated. Microscopically, marked necrosis and inflammation in the entire thickness of the vessel wall is observed. Destruction of the vessel wall predisposes to aneurysm formation. **Etiology** of Kawasaki is not clearly understood. The various possibilities include immunological injury by way of both humoral and cell mediated mechanisms. Autoantibodies to endothelial and smooth muscle cells have been demonstrated which possibly result in acute vasculitis.

Microscopic polyangiitis This is a pauci-immune necrotizing vasculitis that affects the capillaries, venules, arterioles and small arteries in skin (Fig. 13.32), lungs, gastrointestinal tract and kidneys. Microscopically, leukocytoclastic vasculitis in skin, necrotizing glomerulonephritis and pulmonary capillaritis in one or other form may be seen. About 90% patients of microscopic polyangiitis show the presence of p-ANCA in the serum. Immune-complex deposition in blood vessels as seen in other types of cutaneous leukocytoclastic vasculitis are not demonstrated in MPAN.

Henoch-Schönlein purpura This type of vasculitis affects skin, gut, glomeruli and is associated with arthritis/arthralgia. Microscopically, leukocytoclastic vasculitis is seen involving capillaries, arterioles and venules (Fig. 13.33). IgA-dominant immune complexes are demonstrated.

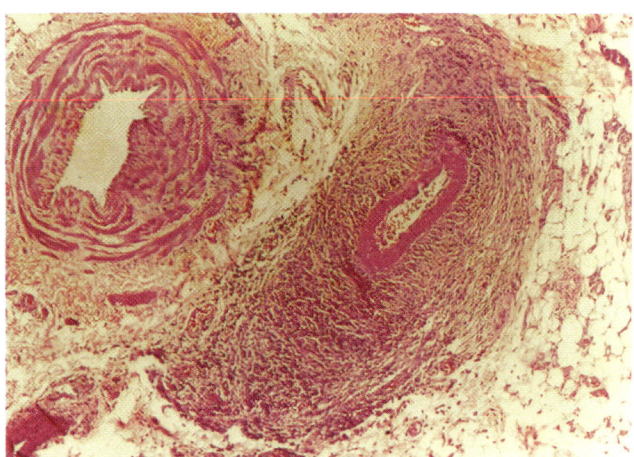

Fig. 13.32a: Nodular vasculitis. Photomicrograph of a tender subcutaneous nodule shows fibrinoid necrosis of the wall of an artery with dense concentric inflammatory cell infiltration composed of lymphocytes and histiocytes. The accompanying vein is uninvolved

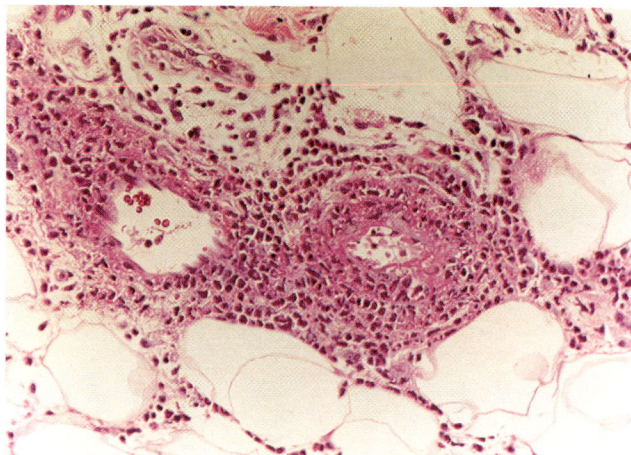

Fig. 13.32b: Vasculitis of small artery in the subcutaneous fat. The wall of the vessel is smudgy and necrotic. Marked infiltration is seen in the perivascular region comprising of lymphocytes and histiocytes. The infiltrate is extending into septae of fat

Cutaneous leukocytoclastic vasculitis (hypersensitivity angiitis) This refers to a broad group of small vessel vasculitis seen in a variety of disorders such as drug induced vasculitis, serum sickness, Henoch-Schönlein purpura, vasculitis associated with collagen vascular disorders, and essential mixed cryoglobulinemia, etc. Characteristically there is involvement of the venules, capillaries and arterioles of the skin without any systemic involvement. It is manifest as palpable purpura of skin. Microscopically leucocytoclastic vasculitis is characterized by fibrinoid necrosis of small vessels, fibrin plugs, extravasation of red blood cells, edema of upper dermis and infiltration predominantly by polymorphs. Prominent nuclear debris is noted (Fig. 13.33). Adequate history and investigations need to be obtained to decipher the cause of vasculitis as a similar histologic picture can be seen in different types of unrelated vasculitis.

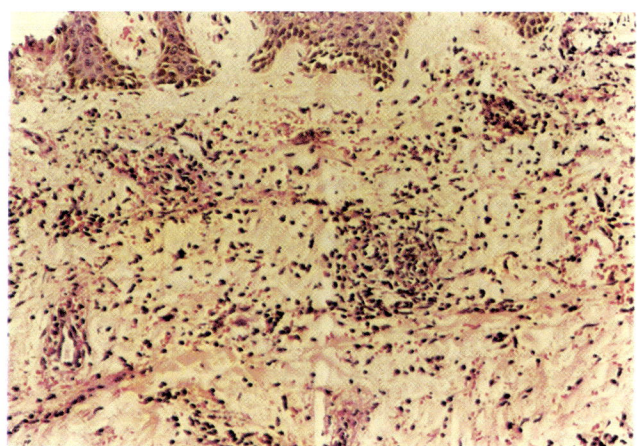

Fig. 13.33a: Leukocytoclastic vasculitis. Inflammatory infiltrate is almost exclusively confined to around capillaries and arterioles in upper dermis. Edema in dermis is also noted. Fibrinoid necrosis of vessel walls and extravasation of red blood cells can be appreciated

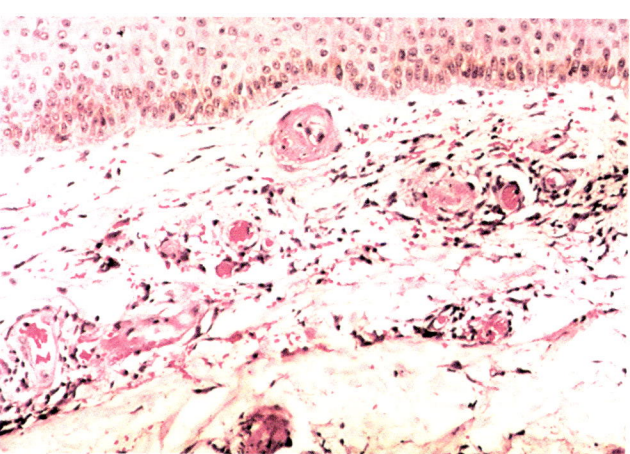

Fig. 13.33b: Leukocytoclastic vasculitis. In contrast to Figure 13.33a the inflammatory component is less. Several capillaries/arterioles show fibrin thrombi. Fibrinoid necrosis extravasation of red blood cells and dermal edema are also noted

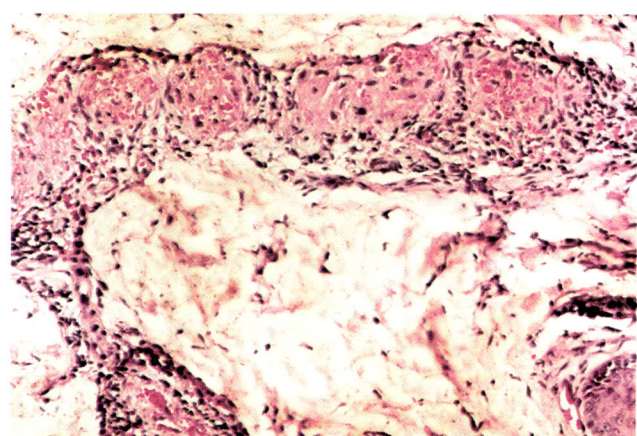

Fig. 13.33c: Leukocytoclastic vasculitis. A row of blood vessels showing fibrinoid necrosis, fibrin, obliteration of vessel lumen and extravasation of red blood cells are observed. Perivascular lymphocytic cuffing is also seen

Primary angiitis of central nervous system This is a rare type of vasculitis and was previously designated as granulomatous angiitis of nervous system or brain and isolated angiitis. Clinical picture of this entity is vague and non-specific. Recurring headaches, multifocal neurological deficits and diffuse encephalopathy with confusion and memory impairment are the predominant features. Patients are usually adults between 30-50 years of age. Demonstration of multiple narrowed segments in cerebral arteries by angiography is essential for the diagnosis but the angiographic findings are not specific to the disease. Arteries are much more frequently affected than veins. It may present in both granulomatous and non-granulomatous forms either separately or co-existing in different parts of the brain in the same patient. The non-granulomatous form may appear as polyarteritis type of necrotizing inflammation. Epithelioid cell granulomas with prominent lymphocyte cuffing are seen in the granulomatous form of the disease (Fig. 13.34). Hemorrhage and infarction of the brain parenchyma may occur. Aggressive immunosuppressive therapy has proved effective. **Etiology** is unknown. However, an infective etiology has been implicated. Association of this entity with Varicella zoster infection as well as Hodgkin's lymphoma has been documented.

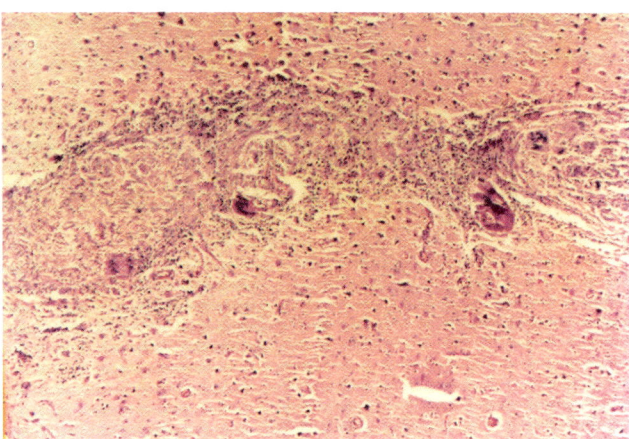

Fig. 13.34a: Primary angiitis of the central nervous system. Numerous epithelioid cell granulomas are seen in the brain parenchyma. These are oriented around small arteries

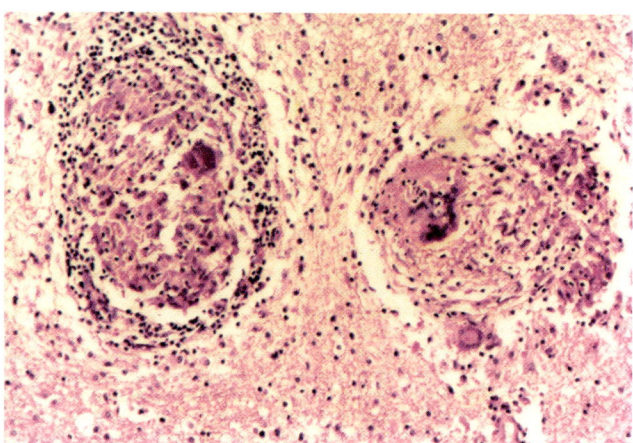

Fig. 13.34b: Primary angiitis of the central nervous system. Two well delineated epithelioid cell granulomas having multinucleated giant cells are seen. Lymphocyte cuffing is observed in one of them

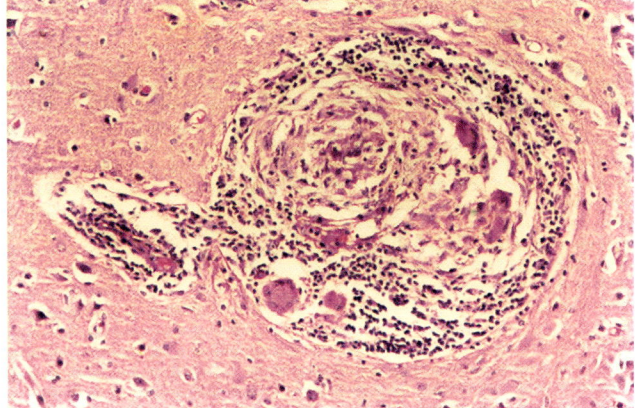

Fig. 13.34c: Primary angiitis of the central nervous system. The lesion is well circumscribed and shows a granulomatous response around a small blood vessel. Lymphocyte cuffing is prominent

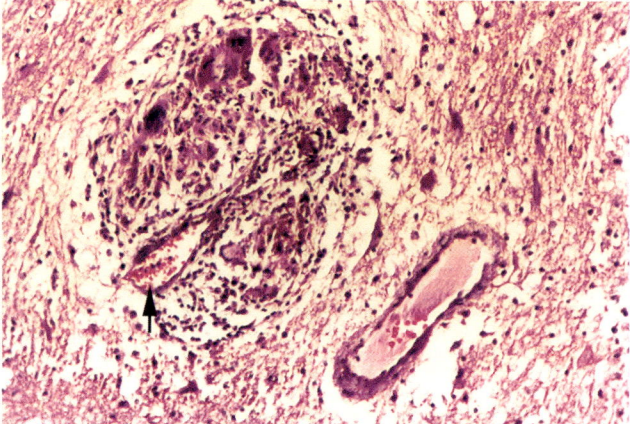

Fig. 13.34d: Primary angiitis of central nervous system. Perivascular (arrow) granulomatous inflammation is striking

Thromboangiitis obliterans (TAO; Buerger disease) is an inflammatory disease of the medium sized and small arteries in the arms and legs involving chiefly the posterior tibial and radial arteries (Fig. 13.35). The adjacent veins and nerves can also be enveloped by the inflammatory process in some cases. Microscopically, acute and chronic inflammation of the vessel wall, occlusive thrombosis with organisation and recanalisation of thrombi is observed. Associated acute phlebitis with prominent intimitis in TAO is present in a number of cases (Fig. 13.36).

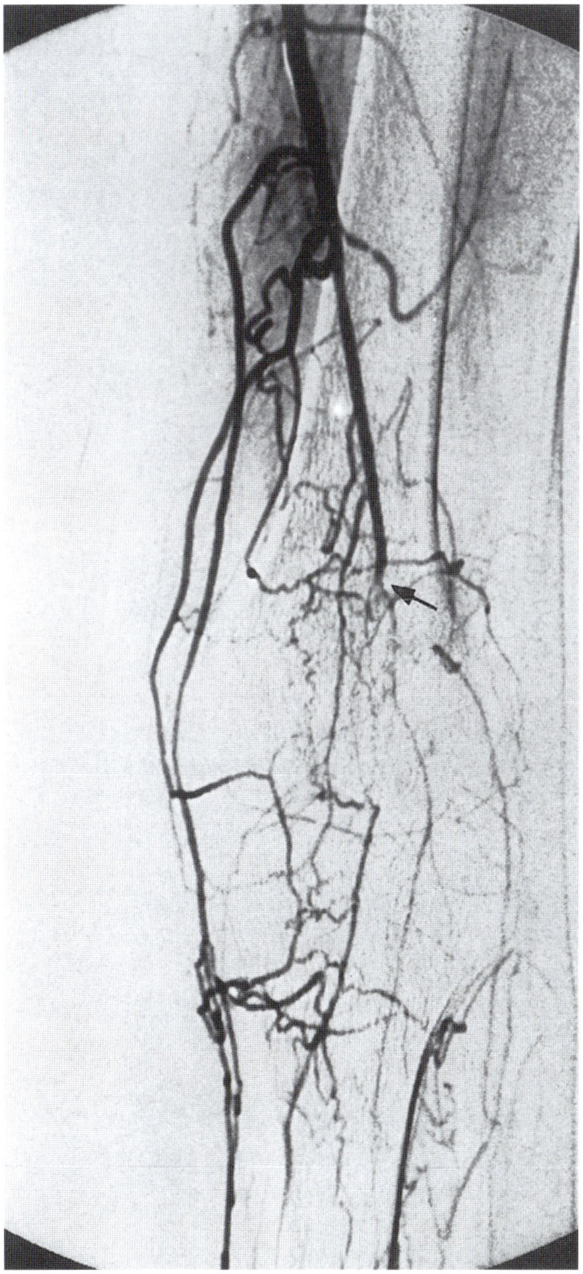

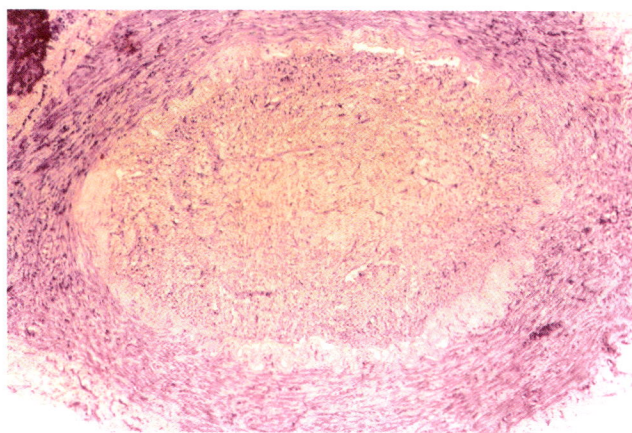

Fig. 13.36a: Thromboangiitis obliterans (Buerger disease). Lumen of the tibial artery is completely obliterated by an organized thrombus. Note that the media does not show any inflammatory infiltrate

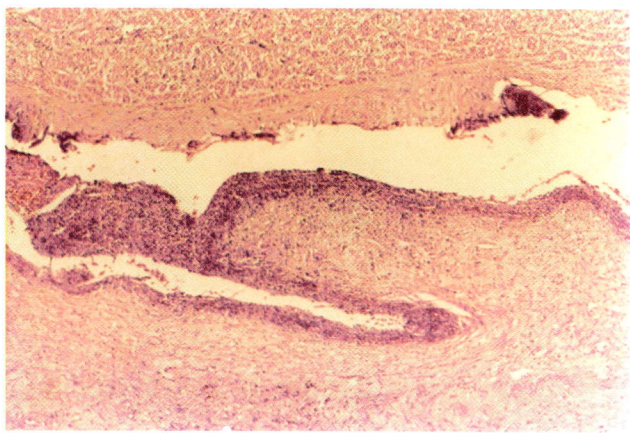

Fig. 13.35: Thromboangiitis obliterans (Buerger disease) in a 30 years old chronic smoker. A selective superficial femoral angiogram shows complete occlusion of the proximal part of popliteal artery (arrow). Multiple collaterals are seen supplying the leg region

Fig. 13.36b: Thromboangiitis obliterans (Buerger disease). Accompanying vein shows fibrin deposition and inflammation. Compare the involved segment with the uninvolved part of the vein which is seen in the upper part of the picture

Etiology of TAO is closely linked with smoking in that cessation of smoking has been reported to be associated with remission of the disease while exacerbation has been observed with smoking. Hypersensitivity to tobacco proteins has been demonstrated in patients of TAO. This is possibly genetically controlled as increased prevalence of HLA-A9 and HLA-B5 haplotypes has been documented in these patients.

Venous involvement in lepromatous leprosy

This is a specific inflammatory condition affecting subcutaneous medium sized veins in the lepromatous leprosy patients. In one study, histologically confirmed cases of leprous phlebitis were defected in 33 out of 36 lepromatous leprosy patients. The degree of infiltration in these cases ranged from early and mild inflammation of intima with AFB in endothelial cells to complete and diffuse infiltration of the whole vessel wall with 90% occlusion of the lumen. The presence of intimal lesions indicates that phlebitis begins with the entry of AFB from blood with subsequent development of granulomata and infiltration of the whole vein wall. The high degree of bacillation in the endothelium could well be a site for release of AFB into the circulation thus perpetuating bacillemia (Fig. 13.37).

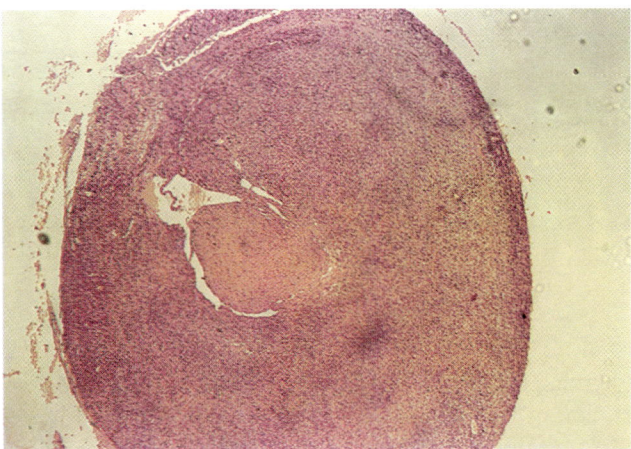

Fig. 13.37a: Lepromatous leprosy, vein. Advanced lesion. The medial muscle fibers although infiltrated are still seen as circularly running bundles

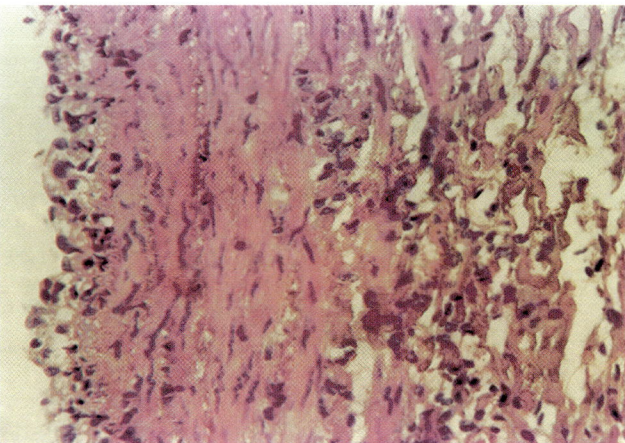

Fig. 13.37b: Lepromatous leprosy, vein. Intima of and wall of the vein of an intermediate lesion show histiocytes/epithelioid cells

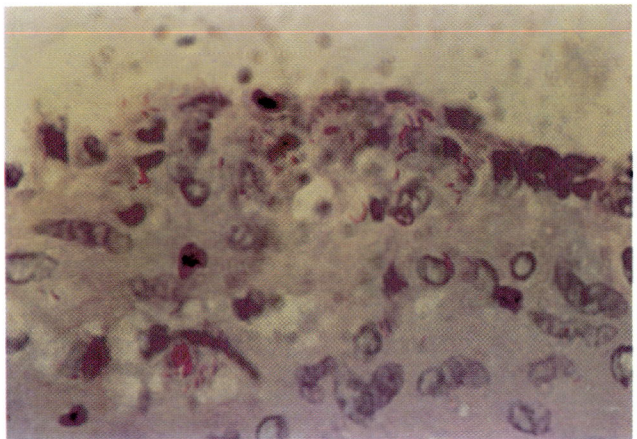

Fig. 13.37c: Lepromatous leprosy, vein. Early lesion showing mild infiltration of inflammatory cells in the intima. Acid-fast bacilli (AFB) were present in the intimal layers

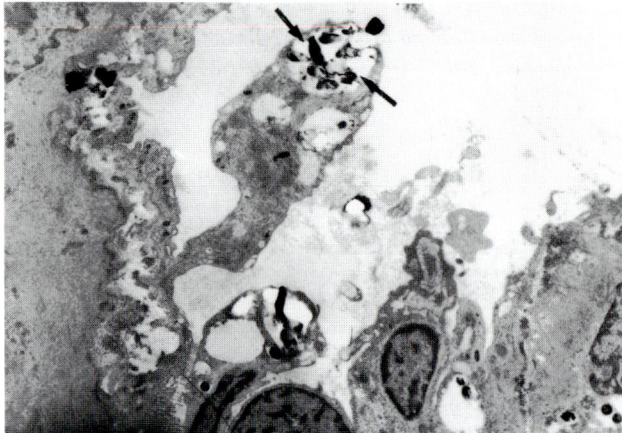

Fig. 13.37d: Lepromatous leprosy, vein. Endothelial cells showing a pseudopod containing a cluster of *M. leprae* at the tip (arrows) *(Figs 13.37a to d Courtesy: Dr Ashok Mukherjee)*

Erythema nodosum leprosum is a type 2 reaction which occurs in lepromatous and borderline leprosy where the mycobacterial antigen load is high. It is characterized by leukocytoclastic vasculitis (Fig. 13.38).

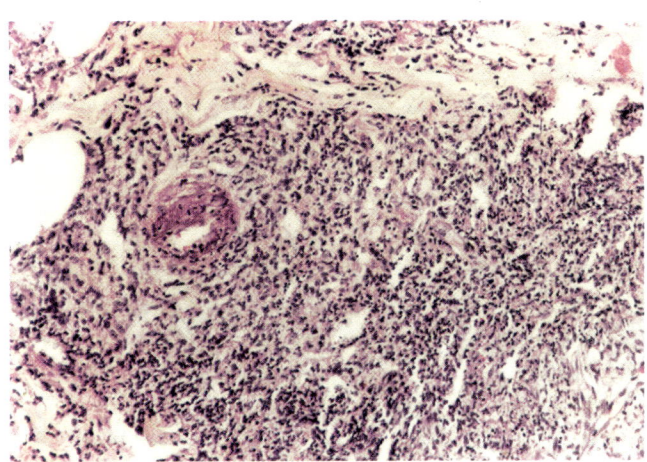

Fig. 13.38a: Erythema nodosum leprosum. Photomicrograph of tender subcutaneous nodule that developed in a case of Hansen's disease on anti-leprosy therapy. Small sized artery shows fibrinoid necrosis of the vessel wall. The dermal collagen reveals a dense inflammatory cell infiltrate consisting of polymorphs, lymphocytes and a large number of foamy macrophages

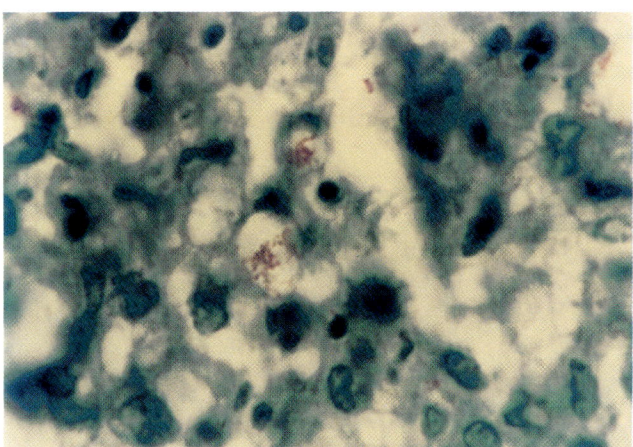

Fig. 13.38b: Erythema nodosum leprosum. Stain for acid-fast bacilli reveals numerous bacilli within macrophages

Tuberculosis of blood vessel It is not uncommon to see involvement of blood vessels by tuberculous leptomeningitis. Granulomatous inflammation along with dense inflammation is seen to involve all layers of the vessel wall (Fig. 13.39). Acid-fast bacilli can be demonstrated in a number of cases.

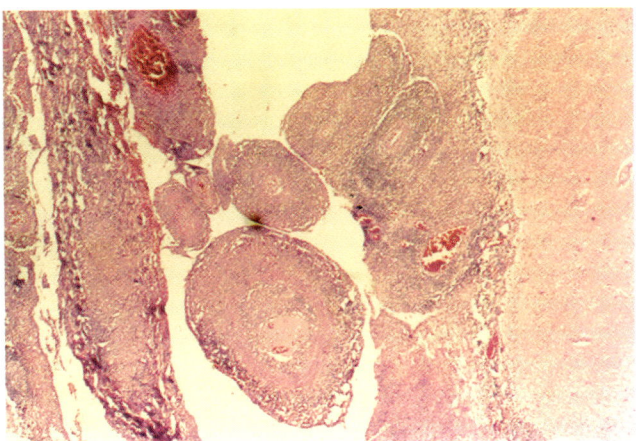

Fig. 13.39a: Tuberculosis leptomeninges. Photomicrograph of leptomeninges over the cerebrum. Numerous prominent blood vessels surrounded by dense inflammation are seen

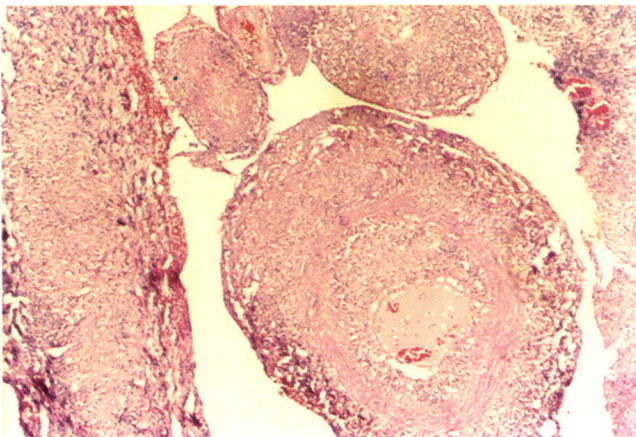

Fig. 13.39b: Tuberculosis leptomeninges. Higher magnification of fig. 13.39a reveals granulomatous inflammation involving all layers of the blood vessel

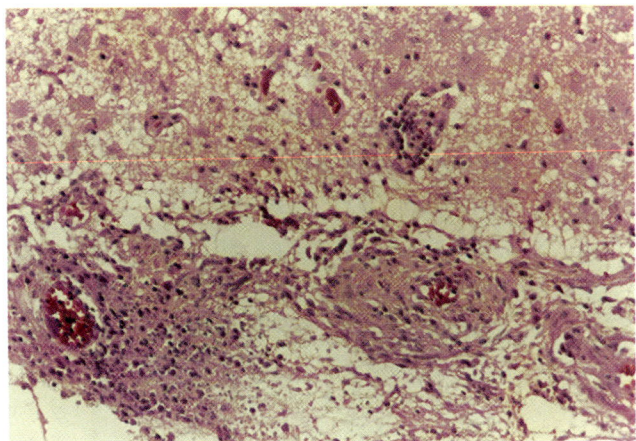

Fig. 13.39c: Tuberculous meningitis. Ill formed epithelioid cell granulomas are seen around blood vessels. Another blood vessel (left lower corner) shows necrosis. Brain parenchyma (upper part of picture) shows features of mild edema

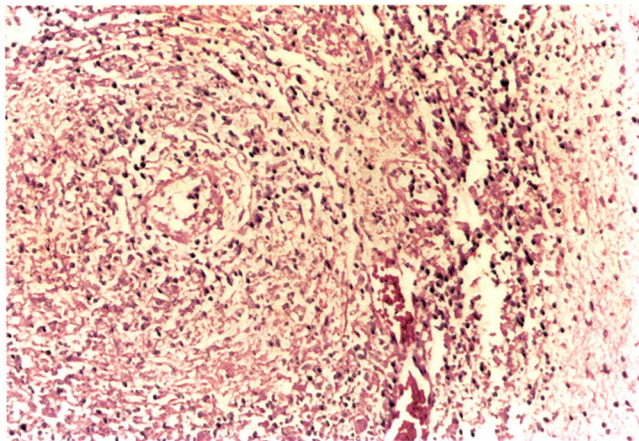

Fig. 13.39d: Tuberculous meningitis. A blood vessel in the leptomeninges shows necrosis and few inflammatory cells including macrophages. No well-defined granulomas are seen. Part of the cerebral cortex is seen in the extreme right of the picture. Stains for acid-fast bacilli were positive

Diseases of Blood Vessels

Aneurysm of blood vessels Aneurysm is an abnormal dilatation of the blood vessel which occurs primarily due to weakness of the vessel wall. Latter may be either congenital or acquired due to various diseases. Aneurysms are either true when its wall is composed of various components of the vessel wall or false when the layers of blood vessel are not recognized and instead fibroconnective tissue is present. Aneurysms are classified depending upon their shape and size, location and etiology.

Atherosclerotic aneurysm Atherosclerosis is the most common cause of aneurysms of the abdominal aorta (Figs 13.40 to 13.43). Atherosclerotic aneurysms can also occasionally affect the ascending and descending thoracic aorta, renal, iliac and popliteal arteries. They occur much more frequently in men and in hypertensives. These aneurysms are classically **fusiform** (ovoid shape parallel to the long axis of the vessel) in shape though **saccular** (outpouching of vessel wall at the site of medial weakening) forms may also occur in some cases. The affected segment shows complicated atherosclerotic lesions, i.e. ulcerated plaques with mural thrombosis. Microscopically, atherosclerotic lesions are seen in the intima which is widened to compress the media. Latter is thinned out and only its remnants can be seen. Varying degree of inflammation and fibrosis of the media and adventitia is observed. The major risk of large abdominal aneurysms (> 5 cm in diameter) is rupture with retroperitoneal hemorrhage which can prove fatal unless it is recognized and managed appropriately.

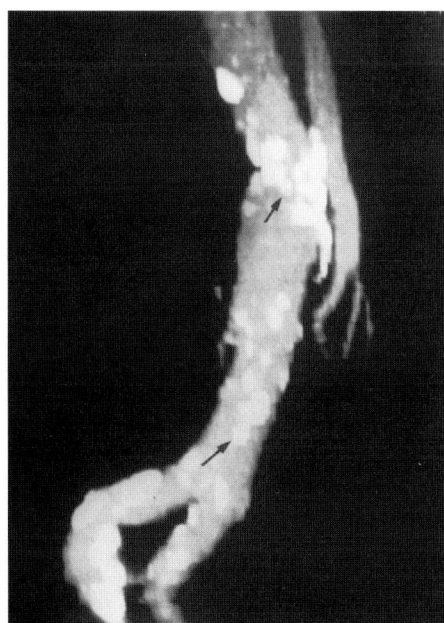

Fig. 13.40: Atherosclerosis of abdominal aorta. A CT angiogram maximum intensity projection image showing a tortuous abdominal aorta and common iliac arteries with mild focal dilatations and numerous high density calcified plaques (arrows)

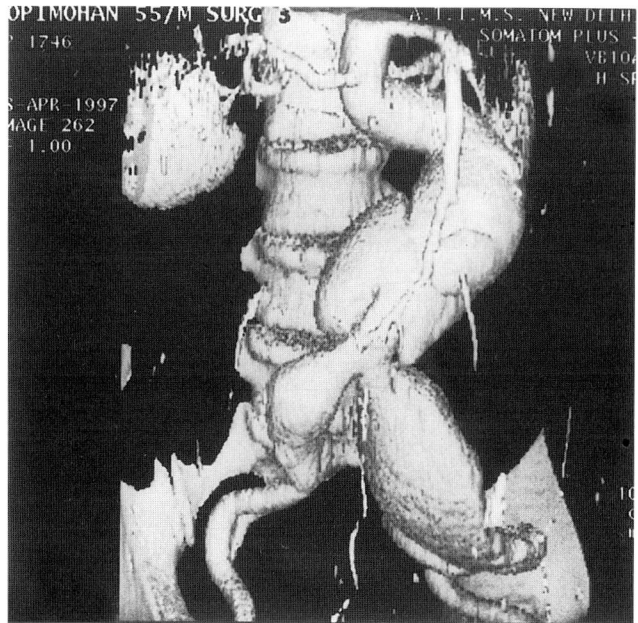

Fig. 13.41: Aortic aneurysm in a 55 years old man. A shaded surface display image obtained by CT angiogram technique showing a large fusiform, tortuous infrarenal aortic aneurysm involving the distal aorta, aortic bifurcation and both common iliac arteries

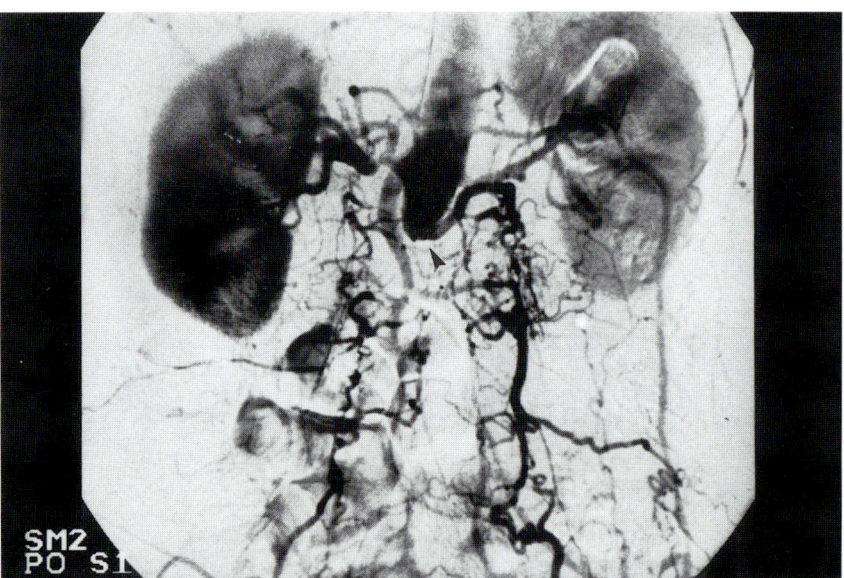

Fig. 13.42: Atherosclerotic disease in a 63 years old diabetic male. Flush aortogram shows complete occlusion of the aorta seen distal to the origin of both renal arteries (arrowhead). Both renal arteries show proximal stenosis. Multiple collaterals are seen in the lower abdomen

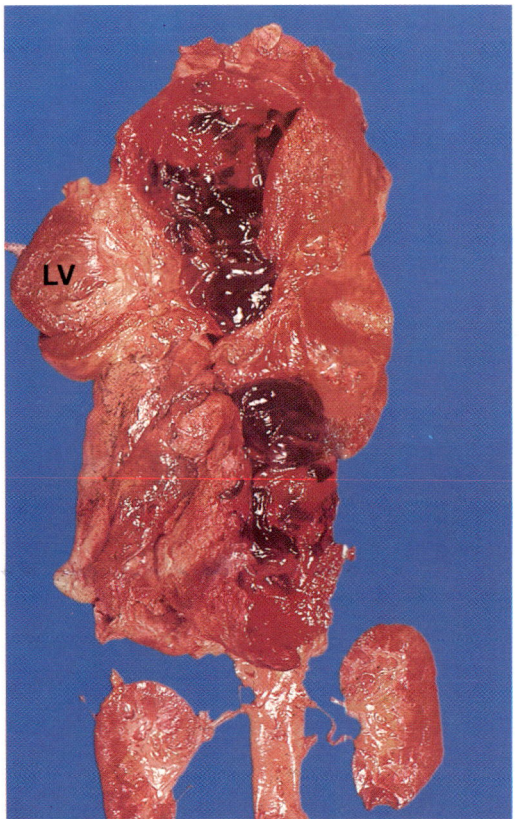

Fig. 13.43a: Atherosclerotic aneurysm of aorta. Extensive aneurysmal dilatation of ascending and descending aorta stopping short at the suprarenal segment of aorta is seen. The aneurysmal sac is filled with a blood clot and an organized thrombus. The aortic valve ring and left ventricle (LV) reveal dilatation

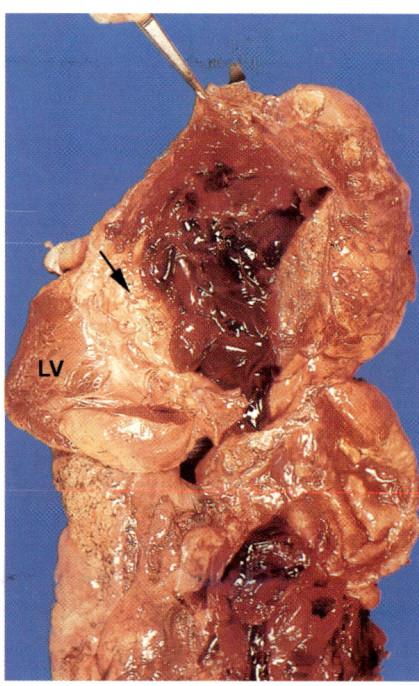

Fig. 13.43b: Aneurysm of aorta. The aneurysmal sac contains blood clot and fresh thrombus. Supravalvular part of ascending aorta shows atherosclerosis (arrow)

Note: A 60 years old male had extensive atherosclerosis involving both the coronary arteries, splenic artery and aorta. Aneurysm of the ascending aorta was eroding anteriorly at the 2nd, 3rd and 4th sternocostal junction while the aneurysm of the descending aorta was detected to be eroding the anterior parts of the 10th, 11th and 12th thoracic and 1st lumbar vertebrae. Left common carotid artery was occluded by an organized and recanalized thrombus

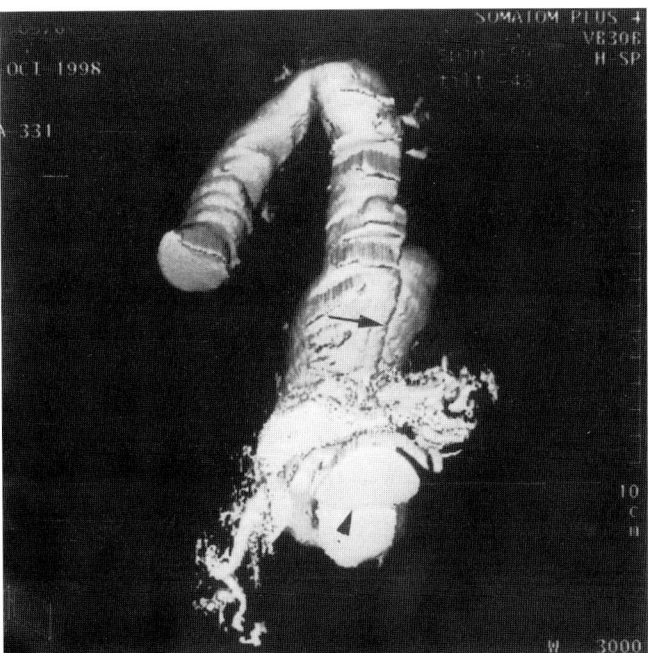

Fig. 13.44: Aortic aneurysm and dissection. A CT angiogram shaded surface display image showing a fusiform dilatation of the distal thoracic aorta with a dissection (arrow). The inferior cut surface shows two lumens and the intimal flap (arrowheads) to good advantage

Dissection hematoma/dissecting aneurysm The word aneurysm for this entity is not correct as truly there is very little dilatation of the aorta and therefore the more appropriate term is dissection hematoma. This is characterized by entry of blood into the wall of the aorta, within the media and its extension along the length of the vessel. It is virtually a parallel column of blood which has dissected the wall (Figs 13.44 to 13.50). A hematoma forms which can undergo organization. This false channel over a period of time becomes endothelialized (Figs 13.49 and 13.50). At times, blood in the parallel channel re-enters the aortic lumen through a second tear in the intima giving rise to a "double-barrelled" aorta. Dissection hematoma occurs commonly in 5th to 6th decades of life and affects men more often than women. A history of hypertension is obtained in a large majority of cases. Dissection hematoma is also well-documented in younger individuals who have abnormality of the connective tissue of aorta. Both localized and generalized forms of the disease can occur.

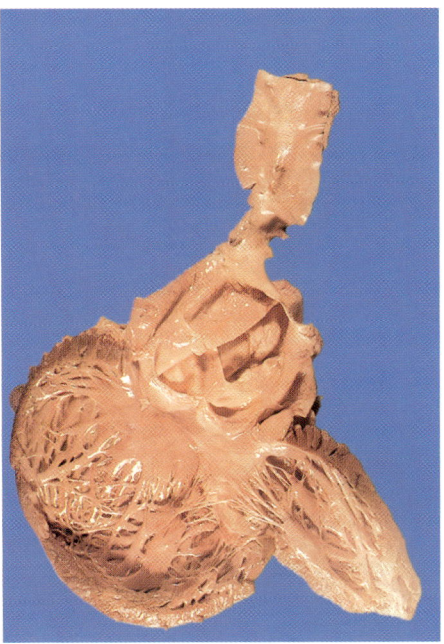

Fig. 13.45a: Aneurysm of aorta. The aorta 2 cm beyond the aortic valve shows a saccular aneurysmal dilatation, measuring 10 cm in diameter. A large intimal tear is present. The intima is seen to be separated from the media. Left ventricle shows marked dilatation and hypertrophy

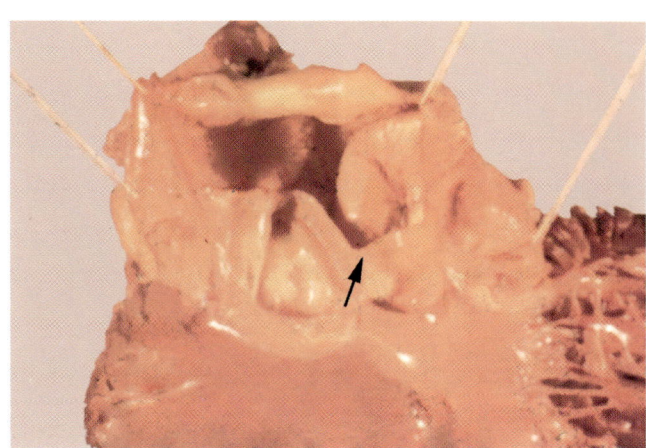

Fig. 13.45b: Aneurysm of aorta. The separated intima stands out as a shelf (arrow). Saccular aneurysmal dilatation of the aorta extends behind the intimal shelf to the aortic valve ring

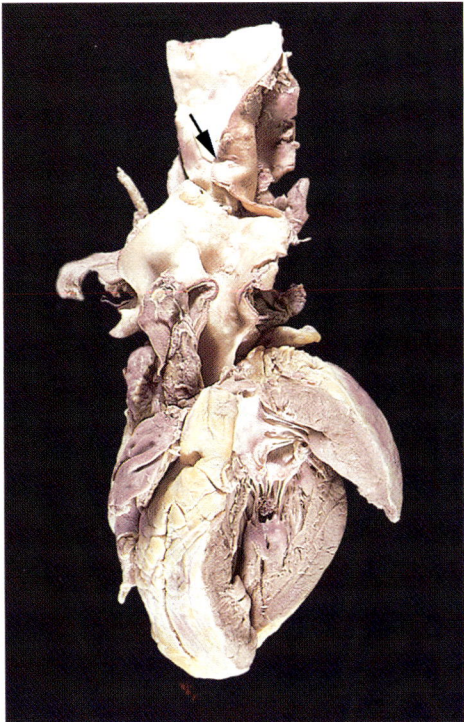

Fig. 13.46a: Dissection hematoma of aorta. The specimen demonstrates split (dissection) of the layers of the aorta (arrow). Left ventricle is hypertrophied

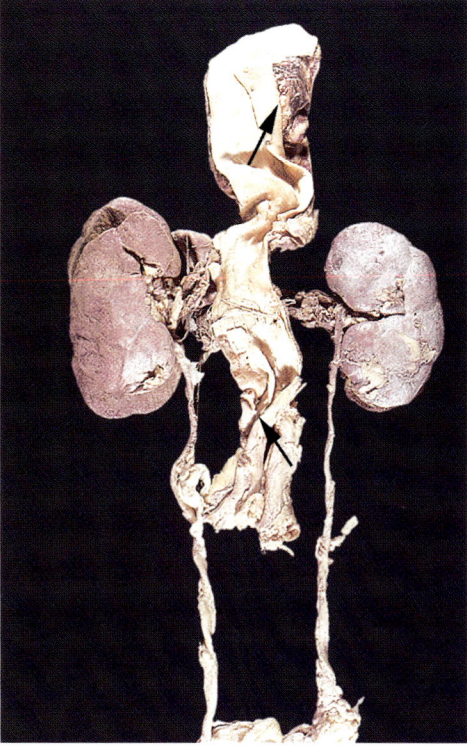

Fig. 13.46b: Dissection hematoma of the abdominal aorta. Split in the wall of the aorta is occupied by a blood clot (arrows)

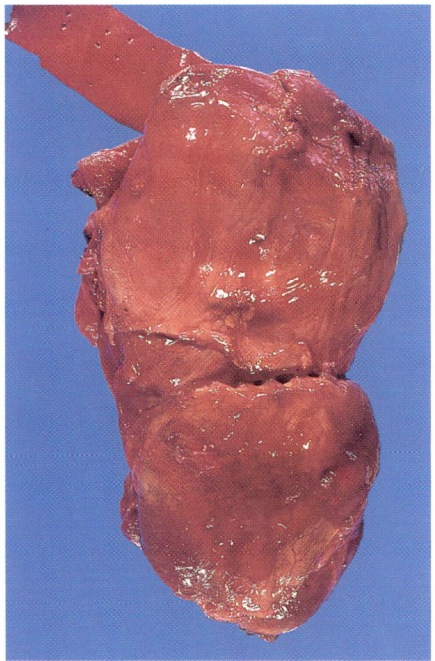

Fig. 13.47a: Aneurysm of ascending aorta which is seen as a globular enlargement. External surface of the heart and part of the normal descending thoracic aorta is also seen in the picture

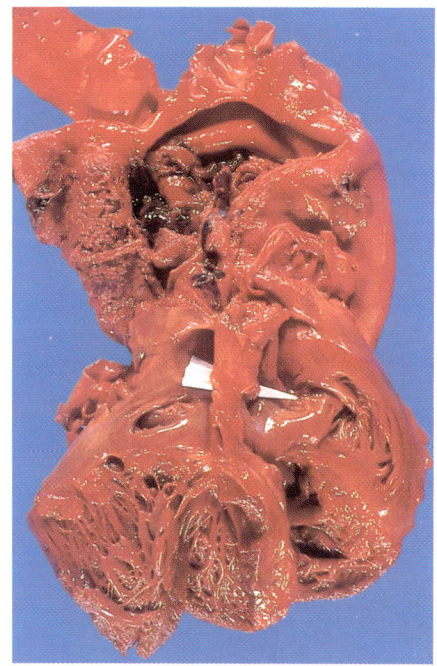

Fig. 13.47b: Opened up aneurysmal sac of the ascending aorta. The sac is filled with extensive fresh hemorrhage. An atrial septal defect (arrow) is also present

Note: Patient was a 21 years old male. Large saccular aneurysm measuring 18 × 15 × 12 cm was present in the ascending and arch of aorta. A transverse intimal tear 4.5 cm in length, 12 cm above the aortic valve was present. Microscopic examination revealed large areas of cystic medial necrosis of the aorta. Fresh and organized thrombi were present within the aneurysmal sac

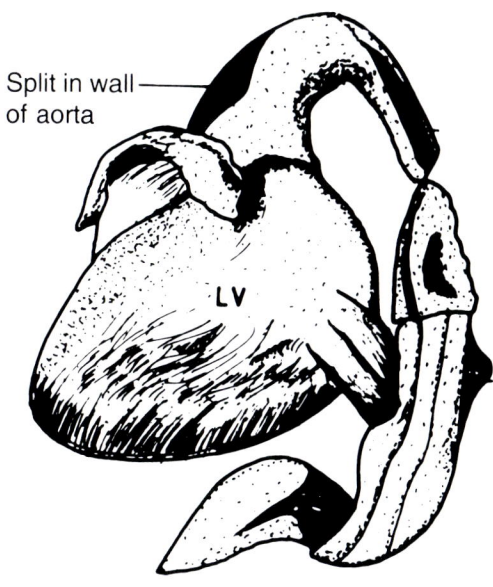

Fig. 13.48a: Diagrammatic representation of dissection hematoma. Split in the wall is seen throughout the length of aorta. LV=Left ventricle

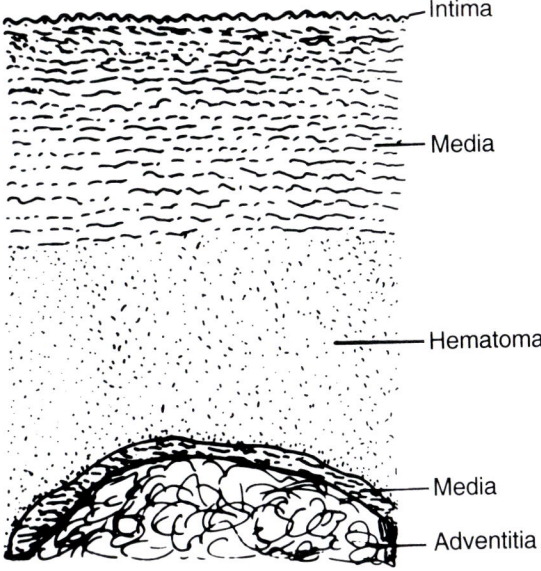

Fig. 13.48b: Diagrammatic representation of dissection hematoma of aorta. Hematoma is shown within the media

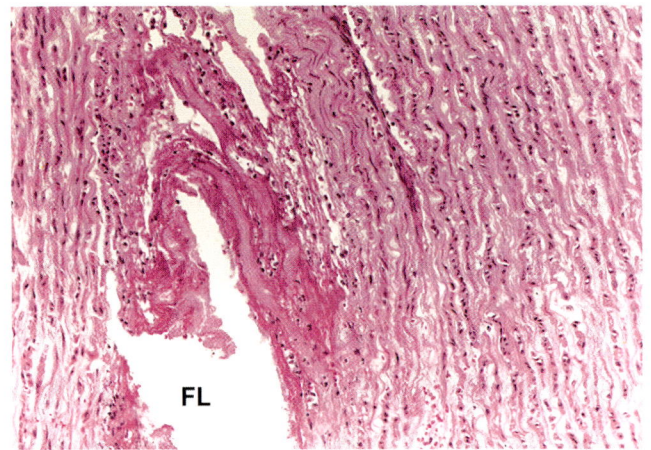

Fig. 13.49: Dissecting hematoma (aneurysm) in early stage. False lumen (FL) is lined by fibrin which merges with the media. No thickened intima is seen

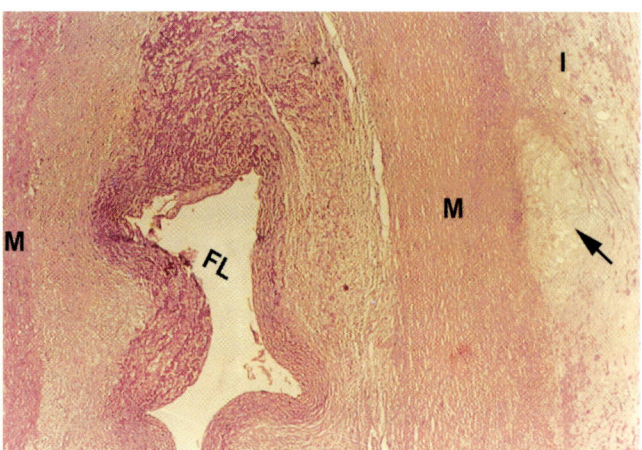

Fig. 13.50a: Dissecting hematoma (aneurysm) showing false lumen (FL) which is lined by dense fibroconnective tissue indicating a dissection of long standing (compare with Figure 13.49). Split media (M) and cholesterol clefts (arrow) in intima (I) are also observed

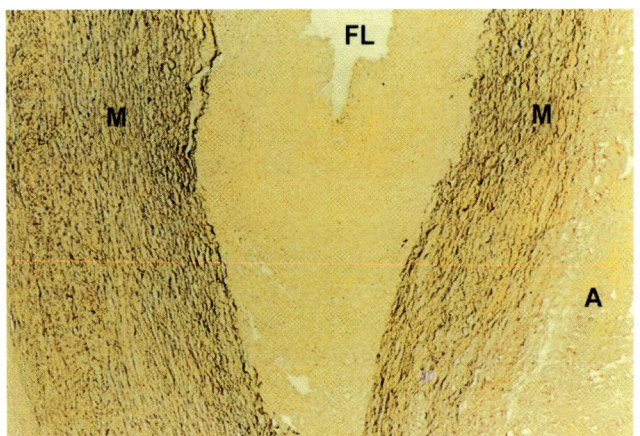

Fig. 13.50b: Chronic dissection of aorta. False lumen (FL) is flanked by fibroconnective tissue split media (M) and adventitia (A) are also included in the picture (VVG)

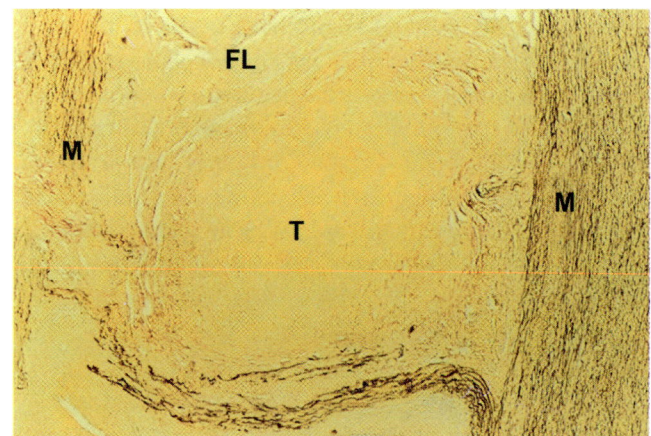

Fig. 13.50c: Chronic dissection. The false lumen shows an organized thrombus (T), FL—False lumen, M—Media

Gross examination of a dissection hematoma of the aorta reveals an intimal tear in the majority of cases. This is generally located in the ascending aorta 1 or 2 cm above the aortic valve ring (Fig. 13.45). The tear is usually horizontal and has irregular margins. This represents the site of entry of blood into the vessel wall. Dissection occurs generally between the layers of the media (Figs 13.48 and 13.46b) and may extend proximally towards the heart and distally into variable lengths of the aorta. At times, dissection may involve the entire length of the aorta including the iliac and femoral arteries. Dissection of the coronary arteries, vessels of the arch of aorta, renal and mesenteric is also described. Microscopically, the media shows disturbed architecture in that the elastic fibers are fragmented and degenerated and enclose pools of metachromatic material which are of variable size (Fig. 13.51). It is likely that disruption of the elastic tissue and presence of myxoid material in the media cause weakening of the vessel wall.

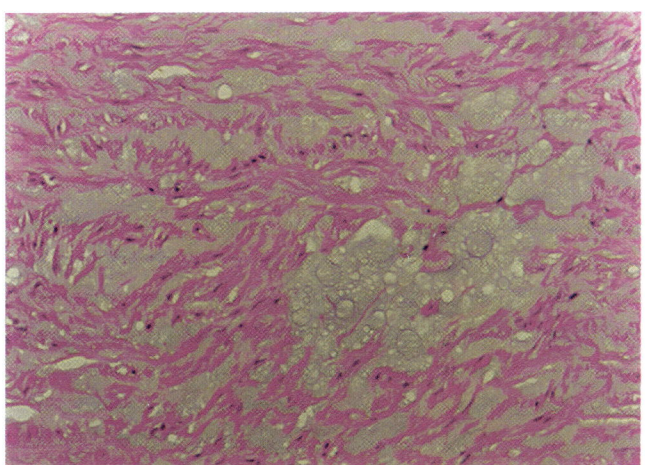

Fig. 13.51a: Section from the excised wall of aorta. It shows disruption of the media with large areas of myxomatous degeneration

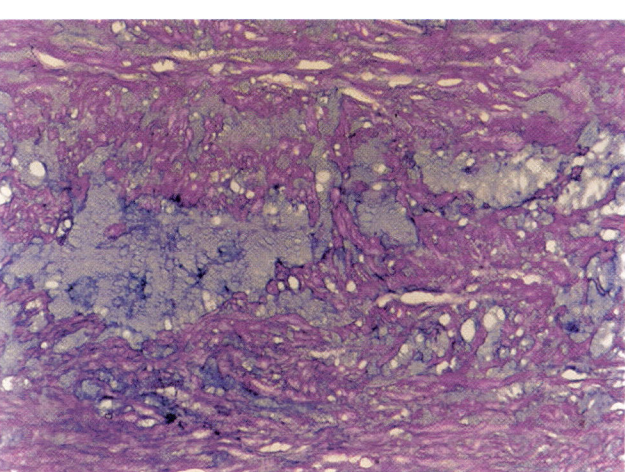

Fig. 13.51b: Alcian blue periodic acid Schiff stain demonstrates large pools of acid mucin which is distorting the medial pattern

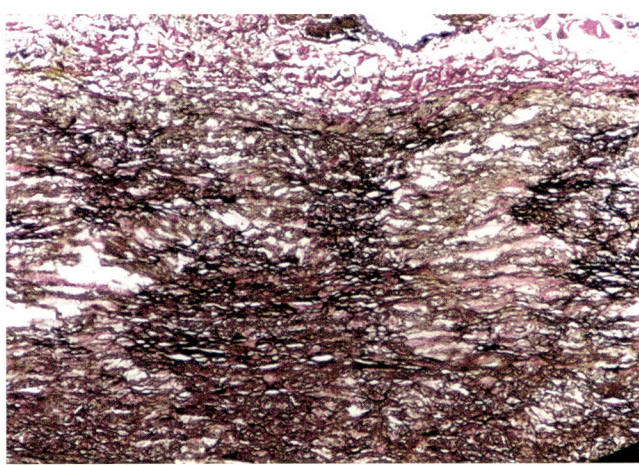

Fig. 13.51c: Verhoeff-van Gieson stain demonstrates disruption of the normal parallel arrays of elastic tissue of the media. Myxomatous degeneration is seen as clear areas of variable shapes and sizes

Note: This patient was a thirty four years female who was diagnosed as a case of aortic ectasia with dilatation of aortic root and annulus. She had features of severe aortic regurgitation. A segment of the aortic wall was excised (Figs 13.51a to c)

Syphilitic aneurysms Cardiovascular system is affected in the tertiary stages of syphilis. Involvement of the ascending and arch of aorta is the favoured site. The lesions include aortitis and aneurysm formation. It must be mentioned that aneurysms consequent to syphilis are uncommon now due to early diagnosis and management of this disease. Grossly the intima is irregular and roughened and has a "tree bark" appearance (destruction and scarring of the media). Microscopically, the striking feature is endarteritis and periarteritis of the vasa vasorum. Perivascular cuffing with lymphocytes, plasma cells and macrophages is observed. Destruction of the elastic tissue, focal necrosis and scarring in the media is seen. These processes lead to weakening of the vessel wall thus predisposing to aneurysm formation.

Aneurysms of cerebral arteries The most common type is the berry aneurysm which arises most commonly from the vessels of circle of Willis either from the arterial branches or at the branching angles of the circle of Willis. It is believed that an inherent weakening of the vessel wall results in an aneurysmal dilatation. These aneurysms assume great significance as they can lead to extensive subarachnoid hemorrhage which is associated with a high mortality.

Mycotic aneurysm Weakening of the vessel wall occurs as a result of infection due to infective organisms (bacteria, fungi etc.) invading the wall. Like in any other type, the aneurysm may rupture and produce hemorrhage (Fig. 13.52).

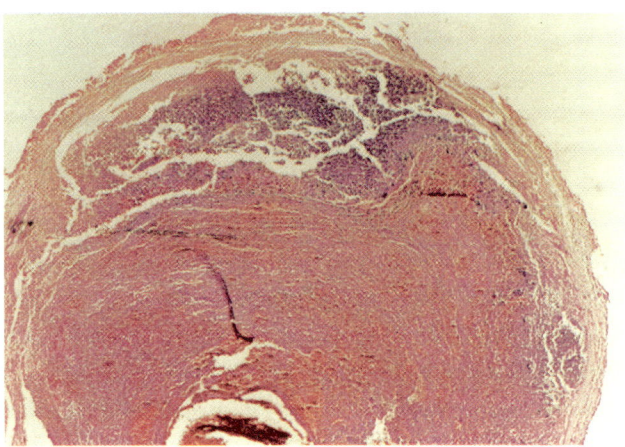

Fig. 13.52a: Photomicrograph from a mycotic aneurysm of the posterior communicating artery of circle of Willis. The artery is occluded by a thrombus. Necrotic material is present in the upper part of picture

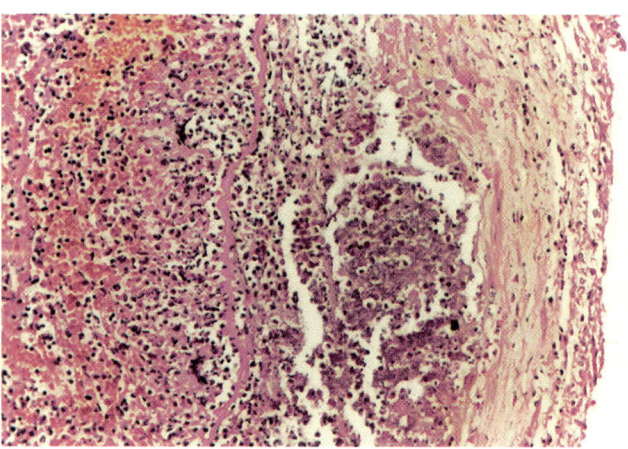

Fig. 13.52b: Higher magnification of the mycotic aneurysm of the posterior communicating artery of the circle of Willis showing destruction of the vessel wall with marked necrosis

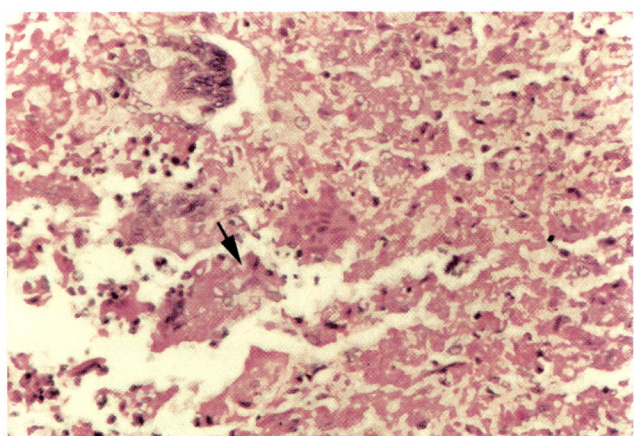

Fig. 13.52c: Mycotic aneurysm. Several multinucleated giant cells are recognized amidst the inflammatory infiltrate. In the cytoplasm of these giant cells fungal hyphae can be seen (arrow)

Diseases of Blood Vessels

Veno-occlusive disease of lung (VOD) is a rare cause of pulmonary hypertension where the involvement is of the pulmonary veins rather than the arteries. It is seen mostly in children and adolescents and may be preceded by a short febrile illness. Clinical features include dyspnea, paroxysmal nocturnal dyspnea with attacks of pulmonary edema. Microscopically, the small and medium sized pulmonary vein radicles show either eccentric or concentric intimal thickening due to fibroconnective tissue proliferation. Recanalization is frequently seen (Fig. 13.53). The pulmonary arteries are essentially unremarkable.

The exact etiology of pulmonary VOD is not known. The suggested possibilities include association with autoimmune disease (association with chronic active hepatitis, celiac disease, systemic lupus erythematosus is described in some cases) genetic predisposition, secondary to chemotherapy/radiotherapy, systemic sclerosis, renal and bone marrow transplants, oral contraceptives, consumption of herbal bush tea containing senacio, crotolaria and heliotropum species, etc.

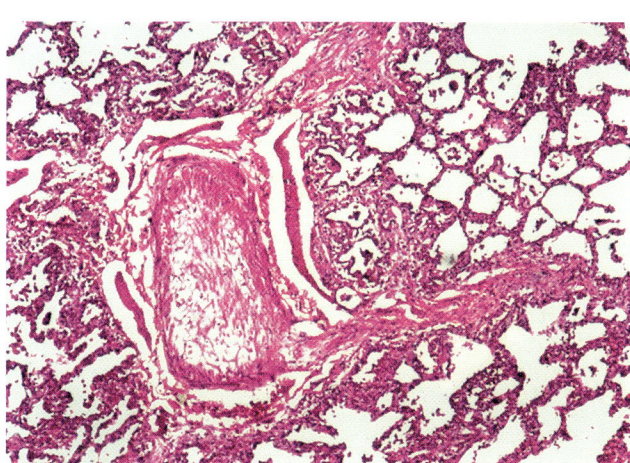

Fig. 13.53a: Veno-occlusive disease of lung. Vein in the interlobular septum of lung shows obliteration of the lumen by loose fibroconnective tissue (organized thrombus)

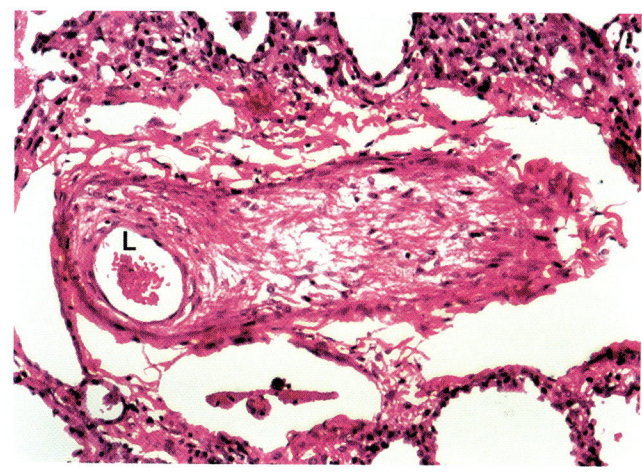

Fig. 13.53b: Veno-occlusive disease of lung. Pulmonary vein is markedly narrowed. Lumen (L) is much reduced in size due to cellular fibroconnective tissue

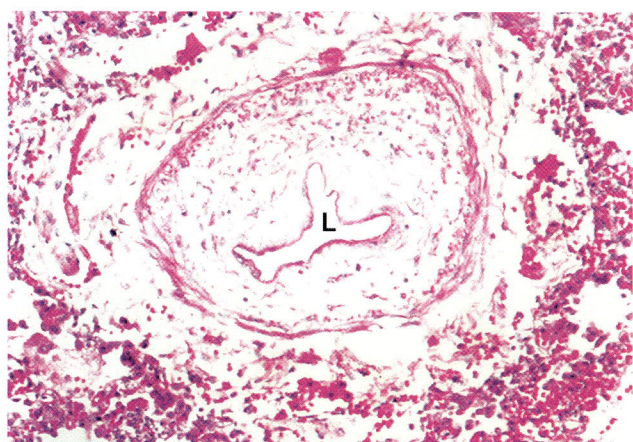

Fig. 13.53c: Veno-occlusive disease of lung. Intima of pulmonary vein is severely thickened by loose fibroconnective tissue. The lumen is markedly narrowed (L)

Note: A seven years old male child presented with breathlessness since 5 months and paroxysmal dyspnea for 3 months. On examination the JVP was raised, liver was palpable 2 cm. Cardiovascular examination revealed a parasternal heave, loud P2 with a narrow split and a pansystolic murmur. Chest X-ray had features of pulmonary hypertension. Echocardiography showed features of severe right ventricular hypertrophy and dilatation with tricuspid insufficiency. The patient went into cardiac arrest and died. At autopsy, the heart weighed 215 gm and showed hypertrophy of both ventricles, with dilatation of right atrium and ventricle. The lungs were firm and subcrepitant

Pulmonary hypertension occurs in patients with congenital cardiac shunts, primary pulmonary hypertension and in left ventricular failure from any cause. Depending upon the type of morphologic changes in the pulmonary arteries, hypertensive changes have been graded (Grades 1-6) (Figs 13.54a to e). Grade 1-medial hypertrophy with muscularization of arterioles; Grade 2-cellular intimal proliferation; Grade 3-intimal fibrosis; Grade 4-plexiform lesions together with dilatation and thinning of pulmonary arteries; Grade 5-rupture of dilatation lesions with parenchymal hemorrhage and hemosiderosis; Grade 6-necrotizing arteritis.

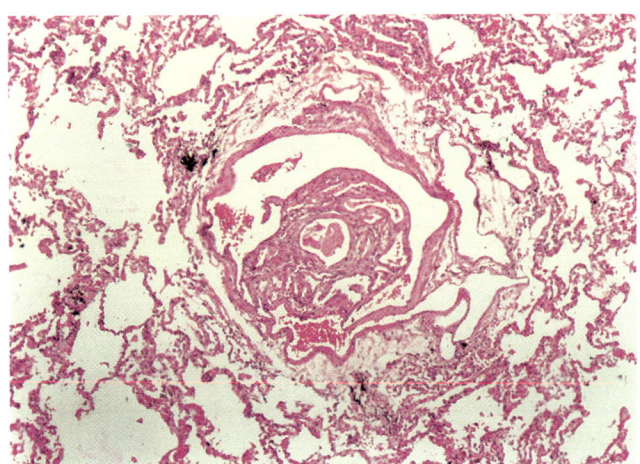

Fig. 13.54a: Pulmonary artery hypertension. The artery shows multiple vascular channels (plexiform lesion). The pulmonary artery is dilated and the wall is thinned out

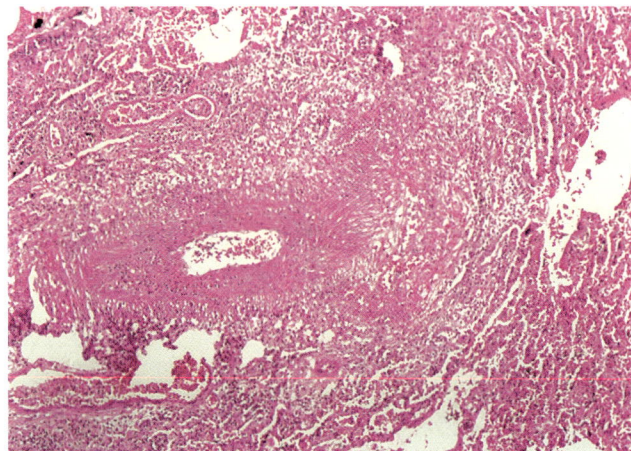

Fig. 13.54b: Pulmonary artery hypertension Grade V. The artery shows necrotizing vasculitis with inflammation of the vessel wall and surrounding area

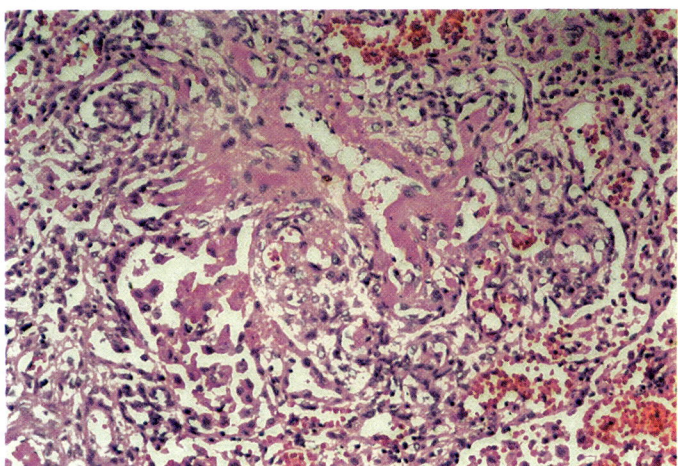

Fig. 13.54c: Pulmonary artery hypertension. Dilatation lesions are observed. In addition the vessel wall shows fibrinoid necrosis

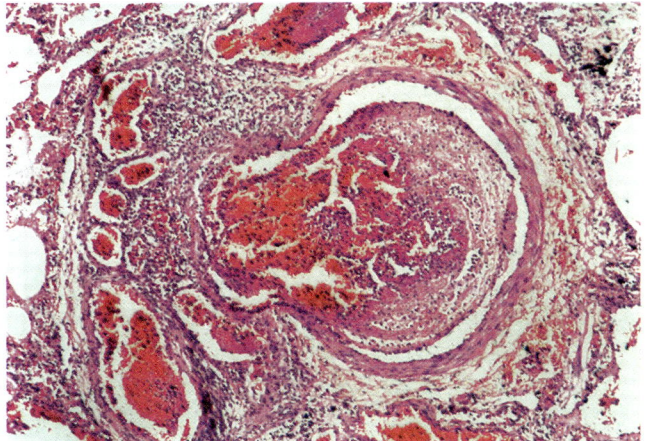

Fig. 13.54d: Pulmonary artery hypertension. Branch of pulmonary artery shows destruction of the vessel wall along with necrotizing vasculitis. Marked inflammation is seen in the perivascular area. The lumen shows a fresh thrombus and hemorrhage. Dilatation lesions are seen in the adjacent zone

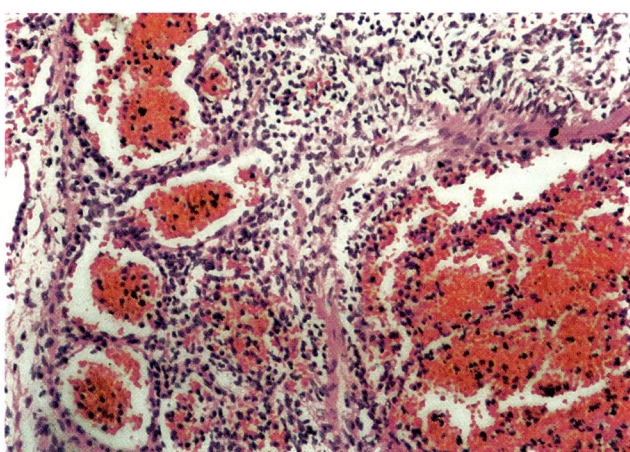

Fig. 13.54e: Pulmonary artery hypertension. Vessel wall shows necrotizing vasculitis. Dilatation lesions are observed in the adjacent area

TUMORS OF BLOOD VESSELS

Tumors of blood vessels may be benign, malignant and of intermediate grade of malignancy.

Hemangioma is the most common tumor of the blood vessels. In fact it has variably been designated as a hamartoma. They usually occur in childhood and in many cases are present at birth. Hemangiomas are generally solitary but they may present as multiple lesions (angiomatosis). Depending upon the histology and the location several types of hemangioma are described.

Capillary hemangioma As the name suggests this type is composed of small sized vascular channels. It may be located in any area/organ but the common sites include skin, subcutaneous tissue, mucous membrane of lip and mouth and internal viscera. Microscopically, numerous capillary spaces are seen amidst spindle shaped stroma. The capillaries appear to emerge from the spindle cells. Some of them contain few red blood cells (Fig. 13.55).

Cavernous hemangioma This lesion consists of large cystically dilated vascular channels filled with blood. Cavernous hemangiomas may occur in the skin (port-wine nevus or nevus flammeus), mucosal surfaces and internal viscera. They may undergo thrombosis, ulceration, infection and intracystic hemorrhages.

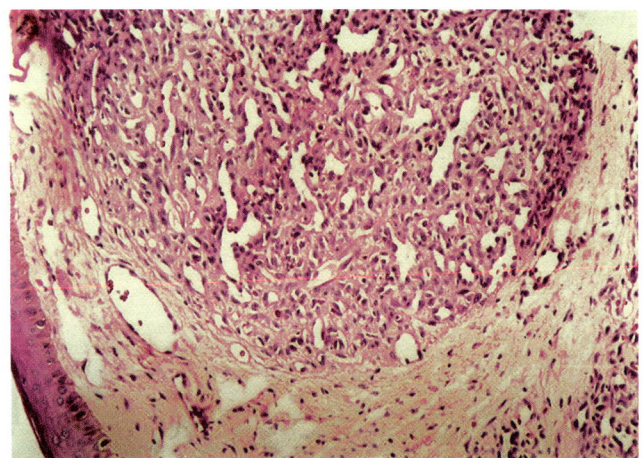

Fig. 13.55a: Capillary hemangioma. Numerous vascular slits are seen amidst spindle shaped cells. The capillaries seem to emerge from the mesenchymal tissue

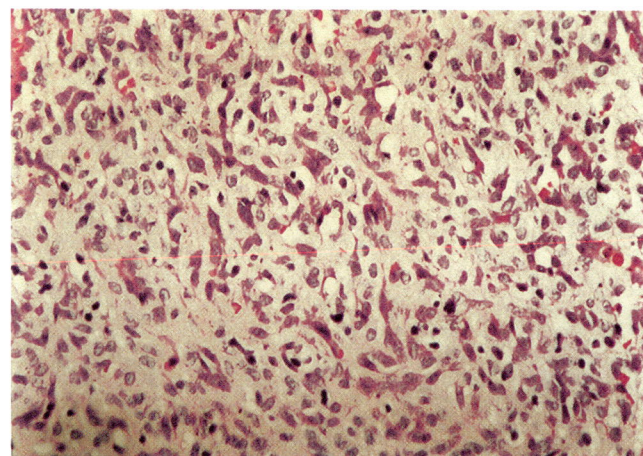

Fig. 13.55b: Capillary hemangioma. Spindle shaped to ovoid mesenchymal cells are seen. These appear as solid capillary buds. Capillary differentiation is also observed

Skeletal muscle hemangioma is a common form of hemangioma of deep soft tissues. These may be capillary, cavernous or mixed type. Capillary hemangioma type, however, is the most common (Fig. 13.56).

Large vessel hemangiomas may arise from the veins (venous hemangioma) or from both veins and arteries designated as arteriovenous hemangioma or malformation, racemose or circoid hemangiomas.

Multiple hemangiomatous syndromes Hemangiomas may occur in two or more tissues. Several syndrome complexes have been recognized. Occurrence of hemangiomas within the cerebellum and retina is termed as **von Hippel-Lindau syndrome**. Vascular hamartomas in the brain and skin characterize the **Sturge-Weber syndrome**. **Maffucci's syndrome** is a rare mesodermal dysplasia featured by multiple hemangiomas and enchondromas.

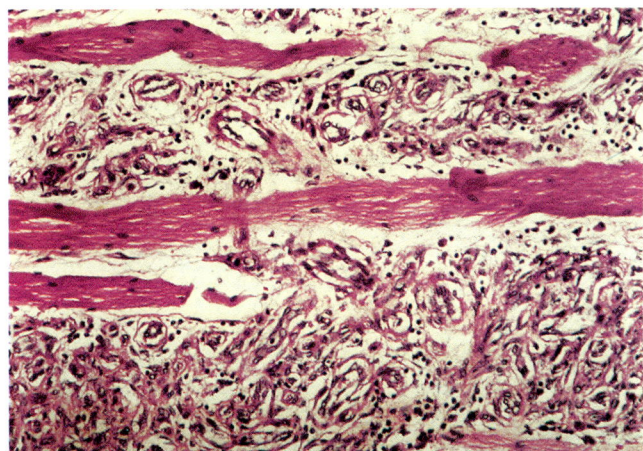

Fig. 13.56: Intramuscular capillary hemangioma. Numerous capillaries, some lined by plump endothelial cells are seen in between the skeletal muscle fibers

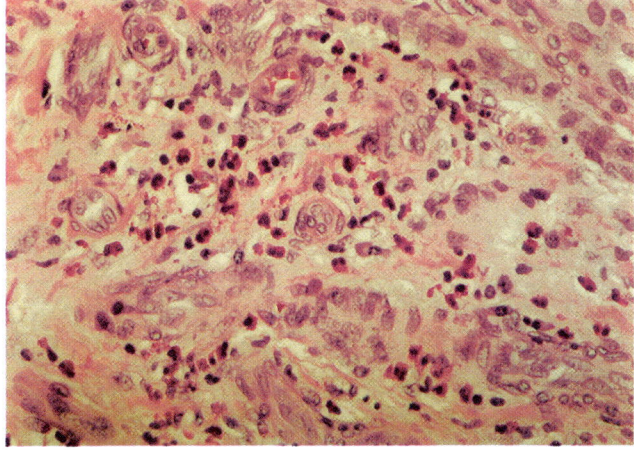

Fig. 13.57: Epithelioid hemangioma (Angiolymphoid hyperplasia). Numerous capillaries lined with plump endothelial cells are observed. The intervening stroma shows striking number of eosinophils

Epithelioid hemangioma is the term used synonymously with angiolymphoid hyperplasia with eosinophilia. Numerous blood vessels lined with plump and vacuolated endothelial cells lie in a fibrous stroma. Latter is rich in eosinophils and lymphoid cells which are often in aggregates (Fig. 13.57). These lesions present most commonly as a lump in the head and neck region.

Glomus tumor (Glomangioma) This is a benign neoplasm of the glomus body (neuromyoarterial receptors which are sensitive to temperature and regulate arterial flow). It occurs in the skin, most frequently in the distal region of the fingers and toes, typically in the subungual location. They are extremely painful. Microscopically, nests of round to polyhedral, monomorphic glomus cells are organized around blood vessels. Variants of glomus tumor include conventional solid type glomangioma, where glomus cells lie in the wall of cavernous vascular channels and glomangiomyoma in which glomus cells terminate as elongated mature smooth muscle cells (Fig. 13.58).

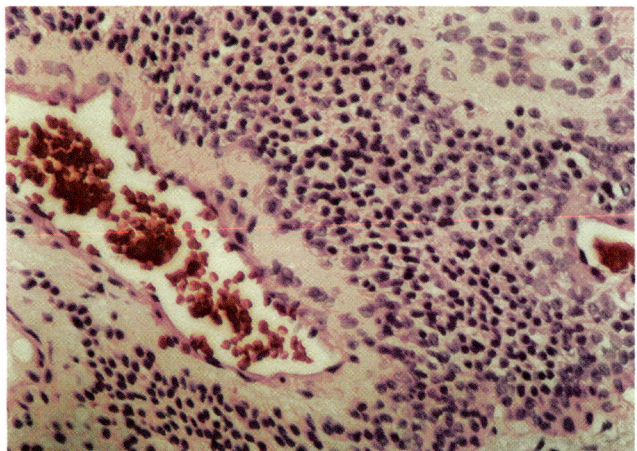

Fig. 13.58a: Glomus tumor. Tumor cells are uniform, round to polyhedral and located in the perivascular area

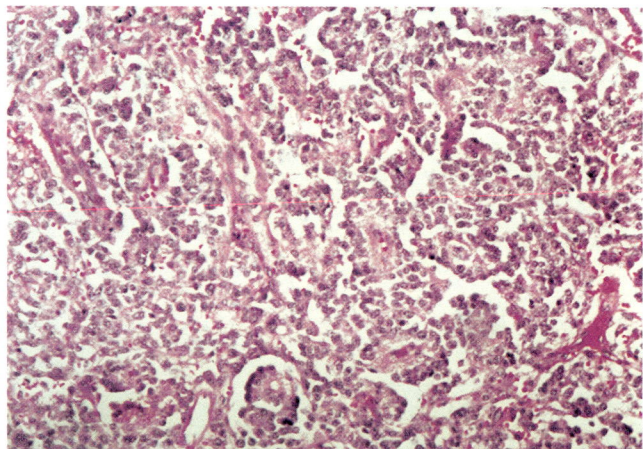

Fig. 13.58b: Glomus tympanicus. Numerous thin walled vascular channels are seen in the wall of which groups of round to polyhedral cells are present

Hemangioendothelioma is a vascular neoplasm of intermediate grade of malignancy. It occurs in skin, soft tissues and internal viscera including lung, liver, bone, pleura, peritoneum, and lymph nodes. It is composed of plump round to ovoid endothelial cells arranged in small groups or small strands. Intracellular lumina are seen as vacuoles or clear spaces within cytoplasm of the endothelial cells. Some of these lumina may contain red blood cells. The stroma shows myxoid and/or hyaline changes. The lesion may be easily confused with adenocarcinoma but markers for endothelial cells—Factor VIII related antigen and Ulex europeans agglutinin help to resolve the issue.

Four different morphologic varieties of hemangioendothelioma have been recognized namely epithelioid hemangioendothelioma, spindle cell hemangioendothelioma, Kaposiform hemangioendothelioma and Dabska tumor (malignant endovascular papillary angioendothelioma).

Angiosarcoma This is a malignant tumor arising from the endothelial cells. Common locations include skin, soft tissues, breast, bone and liver. Microscopically, marked variation in the morphology is observed. This ranges from well differentiated vascular channels which simulate a hemangioma with no pleomorphism or mitosis to highly undifferentiated tumors which show marked pleomorphism, high mitotic activity and areas of necrosis (Figs 13.59a and b). Vascular origin is recognized by vascular channels lined by atypical endothelial cells. In some cases tumor cells are spindle shaped and on close scrutiny formation of vascular channels may be seen. Demonstration of endothelial cells by immunohistochemical stains and/or electronmicroscopy aid in the diagnosis.

Angiosarcoma of the liver deserves a special mention as it is associated with some environmental carcinogens, namely arsenic and vinyl chloride. Angiosarcoma of the liver has also been documented in cases who were administered thorotrast (thorium dioxide) several years earlier. These tumors are highly malignant and aggressive.

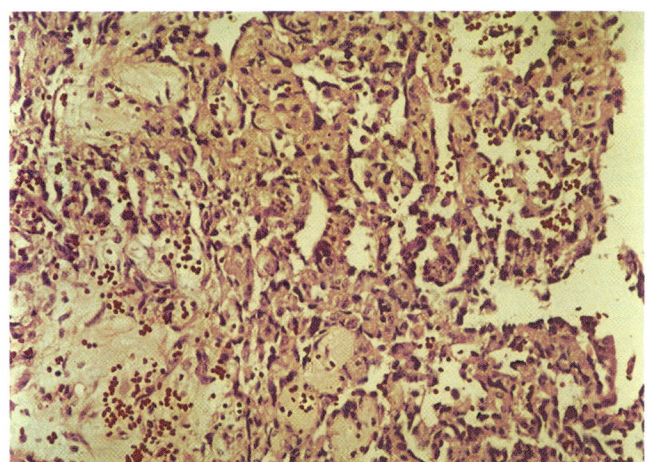

Fig. 13.59a: Angiosarcoma breast. The tumor comprises of anastomosing vascular spaces which are lined by flattened to ovoid cells that show mild pleomorphism. Red blood cells are also present in the lumen

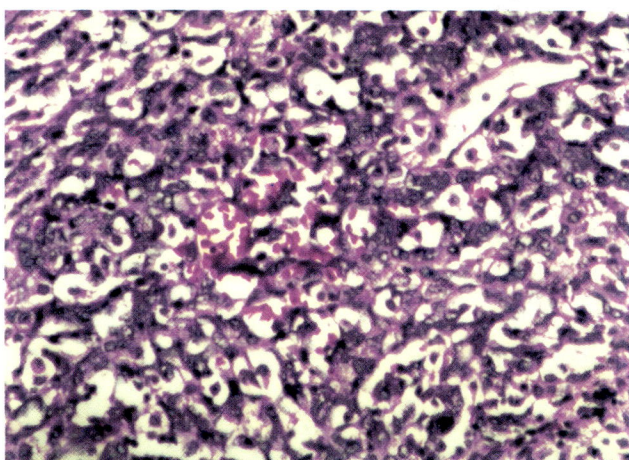

Fig. 13.59b: Angiosarcoma. Tumor cells are round to ovoid and are present in sheets. The cells show pleomorphism and mitotic activity. Vascular differentiation is seen. Red blood cells are present within some vascular spaces

Hemangiopericytoma This is a rare malignant neoplasm of pericytes which are cells that surround the blood vessels. Microscopically groups of polyhedral to spindle shaped cells are seen around slit like vascular channels (Figs 13.60a and b). Ultrastructurally tumor cells have features of both smooth muscle cells and endothelial cells.

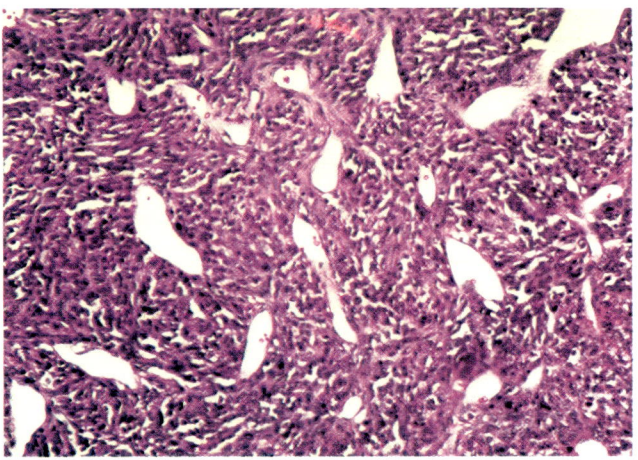

Fig. 13.60a: Hemangiopericytoma. Round to ovoid tumor cells are arranged perivascularly in compact sheets

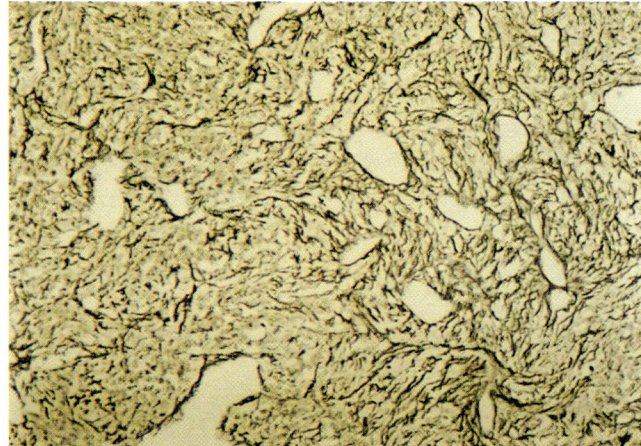

Fig. 13.60b: Hemangiopericytoma. Reticulin stain highlights the blood vessels and the perivascular rich reticulin pattern of the tumor cells

Kaposi sarcoma Is a multicentric, malignant tumor of the endothelial cells affecting the skin and/or internal viscera. It was recognized to occur in a sporadic form in elderly individuals in the 19th century. However, Kaposi sarcoma is present almost in an epidemic form in association with acquired-immune deficiency syndrome (AIDS). The latter is generally a multifocal lesion and is possibly due to low immunity. Microscopically, Kaposi sarcoma is characterized by spindle shaped cells arranged in fascicles within which vascular spaces can be recognized. Latter is often filled with red blood cells. Extravasation of red blood cells and hemosiderin pigment is often encountered. Inflammatory cells may also be seen in the interstitium. In some cases hyaline globules are present both within the tumor cells and extracellularly (Fig. 13.61). Herpesvirus (HHV8) appears to be involved in the genesis of Kaposi sarcoma. This virus has been demonstrated within the tumor cells.

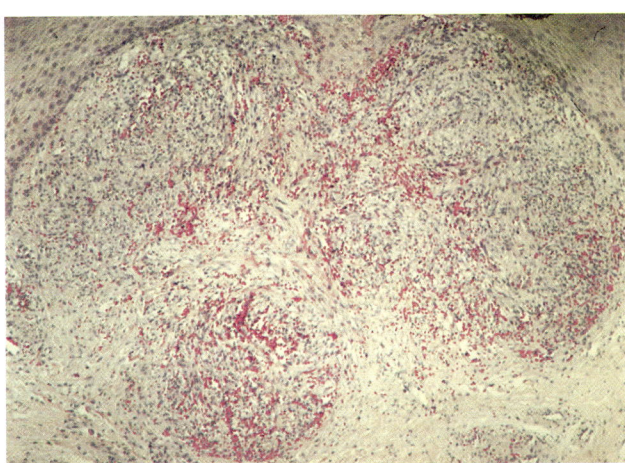

Fig. 13.61a: Kaposi sarcoma. A cellular tumor composed of spindle shaped cells arranged in bundles is seen. Prominent extravasation of red blood cells is observed. Portion of epidermis is seen in the upper part of picture

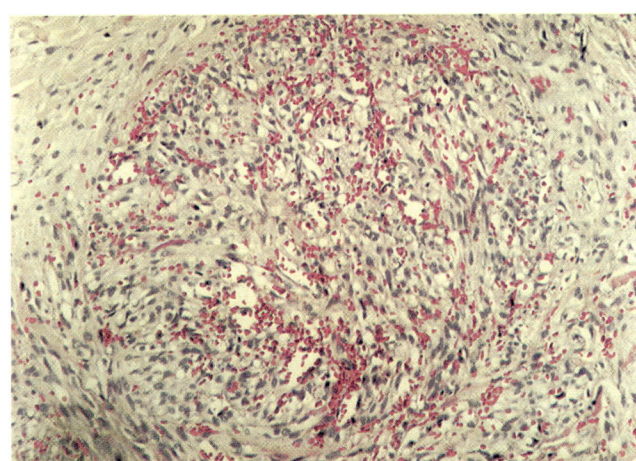

Fig. 13.61b: Kaposi sarcoma. The tumor cells are spindle shaped and seen as whorls. Numerous capillary slits and prominent extravasation of red blood cells are seen amidst the tumor

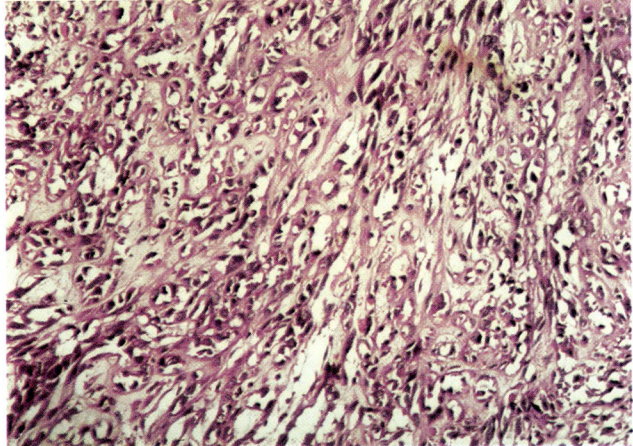

Fig. 13.61c: Kaposi sarcoma. Tumor cells are arranged in flowing bundles. Several capillary slits some of which contain red blood cells in their lumina are seen interspersed

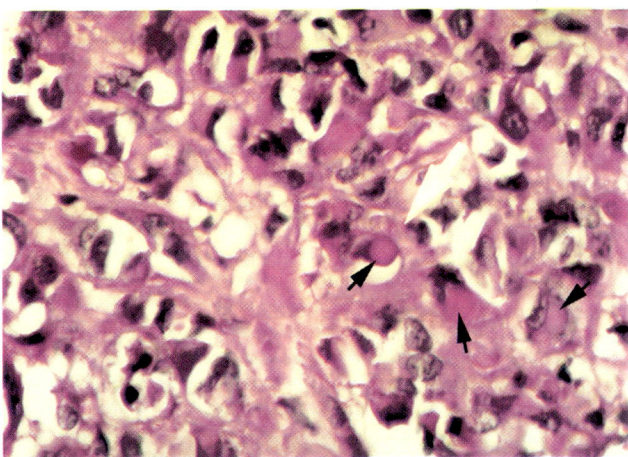

Fig. 13.61d: Kaposi sarcoma. Higher magnification to show hyaline bodies (arrows) amidst the tumor cells. Round to ovoid tumor cells some of which show vacuolation of the cytoplasm, are seen

Tumors of the Lymphatic System

Lymphangioma are common lesions found in the skin of face, lips, chest, extremities, etc. Microscopically, they are composed of small thin walled spaces that are lined by flattened cells and contain homogenous light pink fluid-lymph. At times, lymphangiomas acquire a large size. This type commonly affects the neck and axilla and occasionally the retroperitoneum and mediastinum. Microscopically they consist of large, cavernous/cystic spaces filled with lymph. Lymphocytes are a common accompaniment.

Lymphangiosarcoma is a rare malignant tumor derived from the lymphatics. This develops in patients following radical mastectomy. Histological features are identical to angiosarcoma.

SUGGESTED READINGS

1. Bahl VK, Sengupta PP, Satpathy G, Sharma G *et al*: *Ind Heart J* **54**: 46-49, 2002.
2. Bajema IM, Hagen EC: Evolving concepts about the role of antineutrophil cytoplasm autoantibodies in systemic vasculitides. *Curr Opin Rheumatol* **11(1)**: 34-40, 1999.
3. Chopra P, Datta RK, Das Gupta A, Bhargava S: Nonspecific aortoarteritis: An immunologic study of 50 cases. *Ind J Med Res* **76**: 436-43, 1982.
4. Chopra P, Datta RK, Das Gupta A, Bhargava S: Nonspecific aortoarteritis (Takayasu's disease): An immunologic and autopsy study. *Jap Heart J* **244**: 549-56, 1983.
5. Chopra P, Nayak NC: Aortoarteritis and cardiomyopathy a heretofore undescribed association. *Jap Heart J* **19(3)**: 358-65, 1978.
6. Chugh KS, Sakhuja V, Malik N *et al*: Nonspecific aortoarteritis is a major cause of renovascular hypertension in Asian countries. *Proc Asian Pacific Congr Nephrol*, Beijing, 450-56, 1990.
7. Cid MC, Font C, Coll Vinent B, Grau JM: Large vessel vasculitides. *Curr Opin Rheumatol* **10(1)**: 18-28, 1998.
8. Harper L, Savage Co: Pathologenesis of ANCA-Associated systemic vasculitis. *J Pathol* **190(3)**: 349-59, 2000.
9. Kallenberg CC, Heeringa P: Pathogenesis of vasculitis. *Lupus* **7(4)**: 280-84, 1998.
10. Mukherjee A, Girdhar BK, Desikan KV, Leprous Phlebitis: *Int J Lepr* **48**: 48-50, 1980.
11. Mukherjee A, Girdhar BK, Malaviya GN, Ramu GM, Desikan KV: Involvement of subcutaneous vein in lepromatous leprosy. *Int J Lep* **51**: 1-16, 1983.
12. Neff AG, Greifenstein EM: Giant cell arteritis update. *Semin Ophthalmol* **14(2)**: 109-12, 1999.
13. Nowack R, Flores Suarez LF, van der Woude FJ: New developments in pathogenesis of systemic vasculitis. *Curr Opin Rheumatol* **10(1)**: 3-11, 1998.
14. Rizzi R, Bruno S, Stellaci C, Dammacco R: Takayasu's arteritis: A cell-mediated large-vessel vasculitis. *Int J Clin Lab Res* **29(1)**: 8-13, 1999.
15. Rowley AH, Shulman ST: Kawasaki syndrome. *Pediatr Clin North Am* **46(2)**: 313-29, 1999.
16. Sandhyamani S: Monkey model for mucoid vasculopathy. *Int Angiol* **11**: 256-60, 1992.
17. Sandhyamani S: Mucoid vasculopathy: Vascular lesions in an autopsy study. *Mod Pathol* **6**: 333-41, 1993.
18. Savige J, Gillis D, Benson E, Davies D, Esnault V, Falk RJ *et al*: International Consensus Statement of Testing and Reporting of Antineutrophil cytoplasmic antibodies (ANCA). *Am J Clin Pathol* **111**: 507-13, 1999.
19. Seko Y: Takayasu arteritis: Insights into immunopathology. *Jpn Heart J* **41(1)**: 15-26, 2000.
20. Seko Y, Minota S, Kawasaki A, Shinkai Y *et al*: Perforin secreting killer cell infiltration and expression of a 65-KD heart shock protein in aortic tissue of patients with Takayasu's arteritis. *J Clin Invest* **93**: 750-58, 1994.
21. Sharma S, Rajani M, Talwar KK: Angiographic morphology in nonspecific aortoarteritis (Takayasu's arteritis): A study of 126 patients from North India. *Cardiovasc Intervent Radiol* **15**: 160-65, 1992.
22. Sheller MC, Fauci AS: Pathogenesis of vasculitis syndromes. *Med Clin North Am* **81(1)**: 221-42, 1997.
23. Singh GK: Kawasaki disease: An update. *Indian J Pediatr* **65(2)**: 231-41, 1998.
24. Singhal V, Jain SL, Chopra P: Non-specific aortoarteritis (Takayasu's arteriopathy): An autopsy analysis. *Ind J Med Res* **68**: 322-34, 1978.
25. Vasculitis. Seminars in diagnostic pathology. 18/1 February 2001 Santa Cruz DJ (Ed): Weidner N (Guest Ed): WB Saunders Company.
26. Weiss W Sharon, Goldblum A John, Enzinger & Weiss's Soft Tissue Tumors 4th edition, Chapters 23 to 25.
27. Woolfenden AR, Tong DC, Marks MP, Aali AO, Albers GW: Angiographically delined primary angiitis of the CNS: is it really benign? *Neurology* **51(1)**: 183-88, 1998.

INDEX

A

Acute coronary syndromes 73
Acute myocardial infarction 74
    complications 85, 86
    diagnosis 84
    microscopic changes 77
    morphologic alterations 77
    pathology 74
    serum markers for diagnosis 84
Acute rheumatic fever 28
Allergic granulomatous angiitis 219
Amyloidosis 101, 131
Aneurysm
    atherosclerotic 227
    cerebral arteries 234
    hematoma/dissecting 229
    mycotic 234
    syphilitic 234
Aneurysm formation 86, 87
Aneurysm of aorta 228, 230
Aneurysmal dilatation 62
Angiitis of central nervous system
    etiology 222
Angiosarcoma 241
Angiosarcoma heart 196
Anisonucleosis 120, 121
Ankylosing spondylitis 51
Annulus 43
Anthracycline cardiotoxicity 106
Anthracycline derivatives 124
Antischkow and Aschoff cells 33
Aortic aneurysm 227
Aortic angiography 19
Aortic stenosis 21
Aortic valve 6
Aortic valve disease 50
Aortic valve incompetence/
        regurgitation 51
Aortic valve stenosis 50
Aortoarteritis 201, 202, 207
Arrhythmogenic right ventricular
    dysplasia
        gross examination 136
        pathogenesis 136
Aschoff body/nodule 35
Aschoff cells 37
Aschoff nodules 36
Aspergillosis 70

Atheromatous plaque 74, 81, 82
Atherosclerosis 51, 81
Atherosclerotic disease 228
Atrial fibrillation 47
Atrial septal defect
    management 14
Atrialis 8
Atrioventricular septal defect
    clinical evaluation 18
Atrioventricular valves 43
Autografts 55

B

Bacteremia 57
Bacterial endocarditis 64
Bacterial infection 117
Balanced pattern 8
Bioprostheses 55
Blood cysts 194
Blood vessel
    aneurysm 227
    tuberculosis 226
    tumors 238
Breadloaf technique 2
Bronze diabetes 134
Buerger disease 223
    etiology 224

C

Calcific deposits 50
Capillary hemangioma 238
Cardiac allograft rejection 145, 146
Cardiac amyloidosis 101, 131
Cardiac arrhythmia 85
Cardiac catheterization 24
Cardiac failure 67
Cardiac fibroma 192
Cardiac myocytes 9
Cardiac myxoma 175
    clinical presentation 190
    familial 190
    histogenesis 190
    sporadic 190
    ultrastructure 183
Cardiac tamponade 86
Cardiac transplant rejection 92

Cardiac transplantation 140
    complications 142
        acute cellular rejection 144
        graft rejection 142
        humoral rejection 147
        hyperacute rejection 147
        infections 147
    contraindications 140
    indications 140, 141
    non-rejection pathology 149
        ischemic injury 150
        previous biopsy site 153
        quilty effect 152
Cardiac troponins 85
Cardiac tumors 175
Cardiomyopathy 100, 119
    alcoholic 123
    associated with neuromuscular
        disease 124
    dilated 119
        etiology 123
    drug induced 124
    hypertrophic 135
        etiology 136
    idiopathic restrictive 131
    peripartum 124
    restrictive 124
Cardiovascular disorder 64
Cardiovascular teratogens 12
Central nervous system 41
Chaga's disease 117
Chiari's network 2
Cholestrol clefts 81
Chordae tendinea 43
Chromosomal abnormalities 11
Chronic pulmonary venous congestion
    44
Churg-Strauss syndrome 219
Chylous 162
Circle of Willis 234
Coagulative necrosis 77
Coarctation of aorta 21
Colliquative necrosis 80
Commissural fusion 45
Commissures 43
Conduction system 7
Congenital bicuspid 50

Congenital heart diseases 11
    classification
        acyanotic 13
        cyanotic 13
    etiology 11
        cardiovascular teratogens 12
        chromosomal abnormalities 11
        genetic-environmental interaction 11
        single mutant gene abnormalities 11
        fetal circulation and changes at birth 12, 13
Congestive heart failure 41
Constrictive pericarditis 159
Contraction band necrosis 80
Conventional atherosclerosis 148
Cor bovinum 52
Coronary artery ciculation 7
Coronary cusp 63
Coronary heart disease 73, 80
Coronary thrombosis 81
Creatinine phosphokinase 85
Crista supraventricularis 4
Crista terminalis 2
Cutaneous leukocytoclastic vasculitis 221
Cyanosis 22
Cyanotic heart disease 22
Cysticercosis 114

D

Dacron patch 70
Dallas criteria 108
Dehiscence 55
Dilated cardiomyopathy 93
Double edged sword 84
Double-barrelled aorta 229
Ductal patency 27
Dystrophic calcification 55
Dystrophin gene 123

E

Echo-Doppler 20
Eisenmenger's syndrome 20
Elastic van Gieson's stain 206
Embolic complications 68
Endocardial cushion defect 18
Endocardial fibroelastosis 131
Endocarditis 29
Endocardium 34
Endomyocardial biopsy 91
    cardiomyopathies 100
        amyloidosis 101
        arrhythmogenic right ventricular dysplasia 103
        endomyocardial fibrosis 100
        idiopathic restrictive cardiomyopathy 103
    complications 106
    conditions diagnosed
        cardiac transplant rejection 92
        dilated cardiomyopathy 93
        giant cell myocarditis 96
        granulomatous myocarditis 97
        hypersensitivity myocarditis 99
        lymphocytic myocarditis 93
        rheumatic carditis 98
    indications 91
    interpretation 91
    tumor and tumor-like lesions 106
Endomyocardial fibrosis 100
Endomyocardial fibrosis 125
Endomyocardial fibrosis 100, 125, 126, 128, 129, 130
Eosinophilic myocarditis 99
Erythema nodosum leprosum 225
Explanted heart 141-143

F

Fabry disease 134
Fetal circulation 12
Fibrinoid necrosis 31, 32
Fibrinous pericarditis 163, 164
Fibrocellular crescents 218
Fibrosarcoma heart 195
Fibrous hemorrhagic pericarditis 162
Flea bitten kidney 62
Floppy mitral valve 49
Foam cells 81
Fossa lunata 3
Fossa ovalis 3
Friedreich's ataxia 124
Fungal myocarditis 111, 112

G

Gene abnormalities 11
Genetic-environmental interaction 11
Giant cell myocarditis 96
Glant cell arteirtis 211, 212
Glomangioma 240
Glomus tumor 240
Glomus tympanicus 240
Glycogen storage disease 134
Graft coronary artery disease 148
Graft vascular disease 148
Granulomatous myocarditis 97

H

HACEK organisms 57
Hemangioendothelioma 241
Hemangioma 194
    capillary 238
    cavernous 238
    epithelioid 240
    large vessel 239
    skeletal muscle 239
Hemangiomatous syndromes 239
Hemangiopericytoma 242
Hemochromatosis 134
Hemolysis 55
Hemopericardium 162
Hemosiderosis 134
Henoch-Schönlein purpura 220
High iron diamine stain 183
Histiocytes 31
Hodgkin's lymphoma 172
Homografts 55
Hydatid cyst 115
Hydatid disease 115
Hypertrophic cardiomyopathy 135
Hypereosinophilic syndrome 124
Hypertrophy and dilatation 58
Hypoplastic left heart syndrome 27

I

Immune complex mediated injury 68
Infective endocarditis 41, 51, 57
    acute 57
    bacteremia 57
    changed trends 57
    complications
        cardiac failure 67
        embolic complications 68
        endocarditis in intravenous drug abusers 69
        immune complex mediated injury 68
        Libman-Sacks endocarditis 72
        myocardial abscesses 67
        nonbacterial thrombotic endocarditis 71
        prosthetic valve endocarditis 69
        purulent pericarditis 67
    infective organisms 57
    pathogenesis 67
    pathology 58
    predisposing factors 57
    subacute 57
Infective vegetations 59
International Society for Heart and Lung Transplantation 144
Interruption of aortic arch 26

Index

Interstitium 78
Interventricular septum 5, 6
Intimitis 66
Intravenous drug abusers 69
Ischemic cardiomyopathy 90
Ischemic heart disease 80
Ischemic injury 150
Ischemic myocardium 82

J

Juvenile mitral stenosis 44

K

Kaposi sarcoma 243
Kawasaki syndrome 220

L

Lactic dehydrogenase 85
Lambl's excrescences 190
Lamina fibrosa 8
Lamina spongiosa 8
Left atrium 3
Left to right shunts 13
Left ventricle 5
Leg vein thrombosis 86
Lepromatous leprosy 224
Leukocytoclastic vasculitis 221
Libman-Sacks endocarditis 72
Ligamentum arteriosum 19
Lipomas 194
Loeffoler's endocarditis 124
Lumen 34
Lymphangioma 244
Lymphangiosarcoma 244
Lymphocyte infiltration 49
Lymphocytes 31
Lymphomononuclear cells 44

M

MacCallum's patch 30, 32, 34
Maffucci's syndrome 239
Malaria 116
Marfan's syndrome 51
Masson Trichrome stain 80, 89, 169
Mesenchymal cells 31
Mesenchymal tumors of heart 194
Mesothelial hyperplasia 159
Mesothelioma 159, 173
Mesothelioma of pericardium 197
Mesothelioma of the pericardium 157
Metastatic carcinoma 159
Microscopic polyangiitis 220
Mitral incompetence/regurgitation (MR) 48
Mitral stenosis 43, 44

Mitral valve 6
   apparatus 43
   disease 44
   prolapse 49
Mitral valve replacement 64
Moderator band 4
Molecular techniques 96
Mucocutaneous lymph node syndrome 220
Mucoid vasculopathy 208-210
Mural thrombi 41
Myocardial abscess 113
Myocardial abscesses 67, 113
Myocardial infarction 74
Myocardial infarcts 76
Myocardial ischemia 80
Myocardial rupture 85
Myocardial storage disorders 134
Myocarditis 33, 94, 95, 108
   caused by drugs 109
   caused by infectious agents 108
   Dallas criteria for the diagnosis
      first biopsy 108
      subsequent biopsies 108
   fungal 111
   giant cell 111
   granulomatous 109
   immune-mediated or noninfective 109
   lymphocytic 108
   tuberculosis heart 110
Myocarditis 33, 94, 95
Myocardium 34
Myocytolysis 80
Myofibers 35, 78
Myxoma syndrome 190

N

Nitroblue tetrazolium reaction 76
Non-Hodgkin's lymphoma 172
Normal heart 1
   aortic valve 6
   conduction system 7
   coronary artery circulation 7
   cut by the bread-loaf technique 2
   histology
      atrialis 8
      lamina fibrosa 8, 9
      lamina spongiosa 8, 9
      ventricularis 8
   left atrium
      fossa lunata 3
      fossa ovalis 3
   left ventricle
      inlet, apical trabecular and outlet 5
      interventricular septum 5, 6
   mitral valve 6

   pulmonary valve 5
   right atrium
      coronary sinus 2
      crista terminalis 2
      eustachian valve 2
      fossa ovalis 2
      left atrial appendage 2
      limbus 2
      probe patency of foramen ovale 2
      right atrial appendage 2
      sinoatrial node 2
      sulcus terminalis 2
      thebesian valve 2
   right ventricle
      apical trabecular component 4
      crista supraventricularis 4
      inlet component 4
      moderator band 4
      outlet component 4
      septomarginal trabeculation 4
      septoparietal trabeculations 4
   sequential segmental analysis 1
   tricuspid valve 5
   electron microscopy of cardiac myocytes 9
Obstructive lesions 20, 22
Orthotopic cardiac transplantation 140
Ostium secundum 50

P

Pancarditis 29
Pannus formation 55
Papillary fibroelastoma 190
Papillary muscles 43, 46
Paravalvular leak 55
Patent ductus arteriosus 19
Pauci-immune necrotizing vasculitis 220
Pericardial biopsy 158
Pericardial effusion 156
Pericardial fibroma 169
Pericardial tap 156
Pericardiectomy 156
Pericarditis 29, 162
   adhesive 168
   constrictive 168
   fibrinous/serofibrinous 163
   healed 168
   purulent/suppurative 167
   tuberculous 168
Pericardium 156
Periodic acid-Schiff's reagent 181
Persistent truncus arteriosus 26
Plasma cells 49
Plasmodium 116
Pockets of Zahn 52
Polyarteritis nodosa 213

Polyarthritis 41
Polymorphs 65
Postmyocardial infarction syndrome 89
Preinfarction angina 74
Primary angiitis 222
Prinzmetal variant angina 73
Probe 2
Prostheses 54
Prosthetic heart valves 54
    bioprostheses 55
    mechanical prostheses 54
Prosthetic valve endocarditis 69
Pulmonary artery 25
Pulmonary artery hypertension 236, 237
Pulmonary embolism 86
Pulmonary hypertension 16, 236
Pulmonary infarction 71
Pulmonary valve 5
    insufficiency 54
    stenosis 54
Pulmonic stenosis 20
Pulseless disease 201
Purulent pericarditis 67, 167

Q

Quilty effect 152

R

Rashkind balloon catheter 25
Reperfusion injury 83, 84
Rhabdomyoma 190
Rheumatic carditis 98
Rheumatic heart disease 28
    complications and sequelae
        chronic rheumatic heart disease 41
        congestive heart failure 41
        infective endocarditis 41
        MacCallum's patch 41
        mural thrombi 41
        sudden death 41
        valvular deformities 41
    diagnosis 28
    etiopathogenesis 29
    pathology
        acute rheumatic carditis 29
        central nervous system 41
        endocarditis 29
        myocarditis 33
        polyarthritis 41
        serofibrinous pericarditis 29
        subcutaneous nodule 40
Rheumatic mitral valvulitis 32
Rheumatic valve disease
    pathogenesis 43
Rheumatic valvulitis 49
Rheumatoid arthritis 51
Right atrium 2
Right ventricle 4
Right ventricular dysplasia 103

S

Sarcoidosis 109
Sarcoidosis heart 109
Scanning electron micrograph 38
Semilunar cusps 60
Semilunar valves 43
Senile amyloidosis 132
Senile calcific aortic stenosis 50
Septic infarcts 60
Sequential segmental analysis 1
Serous effusion 156, 158
Serum markers 84
Sinus of Valsalva 43, 63
Spider cells 191
Stable angina 73
Stenosis of the infundibulum 62
Streptococcus 29
Sturge-Weber syndrome 239
Subcutaneous nodule 40
Sudden cardiac death 90
Sulcus terminalis 2
Suppurative arthritis 60
Syphilitic aortitis 51
Systemic embolization 48

T

Takayasu aortitis 51
Takayasu arteritis 201
    etiology 205
    gross examination 205
Tearing of valve 55
Temporal arteritis 211
Tetralogy of Fallot 23
Tetralogy variants 23
Thromboangiitis obliterans 223
Thromboembolism 55
Thrombotic endocarditis 71
Thrombus formation 47
Tissue engineering 55
Total anomalous pulmonary venous connection 26
Toxoplasma gondii 117
Toxoplasmosis 117
Trabeculation 4
Transposition of great arteries
    management 25
    total anomalous pulmonary venous connection
        obstructed 26
        unobstructed 26
Tricuspid regurgitation 53
Tricuspid stenosis 54
Tricuspid valve 5
    insufficiency 53
    leaflets 53
    ring 53
    stenosis 54
Trypanosomacrizi 117
Tuberculosis 109
Tuberculosis heart 110
Tuberculosis leptomeninges 226
Tuberculous meningitis 226
Tuberculous pericarditis 156, 160
Tumor cells 198
Tumors
    fatty tissue 194
    fibrous tissue 192
    heart and pericardium 175
    hematologic 197
    lymphatic system 244
    metastatic 198
    pericardium 169
    vascular 19

U

Unstable angina 74

V

Vaccine for rheumatic fever 41
Valve circumference 10
Valve leaflets 43
Valve orifice 46
Valvular deformitis 41
Vasculitis
    classification/nomenclature 200
Vegetations 58
Veno-occlusive disease of lung 235
Ventricular angiogram 24
Ventricular angiography 17
Ventricular fibrillation 70
Ventricular hypertrophy 21, 47
Ventricular septal defect
    important issues for management 15
    large defects with hyperkinetic pulmonary hypertension 16
    management and timing of surgery 17
    moderate defect 16
    small defect 15
Ventricularis 8
Verhoeff-van Gieson stain 208, 233
von Hippel-Lindau syndrome 239

W

Wegener granulomatosis 217
    etiology 218

X

Xenotransplantation 154

RC
669.9
.C49